HANDBOOK of GASTROINTESTINAL IMAGING

Handbooks of Diagnostic Imaging

Series Editor
RONALD L. EISENBERG, M.D.
Professor and Chairman
Department of Radiology
Louisiana State University Medical Center
Shreveport, Louisiana

Premier Volume

Handbook of Gastrointestinal Imaging, edited by R. Kristina
Gedgaudas-McClees, M.D.

Forthcoming Volumes

Handbook of Head and Neck Imaging, by June M. Unger, M.D., with
contributions by Carl R. Barthelemy, M.D., and Katherine A. Shaffer,
M.D. Illustrated by Carole Russell Hilmer, B.A., A.M.I.

Handbook of Neurologic Imaging, by J. Robert Kirkwood, M.D.

Handbook of Pediatric Imaging, edited by David Kushner, M.D., Robert
H. Cleveland, M.D., and Thomas E. Herman, M.D.

Handbook of Skeletal Imaging, by Daniel Rosenthal, M.D., and Terry
M. Hudson, M.D.

HANDBOOK of GASTROINTESTINAL IMAGING

Edited by

R. Kristina Gedgaudas-McClees, M.D.

Associate Professor
Department of Radiology
Emory University School of Medicine
Emory University Hospital
Atlanta, Georgia

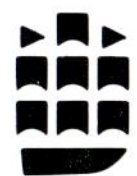

Churchill Livingstone
New York, Edinburgh, London, Melbourne   1987

Library of Congress Cataloging-in-Publication Data

Handbook of gastrointestinal imaging.

(Handbooks of diagnostic imaging; v. 1)
Includes bibliographies and index.
1. Diagnostic imaging—Handbooks, manuals, etc.
2. Gastrointestinal system—Radiography—Handbooks,
manuals, etc. 3. Gastrointestinal system—Diseases—
Diagnosis—Handbooks, manuals, etc. I. Gedgaudas-McClees
R. Kristina. II. Series. [DNLM: 1. Gastrointestinal
System—radiography. WI 141 H236]
RC804.D52H36   1987   616.3'0757   86-34336
ISBN 0-443-08473-4

Distributed in the United Kingdom by Churchill Livingstone, Robert Stevenson House, 1-3
Baxter's Place, Leith Walk, Edinburgh EH1 3AF, and by associated companies, branches, and
representatives throughout the world.

Accurate indications, adverse reactions, and dosage schedules for drugs are provided in this
book, but it is possible that they may change. The reader is urged to review the package
information data of the manufacturers of the medications mentioned.

Acquisitions Editor: *Robert A. Hurley*
Copy Editor: *Leslie Burgess*
Production Designer: *Charlie Lebeda*
Production Supervisor: *Jane Grochowski*

Printed in the United States of America

First published in 1987

Contributors

Michael E. Bernardino, M.D.
Professor, Department of Radiology, Emory University School of Medicine; Director, Abdominal Radiology and Magnetic Resonance Imaging, Emory University Hospital, Atlanta, Georgia

Dina F. Caroline, M.D.
Assistant Professor, Department of Diagnostic Imaging, Temple University School of Medicine, Temple University Hospital, Philadelphia, Pennsylvania

Peter Feczko, M.D.
Clinical Assistant Professor of Radiology, University of Michigan Medical School, Ann Arbor, Michigan; Staff Radiologist, Department of Radiology, Henry Ford Hospital, Detroit, Michigan

Thomas S. Forrest, M.D.
Assistant Professor of Radiology, Creighton University School of Medicine; Chief, Department of Ultrasound, Creighton University Health Sciences Center, Saint Joseph Hospital, Omaha, Nebraska

Mathis P. Frick, M.D.
Professor and Chairman, Department of Radiology, Creighton University School of Medicine, Creighton University Health Sciences Center, Omaha, Nebraska

R. Kristina Gedgaudas-McClees, M.D.
Associate Professor, Department of Radiology, Emory University School of Medicine, Emory University Hospital, Atlanta, Georgia

Robert Halpert, M.D.
Associate Professor of Radiology; Director, Ambulatory Care Radiology, and Chief, Division of Gastrointestinal Radiology, University of Texas Medical Branch at Galveston, Galveston, Texas

Roger K. Harned, M.D.
Professor, Department of Radiology, University of Nebraska College of Medicine, University of Nebraska Medical Center, Omaha, Nebraska

Dean D.T. Maglinte, M.D.
Clinical Professor of Radiology, Indiana University School of Medicine; Chief of Gastrointestinal Radiology, Methodist Hospital of Indiana, Indianapolis, Indiana

Eric C. McClees, M.D.
Clinical Assistant Professor, Department of Radiology, Emory University School of Medicine; Staff Radiologist, Department of Radiology, Piedmont Hospital, Atlanta, Georgia

Harvey V. Steinberg, M.D.
Assistant Professor, Department of Radiology, Emory University School of Medicine, Emory University Hospital, Atlanta, Georgia

William E. Torres, M.D.
Associate Professor, Department of Radiology, Emory University School of Medicine, Emory University Hospital, Atlanta, Georgia

Susan M. Williams, M.D.
Associate Professor, Department of Radiology, University of Nebraska College of Medicine, University of Nebraska Medical Center, Omaha, Nebraska

Foreword

When I was approached by Churchill Livingstone to organize a new series in Radiology, my initial reaction was that with all the books currently available, why do we need any new ones? However, as we examined the list of published books, it became clear that although there were both large comprehensive texts as well as simple introductory works in each subspecialty area, there was no series specifically aimed at the level of radiology residents preparing for their oral board examinations.

Handbooks in Diagnostic Imaging is a series designed to fill that gap. Each book is devoted to a single organ system and focuses on that information essential to passing the board examination dealing with that subspecialty area.

I was fortunate to enlist a number of gifted radiologists to write or edit the individual volumes. Although each editor has been free to organize his or her book based on the nature of the subject and the approach that has proven to be effective in teaching residents, all of the volumes are based on the original goal of meeting the needs of radiology residents preparing for their board examinations.

Each volume should also be useful to those residents in related medical and surgical subspecialties who are preparing for their boards or, indeed, to any radiologist interested in a practical review of imaging in a particular organ system.

Ronald L. Eisenberg, M.D.
Professor and Chairman
Department of Radiology
Louisiana State University Medical Center
Shreveport, Louisiana

Preface

Our purpose in writing this book is to provide radiologists, particularly those preparing for examination by the American Board of Radiology, but also those who have been in practice for a number of years, with a concise and complete review of gastrointestinal radiology. All areas of abdominal imaging have been included in this text. Each chapter systematically reviews diseases involving the various organ systems and their radiographic interpretation, with clinical and pathologic discussions.

This book is not an encyclopedic tome on gastrointestinal radiology. It does, however, present in sufficient detail, and with carefully selected illustrations, pathologic processes involving the esophagus, stomach, small bowel, colon, biliary system, liver, and pancreas. All the contributing authors are respected authorities in gastrointestinal radiology. They discuss all state-of-the-art diagnostic modalities currently used to evaluate the various organ systems, and attempt to elucidate the relationship between the various imaging techniques and the appropriate diagnostic approach for particular disease entities. Each chapter serves as an excellent reference source for radiologists and other clinicians to gain rapid access to radiographic diagnostic information.

R. Kristina Gedgaudas-McClees, M.D.

Contents

HANDBOOK of GASTROINTESTINAL IMAGING

1

Radiology of the Esophagus

William E. Torres

During the course of an upper gastrointestinal (UGI) examination on an adult, the esophagus is often superficially evaluated by the radiologist. In the past few years, there have been refinements in the radiographic techniques available to evaluate the gastrointestinal tract; these techniques have enabled us to view the esophagus from a slightly different perspective. To effectively evaluate the esophagus, both an understanding of its pertinent anatomy and the ability to assess the esophagus using a variety of techniques are required.

RADIOGRAPHIC EXAMINATION

The proper use of the multiple techniques available to the radiologist for studies of the esophagus is crucial in obtaining optimum information. Full-column, mucosal-relief, double-contrast, and motion-recording studies are all useful. Each has its own value in the evaluation of various portions of the esophagus.

Full-Column Technique

In the full-column technique, a single-column study is performed as with any hollow viscus. Barium is used to fill the esophagus, which is observed fluoroscopically and then radiographed in at least two dif-

ferent positions. The study is best performed with the patient in the recumbent position and drinking barium. To obtain maximum distension, the patient drinks the barium rapidly while performing the Valsalva maneuver. Use of these techniques together helps to suppress primary peristalsis by exerting a pinchcock effect at the level of the diaphragm. This results in the accumulation of barium in the esophagus and therefore, better visualization of the gastroesophageal junction.

Barium swallow after-studies should include a minimum of at least two views of the esophagus, although some controversy exists as to the appropriate views; combinations of AP, lateral, and oblique views should be obtained. With the use of dense barium, circumferential and many noncircumferential lesions can be seen as contour defects; the shortcoming of the full-column technique lies in its poor ability to detect small lesions not seen in profile. This necessitates additional studies using mucosal relief or double contrast in an attempt to avoid overlooking small lesions (Fig. 1-1).

Mucosal-Relief Technique

In the mucosal-relief examination barium is introduced to coat the esophageal mucosa without dis-

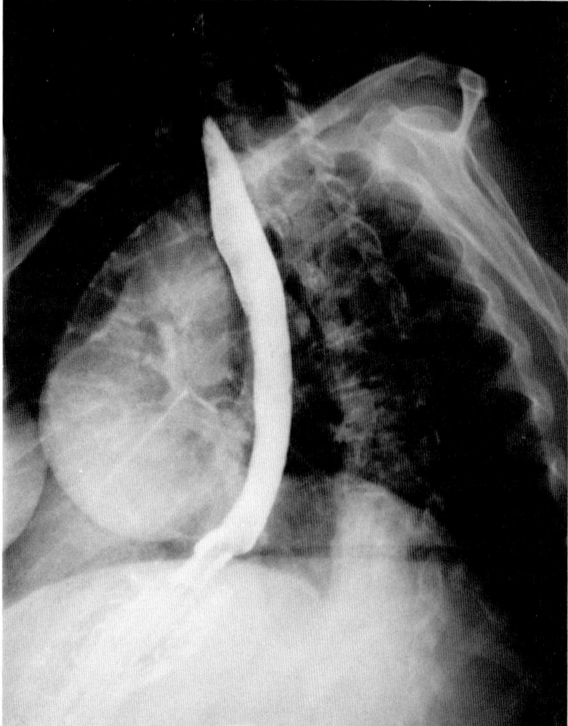

Fig. 1-1 Oblique view of a distended thoracic esophagus filmed using the full-column technique.

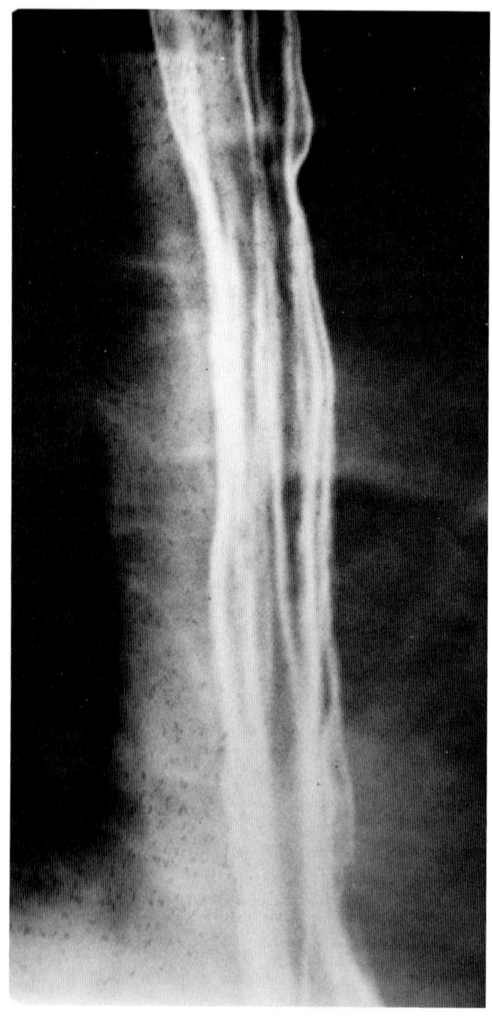

Fig. 1-2 AP view of thoracic esophagus using the mucosal-relief technique. Note smooth, longitudinal esophageal folds.

tending the lumen so as to demonstrate the smooth, longitudinal folds of nondistended esophagus. This effect is achieved by having the patient drink a dense barium solution; in the past a dense barium paste was used. The viscosity of the barium must be sufficient to withstand peristaltic waves and several swallows may be required before adequate coating is achieved (Fig. 1-2).

Lesions that can be seen when the mucosal-relief technique is used include varices, neoplasms, and, to a lesser extent, ulcers and esophagitis. Any lesion that must be distended to be seen (e.g., strictures) is often invisible in mucosal-relief studies.

Double-Contrast Technique

The strength of the double-contrast technique lies in its ability to show small mucosal irregularities. This technique is especially good for examining the hypo-pharynx, but is of little use in the cervical esophagus. Each of the different esophageal areas — hypo-pharynx, proximal thoracic esophagus, and distal esophagus — require different techniques. The type of barium used is of paramount importance and must be chosen for its ability to densely coat the esophagus. We use the higher weight barium (250% W/V). A single swallow of this dense barium usually coats the hypopharynx adequately. In the resting state, air is also present, creating the double-contrast effect (Fig. 1-3). The thoracic esophagus is examined in the upright position. Patients place effervescent

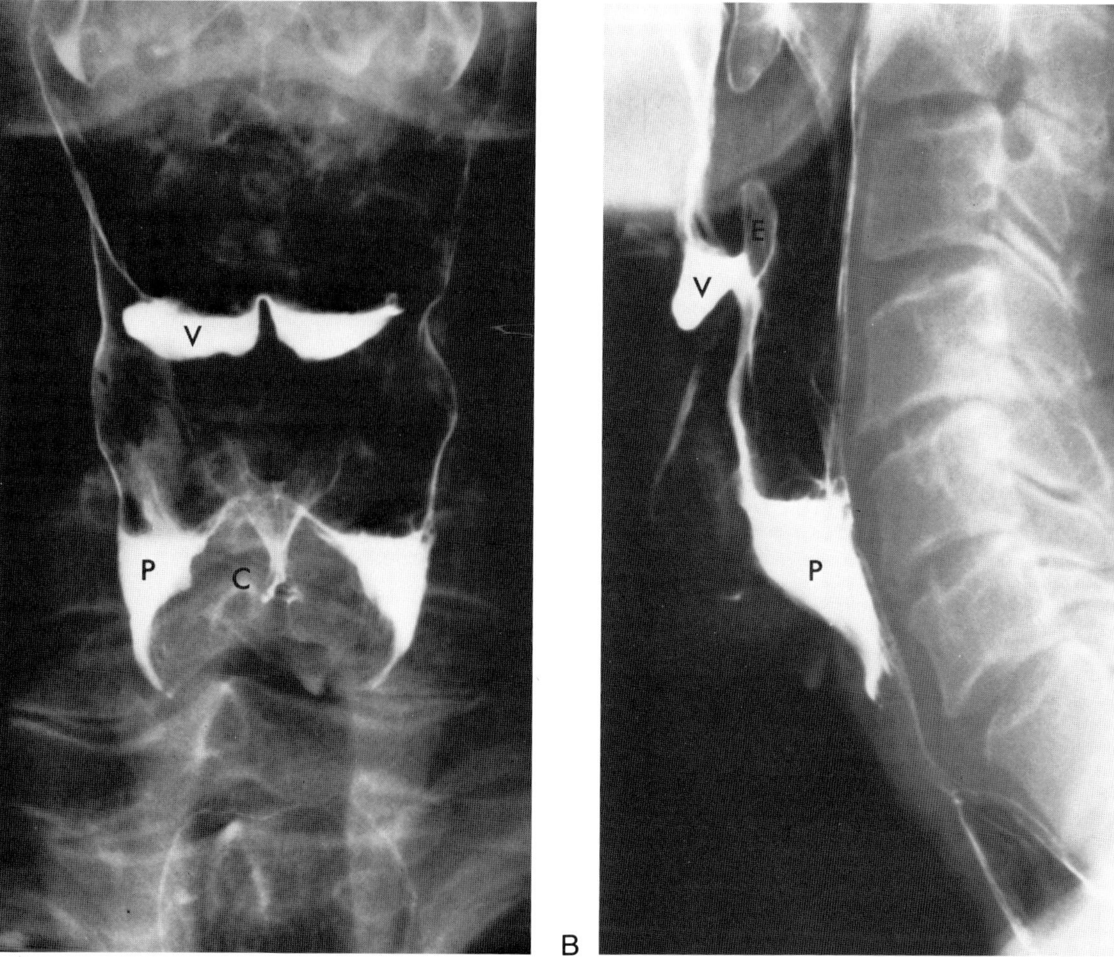

Fig. 1-3 (**A**) AP view of hypopharynx using air-contrast technique (V = vallecula, P = pyriform sinuses, C = vocal cords). (**B**) Lateral view of hypopharynx using air contrast. (V = vallecula, P = pyriform sinuses, E = epiglottis).

granules in the mouth and swallow barium as quickly as possible. Excellent distension of the entire thoracic esophagus is obtained, down to and including the esophagogastric junction (Fig. 1-4). The double-contrast effect is shortlasting, and radiographs should be taken as quickly as possible. Additional radiographs are taken in the prone oblique position to assess esophageal motility, which is best appreciated in recumbancy. In most cases a 12.5 mm barium tablet, the lower limits of the normal diameter of the esophageal lumen, is given to patients, especially those with suspected stricture or narrowing. Double-contrast evalu-

ation of the esophagus demonstrates esophageal neoplasms, small erosions and ulcers, as well as esophagitis.

Motion-Recording Techniques

A variety of techniques are available to record the motion of the gastrointestinal tract and these have been especially useful in the esophagus. These techniques, especially rapid-sequence spot-filming and videotape recording, have been particularly helpful in evaluating the pharynx and cervical esophagus. Care-

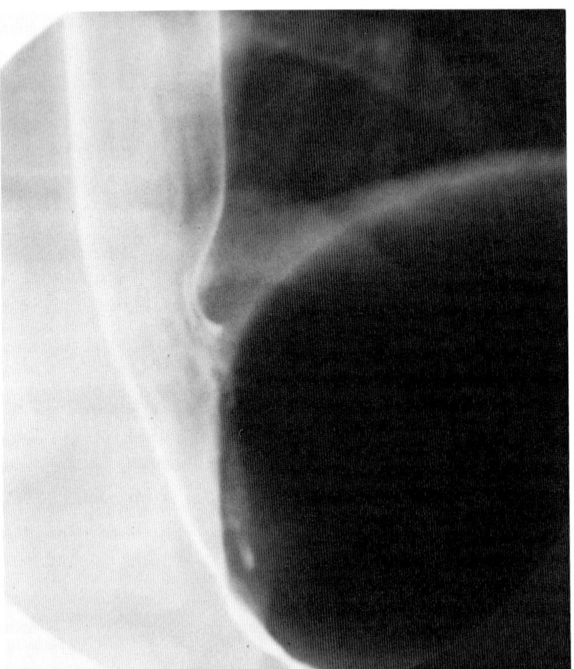

Fig. 1-4 AP air-contrast view of normal gastroesophageal junction.

ful study is often necessary to analyze various components in the act of swallowing.

Barium-Swallow Technique

The esophagogram or barium swallow can be done separately or in conjunction with an upper gastrointestinal examination. In each case, some modifications need to be made in the actual performance of the study. In the case of the esophagogram as a separate study, the examination requires 6 to 8 ounces of a dense 250% W/V barium suspension and spot-film capability. The patient, upright, is turned into the left posterior oblique position, places effervescent granules in the mouth, and rapidly drinks the dense barium, washing the granules down at the same time. This provides distension of the esophagus as well as a good coating of barium. The entire esophagus, excluding the cervical esophagus, can be evaluated well in the double-contrast manner.

The patient is now placed in the prone right-anterior oblique position and again drinks barium as its descent is watched fluoroscopically. To evaluate peristalsis, the examiner tells the patient to take a single swallow. The barium suspension is then drunk as the patient holds his or her breath in an attempt to achieve maximum distension. The lower esophagus is then radiographed, paying special attention to the hiatus. The process is then repeated in the prone or supine position. At this point the patient is given a 12.5 mm barium tablet, with a small amount of water and is told to swallow the tablet. The tablet's descent is watched under the fluoroscope. In patients with dysphagia, we evaluate the cervical esophagus in the erect, AP, and lateral positions, as well as in the supine or prone position, using either rapid sequence-filming or videotape recording.

If the barium swallow and UGI examination are done in conjunction, the thoracic esophagus is evaluated in the upright position, as previously mentioned, but the prone films are delayed until the UGI examination is completed.

PHARYNX

Even though the pharynx is easily examined clinically, radiographic studies can supply physiologic information and an accurate assessment of both the presence and extent of disease. The pharynx is an area often ignored or, at best, incompletely studied by the radiologist during a routine UGI. Radiographic evaluation of the pharynx should be routine on all patients. In those presenting with dysphagia, extra care is required when evaluating the pharynx; often, rapid-sequence filming or video recording is used.

Pharyngeal anatomy, as described previously, is best seen with double-contrast studies. When the pharynx is distended with thick barium, only margins in profile can be seen; intraluminal masses may be hidden by dense barium. The hypopharynx, as has been described, is examined by having the patient take a single swallow of dense barium (250% W/V) to get good mucosal coating. Along with the air usually present in the resting state, there is a double-contrast effect. Films are taken in frontal and lateral positions as necessary, mainly with oblique views. The modified Valsalva maneuver is optional in distending the pharynx. This, plus phonation to assess motion of the vocal cords, is important in evaluating this area for early inflammatory or neoplastic disease.

Anatomy

Classically, the pharynx has been divided into three parts — the nasopharynx, the oropharynx, and the hypopharynx. The function of the nasopharynx is respiratory, contrasted with the oropharynx where food and air intermix; the hypopharynx is solely concerned with swallowing. Anatomically, the oropharynx extends from the free border of the soft palate to the tip of the epiglottis, whereas the hypopharynx begins at the level of the hyoid bone and extends to the level of the cricopharyngeal muscle. The pharynx is a tubular structure, beginning at the base of the skull and ending at the lower border of the cricoid cartilage where it merges with the esophagus. Five pairs of voluntary muscles are present in the pharynx. The outer coat of circular muscles is formed by three pairs of constrictors — the superior, middle, and inferior pharyngeal. An inner, longitudinal layer of muscles is formed by fibers of the stylopharyngeus and palatopharyngeus muscles.

The anatomy of the hypopharynx is best viewed in the frontal projection (see Fig. 1-3A). The epiglottis is seen as a smooth, arched barium-coated structure superior to the valleculae. The valleculae, themselves, are symmetric, often containing filling defects that represent lymphoid tissue of the lingual tonsils. The outer margins of the hypopharynx are the lateral aspects of the pyriform sinuses. They are connected inferiorly by an arched line, representing the posterosuperior aspect of the larynx and the posterior wall of the hypopharynx.

The hypopharynx merges into the cervical esophagus at the level of the sixth cervical vertebral body. It is bounded anteriorly by the larynx, cervical lymph nodes, parathyroid, and thyroid gland laterally, and the cervical spine posteriorly.

In the lateral view of the hypopharynx, structures are superimposed. The two valleculae overlie each other superiorly, and the superimposed aryepiglottic folds extend obliquely from the epiglottis to the arytenoid cartilage. The pyriform sinuses are also superimposed. Laterally, the epiglottis is well seen in profile, and the posterior pharyngeal wall is easily evaluated.

The cricopharyngeus muscle is the lower, more horizontal portion of the inferior pharyngeal constrictors (Fig. 1-5). The fibers of the cricopharyngeus arise from the lateral surface of the cricoid cartilage and extend backward horizontally without interlinking dorsally into a raphe, thus forming a sphincter. The transverse fibers separate from the lower oblique fibers, leaving a triangular-shaped area relatively devoid of muscle fibers. This area is a potential weak spot, known as Killian's dehiscence or the triangle of Lannier, where Zenker diverticula occur in response to a rise in pressure during swallowing.

The act of swallowing is a coordinated effort between the tongue, palate, and pharynx. The tongue begins the swallowing process by transferring the bolus to the back of the mouth, at which point the uvula apposes the posterior pharyngeal wall to prevent nasal regurgitation. Laryngeal aspiration is prevented by the epiglottis, which covers the entrance to the lar-

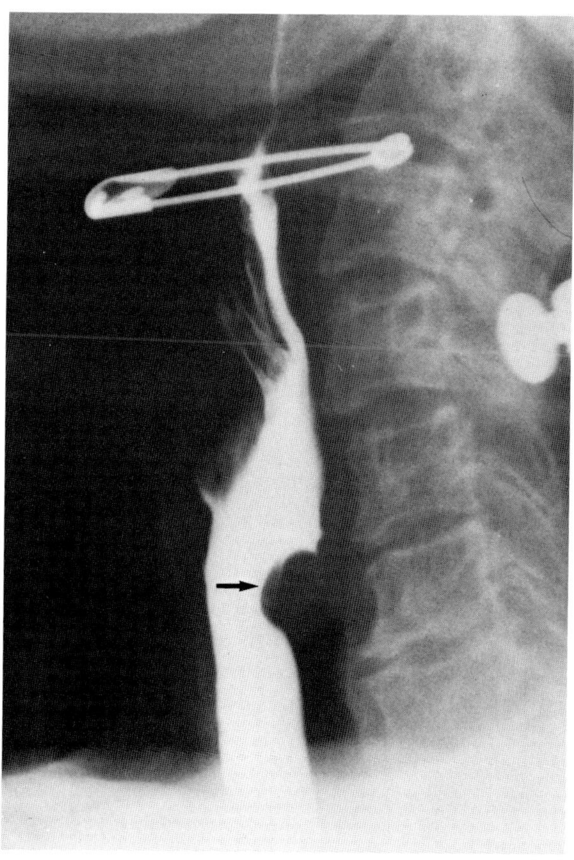

Fig. 1-5 Lateral view of cervical esophagus demonstrating a prominent cricopharyngeus muscle *(arrow)*.

ynx. The cricopharyngeus muscle relaxes, allowing the bolus to pass into the esophagus. Since the pharynx is composed of striated muscle, any disease involving these muscles can cause a swallowing abnormality, as in patients with myasthenia gravis or dermatomyositis.

CERVICAL ESOPHAGUS

The cervical esophagus begins at the level of the sixth cervical vertebra, blending into the thoracic esophagus at the thoracic inlet. Peristalsis is extremely fast through the cervical esophagus, making routine radiography difficult. The posterior wall of the pharyngeal esophagus runs parallel to the spine and is straight and featureless (Fig. 1-6); it can, in older individuals, be indented by vertebral osteophytes. In the postcricoid area on the anterior wall, a small inconstant triangular irregularity, the postcricoid defect, can be seen. This defect is thought to represent prolapse of the mucosa over submucosal veins and should not be confused with a web or neoplasm.

Diverticula

Esophageal and pharyngeal diverticula are classified as congenital or acquired and are located anterior, lateral, or posterior. Anterior pharyngeal pouches represent nothing other than overdeveloped vallecular fossae. True lateral pharyngeal diverticula are rare; protrusion of the lateral pharyngeal wall often can be observed on frontal views when the pharynx is distended (Fig. 1-7). There is increased intraluminal pressure in the anterolateral portion of the pyriform

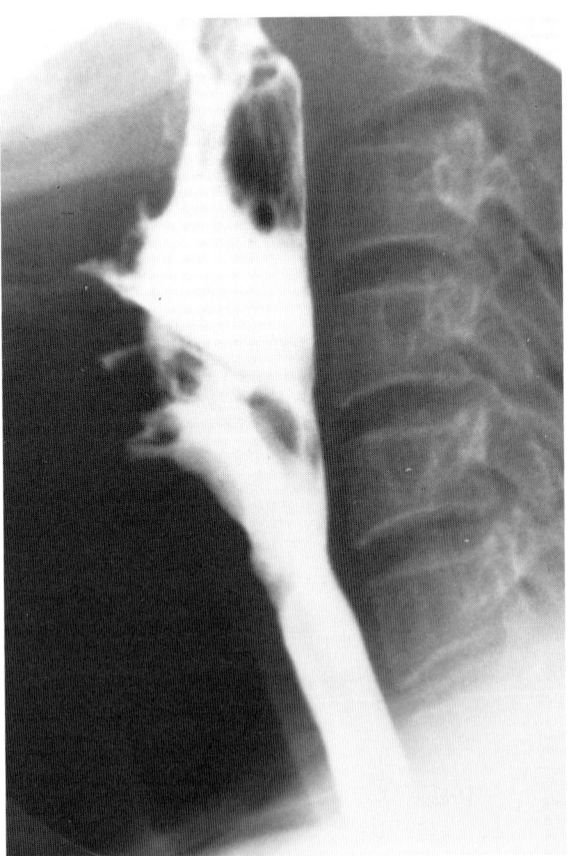

Fig. 1-6 Lateral view of barium-filled cervical esophagus. Note straight, featureless posterior wall.

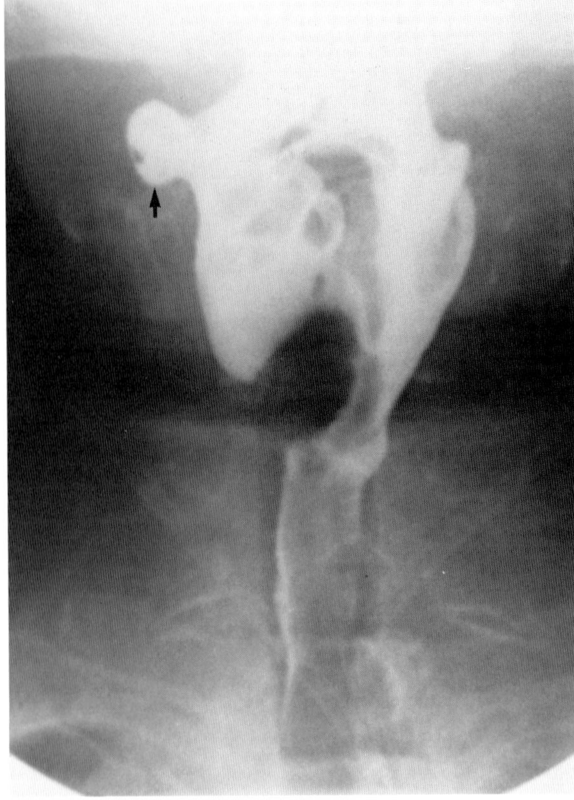

Fig. 1-7 AP view of hypopharynx demonstrating lateral pharyngeal diverticula *(arrow)*.

sinus at the vallecular level; this region, between the hyoid and thyroid cartilage, is relatively weak because it lacks supporting cartilage or bone. Protrusion of the lateral pharyngeal wall in this area is frequent in older individuals and has been referred to by multiple names, including hypopharyngeal pouches, hypopharyngeal ears, and pharyngoceles. Some controversy exists as to whether the lateral pharyngeal diverticula, reported in the literature, represent lateral pouches or are, in fact, a pulsion type diverticulum.

Posterior diverticula, also known as posterior hypopharyngeal pouches, Zenker, pulsion, or pharyngoesophageal diverticula are the most common in the pharynx. These diverticula always form in the midline on the posterior wall. They occur at the site of an anatomic weak point, Killian dehiscence or the triangle of Lannier, which is formed as the result of divergence of the fibers of the cricopharyngeus muscle from the inferior pharyngeal constrictor.

Although the exact cause of these diverticula has not been determined, an acquired origin is favored. These posterior diverticula are classified as pulsion type, arising as the result of pressure from within. The cricopharyngeus muscle is felt to close too soon on swallowing, and the resultant pressure forces the mucosa to herniate into the anatomic weak spot. When small, the diverticula are directed backward, moving to one side or the other as they become larger. These diverticula are easily seen on barium studies and at times are visible on plain radiographs of the neck. On plain radiographs, a Zenker diverticulum may appear as a widened retrotracheal soft tissue structure, often with an air-fluid level. With barium, the diverticulum is seen as a saccular outpouching that extends posteriorly from the upper esophageal lumen and is best identified in the lateral projection (Figs. 1-8 and 1-9). With enlargement, the sac extends downward and posteriorly, displacing and narrowing the adjacent lumen.

Webs

Cervical webs are usually found on the anterior wall of the esophagus just below the level of the cricopharyngeus muscle. Webs are easiest to see when the esophagus is fully distended; often, they are not recognized with small amounts of barium (Fig. 1-10).

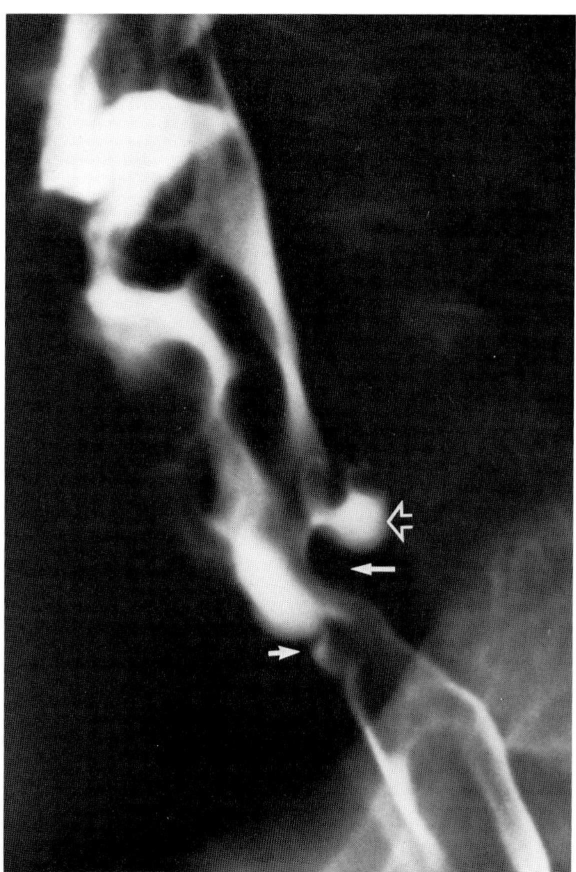

Fig. 1-8 Lateral view of cervical esophagus demonstrating a prominent cricopharyngeus muscle *(white arrow)* with a Zenker diverticulum *(open white arrow)* and small cervical esophageal web *(small white arrow)*.

Webs are most commonly found in asymptomatic patients and can be associated with the Plummer–Vinson syndrome. Webs should not be confused with a normal triangular defect — the postcricoid defect — on the anterior wall above the level of the cricopharyngeus muscle. Webs have also been described in association with certain dermatologic diseases.

THORACIC ESOPHAGUS

The thoracic esophagus is the area most often affected by serious intrinsic pathology. The thoracic esophagus is anterior to the spine and lies to the left of

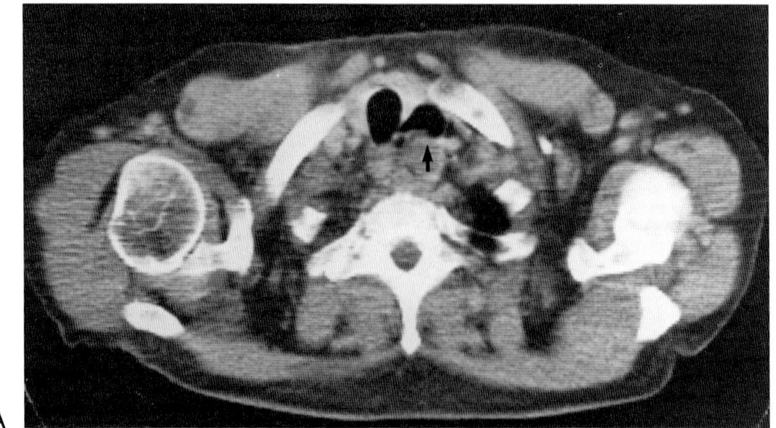

A

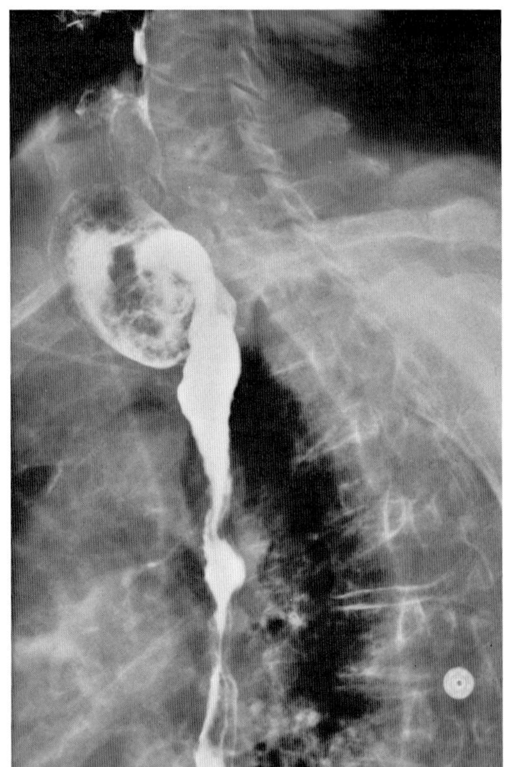

B

Fig. 1-9 (**A**) CT through the upper mediastinum demonstrating tracheal displacement to right by an irregular air-containing structure *(arrow)*. (**B**) Barium swallow showing a Zenker diverticulum displaced to side.

the midline; it deviates to the right at the level of the aortic arch and extends posteriorly at the cardiac level. The thoracic esophagus is tubular in shape, with a smooth lumen. When the esophagus is collapsed, thin smooth longitudinal folds are seen along its course. Distally, the esophagus enlarges at the vestibule or phrenic ampulla, an area just proximal to the gastric orifice.

Anatomy

The muscular coat is composed of smooth muscle, except in its most proximal portion, which contributes to its slower peristalsis. In the esophagus, three main types of peristaltic waves are seen. (1) The primary wave is initiated at the time of swallowing, pushing the esophageal contents toward the gastro-

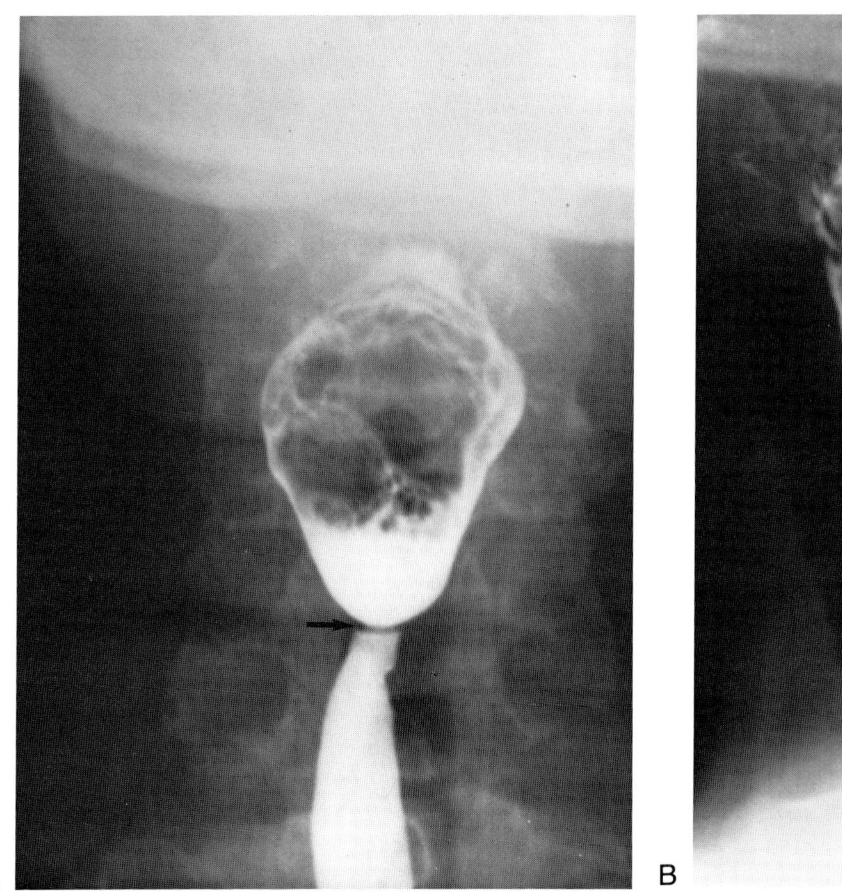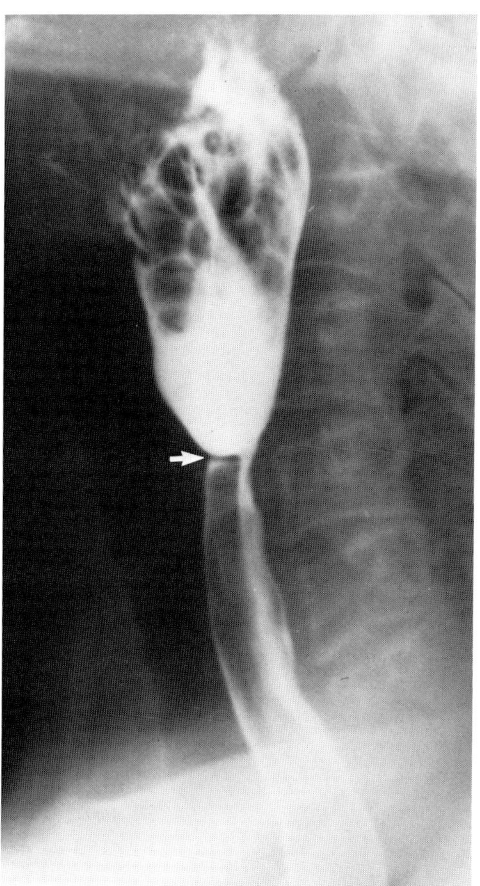

Fig. 1-10 **(A)** AP view of cervical esophageal web *(arrow)*. **(B)** Lateral view of the cervical esophagus demonstrating a cervical esophageal web *(white arrow)*.

esophageal junction. (2) Secondary waves result from distension of the esophagus and begin at the level of the remaining bolus, and (3) uncoordinated, nonpropulsive waves, known as tertiary waves or contractions, occur with increasing age and are usually of little clinical significance.

In evaluating esophageal peristalsis, the patient should be in the recumbent position. True peristalsis can only be assessed in the horizontal position; gravity helps to empty the esophagus in the upright position.

Motility Disorders

A variety of classifications of esophageal motility disorders have been proposed. Zboralske and Dodds (1969) divided motility disorders into primary and secondary causes. The primary motility disorders are achalasia, diffuse esophageal spasm, and presbyesophagus. Secondary esophageal motility disorders include collagen vascular diseases, chemical irritants, physiologic disorders, and physical causes such as vagotomy and other miscellaneous entities, including metabolic, neurologic, and endocrine diseases.

In esophageal motility disturbances, peristalsis, sphincter function, or both are altered. Relaxation of the sphincter is evaluated radiographically. Barium retained above the sphincter for longer than 2.5 seconds suggests failure of sphincter relaxation. With incomplete sphincter relaxation, the lumen does not open as widely as in the normal subject. It is often difficult to determine whether a narrowed sphincter is the result of incomplete relaxation, failure of relaxation, or stricture.

During radiographic evaluation of esophageal motility, the patient should be instructed to take single swallows of barium to avoid initiating additional peristaltic waves; the aim is to evaluate a single swallow.

ACHALASIA

A disease of the young, achalasia is associated with the gastroesophageal junction's failure to relax. Two prerequisites must be present to diagnose this entity: (1) primary and secondary peristalsis must be completely absent in esophageal smooth muscle and (2) the lower esophageal sphincter (LES) must fail to relax completely on swallowing. The result of this absence of smooth muscle peristalsis and the sustained high pressure at the gastroesophageal junction is retention of food materials in the body of the esophagus. Over a period of time, the esophagus will exhibit loss of tone and progressive dilatation of the body of the esophagus. The diagnosis of achalasia can be made either with barium swallow or by manometric testing, where a characteristic pattern of gastroesophageal sphincter hypertension and incomplete relaxation on swallowing is seen.

Clinically, patients with achalasia uniformly have dysphagia for both liquids and solids. Chest pain can be a presenting problem early in the disease in patients with so-called "vigorous achalasia," which is associated with tertiary peristalsis.

Pathologically, achalasia is thought to be caused by a decrease in neural elements, especially the ganglion cells of the myenteric plexus in the LES and in the dilated segment of the esophageal body.

Radiologically (Fig. 1-11), the esophagus above the diaphragm is dilated. Often, a chest radiograph shows a large paramediastinal mass with an associated air-fluid level. Classically, primary peristalsis is absent throughout the entire esophagus; in some patients, however, peristalsis has been seen to the level of the aortic arch. The radiograph shows an elongated, tortuous, or angulated esophagus. The distal portion of the esophagus curves to the right and then back to the

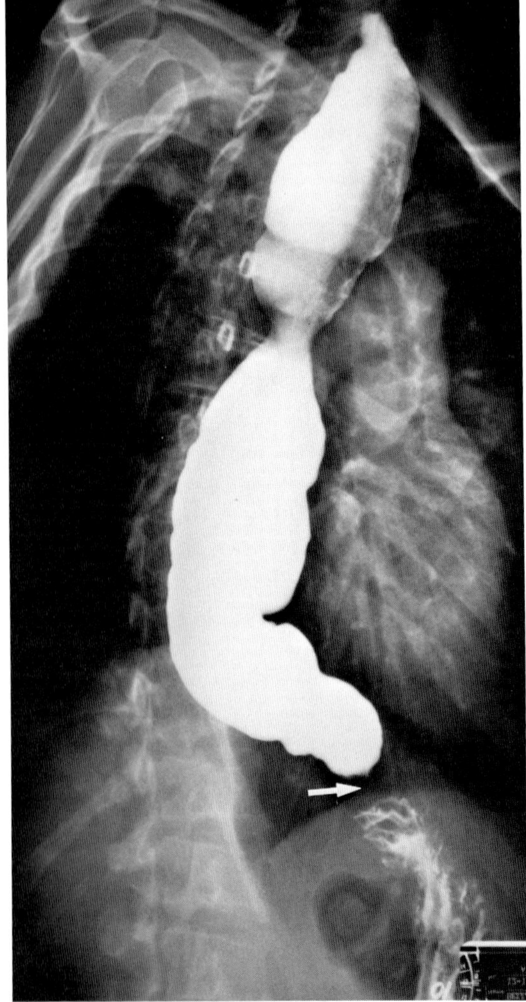

Fig. 1-11 AP view of gastroesophageal junction in patient with achalasia. Note dilatation of esophagus with focal narrowed distal esophagus *(arrow)*.

midline before passing through the diaphragmatic hiatus. The narrowed distal portion of the esophagus takes on an elongated V-conformation that has been likened to a bird beak. In the upright position, the LES does not relax normally but fails to open after a swallow. Esophageal material, whether liquid or food, does not pass until the pressure transmitted through the column by nonperistaltic esophageal contractions, or by hydrostatic pressure, overcomes the unrelaxed sphincter. At this point, esophageal material can slowly flow into the stomach. In the supine position, the esophagus does not empty. When the esophagus is mildly to moderately dilated, nonperistaltic esophageal contractions can occur after swallowing and are known as "vigorous achalasia." With severe esophageal dilatation (megaesophagus), the esophagus is usually atonic.

In achalasia, progressive dilatation of the esophagus is caused by the functional distal obstruction; recurrent aspiration can occur in the recumbent position and cause pulmonary infections from overflow of esophageal contents. It has been shown that patients with achalasia have an increased incidence of esophageal carcinoma, apparently the result of continued chronic inflammation secondary to stasis. In older patients the onset of achalasia-type symptoms should be viewed with suspicion, since cancer of the gastroesophageal junction can mimic achalasia. The narrowing of the distal esophagus does not change and is not relieved with the hydrostatic pressure of barium in patients with carcinoma (Fig. 1-12).

SCLERODERMA

A collagen-vascular disease that affects smooth muscle, scleroderma involves the middle and distal third of the esophagus. However, any portion of the gastrointestinal tract can be involved, resulting in poor motility, dilatation, and sacculation (pseudodiverticula). In the esophagus, the gastroesophageal junction is widely patent (Fig. 1-13); gravity helps to empty the esophageal contents into the stomach in the upright position. In the supine position, the esophagus is aperistaltic and the esophagus remains filled throughout the study. Reflux esophagitis, a frequent occurrence in these patients, results in strictures secondary to the widely patent gastroesophageal junction. Although patients with scleroderma usually have peripheral signs and symptoms before gastrointestinal manifestations, esophageal motility problems can be the presenting complaint.

Diffuse esophageal spasm, the so-called corkscrew esophagus, is characterized by (1) chest pain and intermittent dysphagia; (2) forceful, repetitive, simultaneous contractions on manometry; (3) segmental contraction on barium swallow; and (4) esophageal wall thickening. Occasionally, diffuse esophageal spasm can occur secondary to esophagitis. In this en-

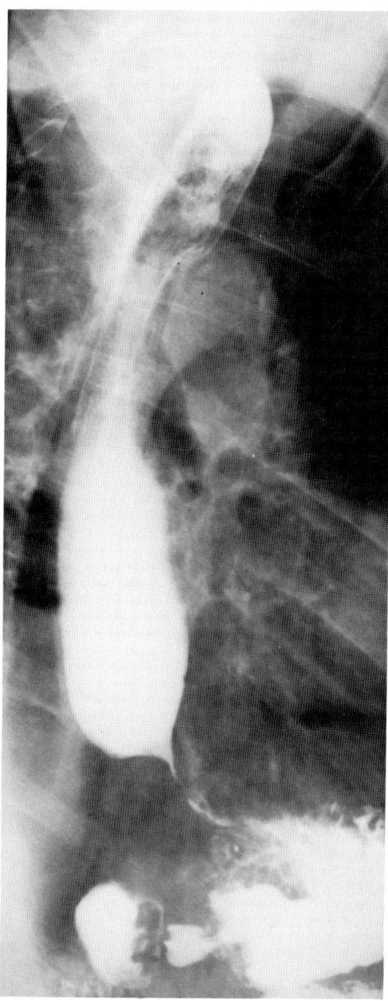

Fig. 1-12 Oblique view from barium swallow. Mild dilatation of the proximal and midesophagus are seen. Marked abrupt narrowing and eccentricity are present in this malignant stricture caused by invasion of the esophagus by a carcinoma in the gastric fundus. Compare this with the achalasia case of Figure 1-11.

tity there is no sex predilection and patients are usually middle-aged. The chest pain is often described as moderate substernal discomfort, but it can be severe enough to mimic angina. The chest pain and dysphagia are intermittent and can be elicited by eating, especially after a large bolus. These patients often are referred to a cardiologist for evaluation of coronary heart disease; many times, it is only after cardiac catheterization that another etiology of the pain is sought.

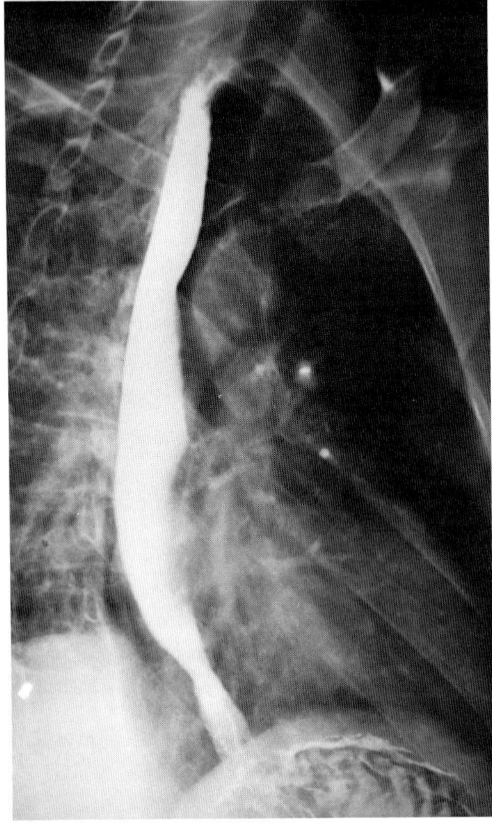

A

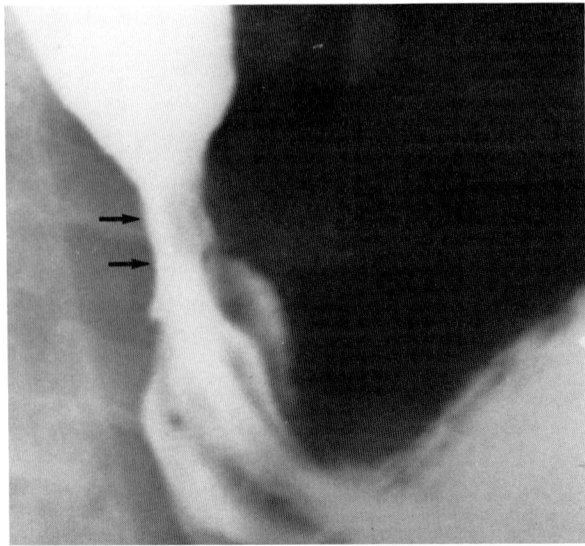

B

Fig. 1-13 **(A)** Oblique view of thoracic esophagus in a patient with scleroderma. An aperistaltic esophagus that narrows near the gastroesophageal junction is present. **(B)** AP view of gastroesophageal junction in a patient with scleroderma. A stricture is present *(arrows)* above a hiatal hernia.

Pathologically, thickening of the esophageal wall occurs; measurements as large as 2 cm have been recorded (normal wall is approximately 5 mm). In the upper third of the esophagus, peristalsis is normal; in the lower two-thirds of the esophagus, nonpropulsive contractions occur after swallowing.

Radiographically, nonpropulsive contractions occur in the smooth muscle portion of the esophagus (Fig. 1-14). Conditions that obliterate the lumen give the esophagus a corkscrew appearance and result in functional obstruction. As the contractions relax, the esophagus regains its tubular shape; when the repetitive contractions resume, the normal configuration of the esophagus is again disrupted.

Some authors feel that diffuse esophageal spasm is part of a spectrum that includes achalasia. In some patients, the transition from esophageal spasm to achalasia occurs with the demonstration of a hypersensitive esophageal response to methacholine. In contrast, electron microscopic evaluation of surgical and postmortem specimens from patients with esophageal spasm and achalasia suggested that the two entities are, in fact, separate diseases. The authors in this second study concluded that esophageal spasm is caused by a primary abnormality of vagal sensory nerves, whereas vagal motor pathways are involved in achalasia.

PRESBYESOPHAGUS

A motor disturbance associated with aging, presbyesophagus is usually limited to individuals in their later years of life, although it can occur in middle-age. Not all geriatric patients exhibit physiologic and radiographic changes, although most reveal some abnormality. Dysphagia is present occasionally, but most patients tend to be asymptomatic.

Manometrically, there is a defect in initiating primary peristalsis, as well as a defect in relaxation of the lower

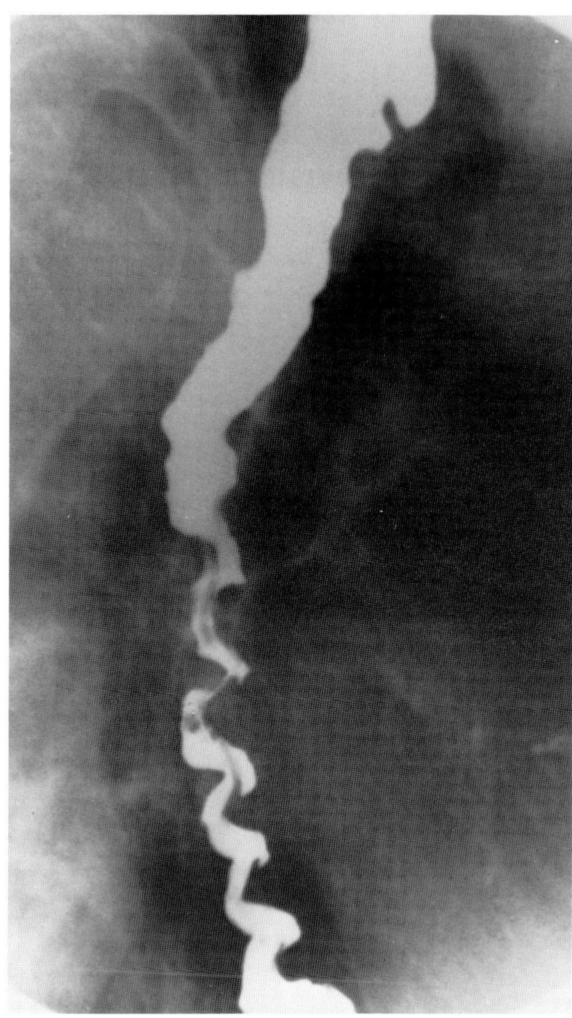

Fig. 1-14 Lateral views of the esophagus in a patient with chest pain, demonstrating marked esophageal spasm.

esophageal sphincter. Radiographically, a variety of peristaltic abnormalities are present, ranging from absent peristalsis to tertiary contractions, the most common abnormality seen. Similarly, the lower esophageal sphincter can exhibit a variety of changes, from normal or diminished relaxation to complete absence of relaxation. Uniform, usually moderate dilatation of the esophagus can occur in these individuals, with either total or partial failure of relaxation.

The radiographic features of presbyesophagus vary and can resemble a variety of other motility disorders. In these instances, other procedures may be required to establish a definitive diagnosis.

Hiatus Hernia

The most overdiagnosed abnormality in UGI studies is the hiatus hernia. The overdiagnosis results from confusion with the phrenic ampulla or esophageal vestibule, the normal saclike dilatation in the distal esophagus. To diagnose a hiatus hernia either the gastroesophageal junction or gastric folds must be identified above the diaphragm.

Although the exact etiology of a hiatus hernia is uncertain, it probably results from a combination of weakening of the phrenicoesophageal ligament and diaphragmatic hiatus widening.

Two types of hiatus hernia are seen: the sliding (Fig. 1-15) and the paraesophageal (Fig. 1-16), each having a different presentation, treatment, and prognosis.

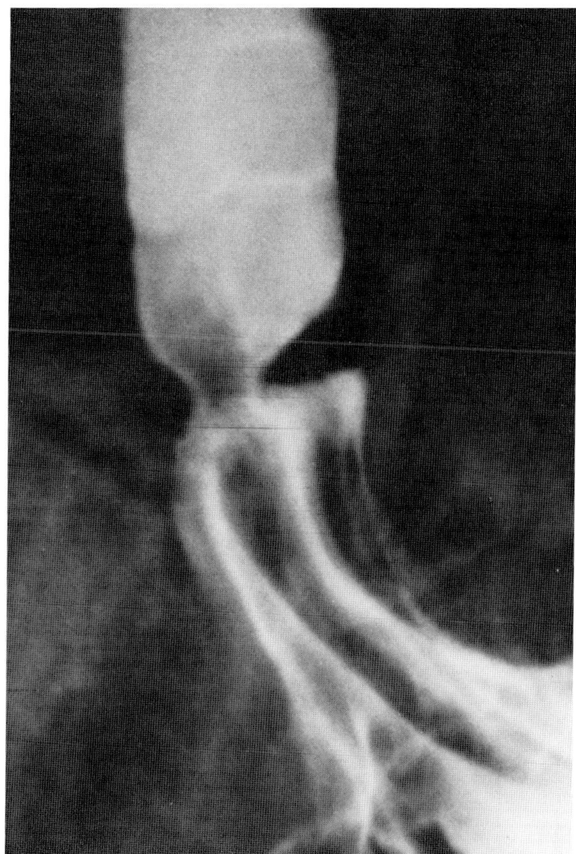

Fig. 1-15 Sliding hiatal hernia with narrowed, lower esophageal sphincter or Schatski ring.

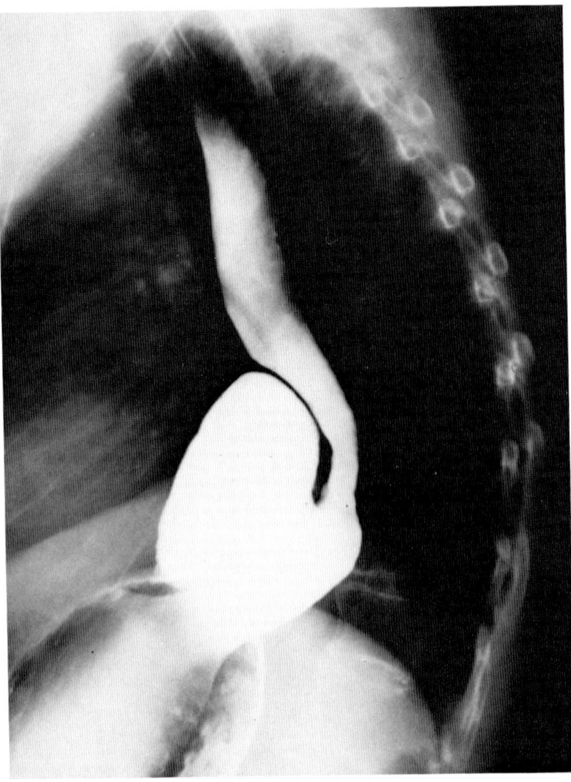

Fig. 1-16 Lateral view from barium swallow demonstrates a paraesophageal hiatal hernia.

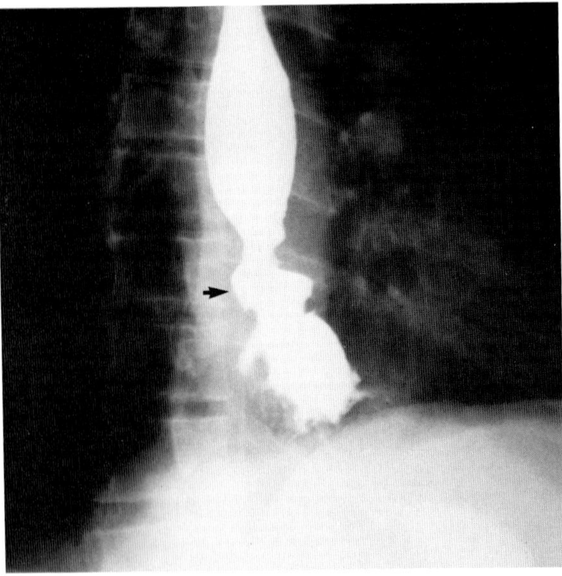

Fig. 1-17 AP view of gastroesophageal junction showing marked irregularity of distal esophagus with an ulcer *(arrow)* from reflux esophagitis.

The more common is the sliding type, where the patient's usual symptoms are caused by reflux with "heartburn" related to poorly functioning antireflux mechanisms. Radiographically, the gastroesophageal junction rises into the chest and is seen above the diaphragm on a UGI series. In the paraesophageal type, the gastroesophageal junction is in its normal position, but a portion of the stomach herniates through the diaphragm next to the esophagus. Usually, the patient has no symptoms, unless the hernia becomes incarcerated or strangulated.

Reflux of acid material into the esophagus results in esophagitis, which can produce a variaty of radiographic changes ranging from spasm to ulceration (Fig. 1-17) and subsequent stricture formation. With the formation of a stricture, the symptoms usually change from reflux to dysphagia. Many other causes of esophagitis, e.g., lye ingestion, candidiasis, herpes, and radiation, can produce an appearance similar to reflux. Another condition can occur in the esophagus, wherein the normal squamous epithelium is replaced by columnar epithelium — Barrett esophagus. The appearance varies, but focal ulceration, stricture formation (Fig. 1-18), or a granular or reticular mucosal pattern (Fig. 1-19) high in the esophagus should suggest the diagnosis. The importance of this entity lies in its association with an increased incidence of esophageal cancer (10 percent). Histologically, the metaplastic columnar epithelium extends from the gastric cardia to the site of esophageal abnormality. Reversion to squamous epithelium can occur after antireflux surgery.

Gastroesophageal Junction

There has been a great deal of controversy as to the exact location of the junction of the esophagus and the stomach. Many authors have used the squamocolumnar mucosal junction, or Z-line, as the dividing point. However, recent evidence, both anatomic and histologic, disputes the Z-line. The gastric sling, which delineates the left lateral margin of the esophagogastric junction, is now believed to be the most reliable landmark for the junction. This area is approximately

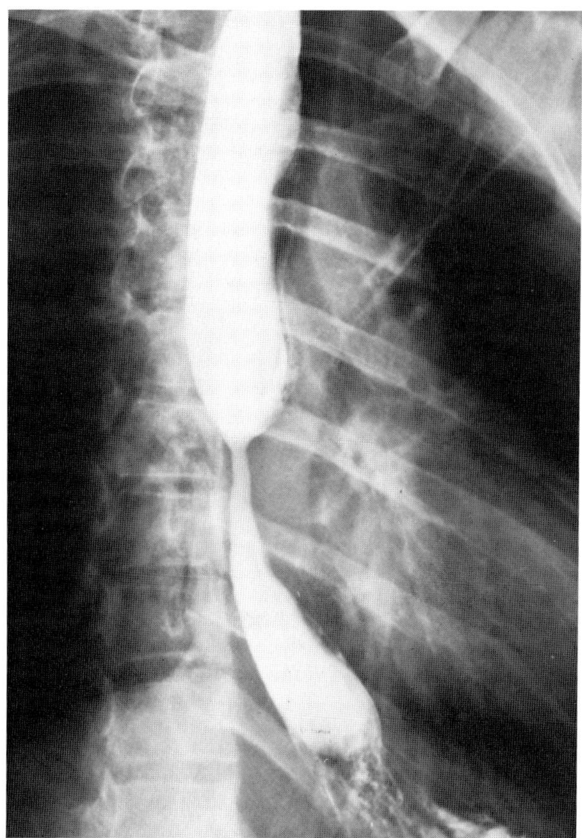

Fig. 1-18 Oblique view of barium swallow with a focal lower esophageal stricture secondary to Barrett esophagus.

1 to 2 cm below the squamocolumnar junction (Z-line).

Three common esophageal rings are seen at the gastroesophageal junction. The muscular, or A ring occurs at the upper border of the esophageal vestibule or ampulla, whereas the mucosal or B ring is located at the lower border of the vestibule. The annular peptic ring occurs at virtually the same level as the mucosal ring (Fig. 1-20).

The lower esophageal mucosal ring, also known as the Schatski ring, is the most common ringlike narrowing seen in the esophagogastric region. This ring, located at the distal end of the esophageal vestibule, is felt to be at, or just distal to, the squamocolumnar mucosal junction. Its exact etiology is uncertain, but most authors feel it is part of the spectrum of reflux esophagitis. Radiographically, the ring is seen only when it is displaced above, or located at, the diaphragmatic esophageal hiatus. When present, the lower mucosal ring is seen as a thin, transverse, circumferential structure with smooth margins. Its internal caliber is fixed, unchanging from exam to exam, and the ring should only be called a Schatski ring when the internal diameter is less than 12.5 mm, the size of the barium tablet.

The great majority of patients with lower esophageal rings are asymptomatic; however, the clinical significance of the ring depends on its relationship to the hiatus hernia and on the internal caliber of the ring. Since it localizes the junction between the esophageal vestibule and the stomach, some believe that the location of the mucosal ring can be used as an indication of a sliding hiatal hernia, if it is located above the dia-

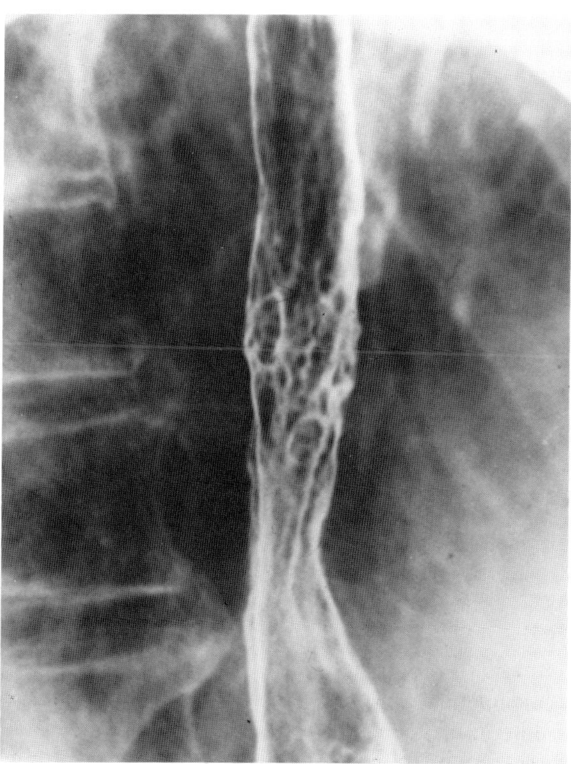

Fig. 1-19 Air-contrast view of midesophagus in patient with midsternal discomfort. Distensibility and peristalsis were normal. Note the irregular nodular mucosa secondary to Barrett esophagus.

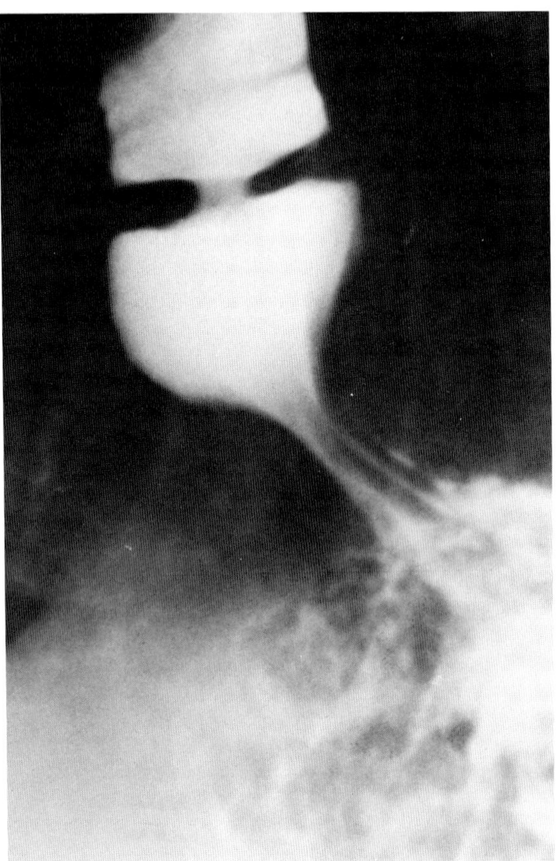

Fig. 1-20 View of gastroesophageal junction demonstrating a narrowed lower esophageal mucosal ring (Schatski ring).

phragmatic hiatus. Other authors have argued that the ring must be located 1 to 2 cm above the level of the diaphragmatic hiatus to be considered a valid sign; normally, some orad motion of the esophagogastric region occurs on swallowing. Some physiologic herniation is possible as individuals age.

If the internal caliber of the mucosal ring is greater than 20 mm, symptoms rarely develop; on the other hand, patients with rings less than 13 mm in internal caliber usually are symptomatic. Although most mucosal rings remain stable in size, a significant number of both symptomatic and asymptomatic rings decrease in size over a period of time. The use of a 12.5 mm barium tablet, as mentioned, is useful in assessing the size of the lower esophageal mucosal ring.

Esophageal Diverticula

The two types of esophageal diverticula seen are (1) traction, which contain all layers of the esophagus; and (2) pulsion, which are composed of mucosa and submucosa which herniate through the muscularis.

In the thoracic esophagus, traction diverticula can arise opposite the bifurcation of the trachea in the hilar region. Usually, traction diverticula result from fibrous adhesions following mediastinal node infection. Radiographically, a barium-filled sac is seen to extend horizontally or slightly inferiorly from the midesophagus (Fig. 1-21).

Epiphrenic diverticula are pulsion-type diverticula that occur in the distal 10 cm of the esophagus and result from increased intraluminal pressure (Fig. 1-22). In the lower esophageal segment, there is no coordination between sphincter relaxation and esophageal peristalsis. Dysphagia can occur if the diverticula are large enough to displace the adjacent esophagus.

Intramural esophageal diverticulosis simulates diverticular involvement of the esophagus. It is a rare disorder, with 1 to 3 mm saclike outpouchings that, in fact, represent dilated ducts from submucosal glands (Fig. 1-23). An extremely high association (93 percent) with esophageal strictures is present. The etiology of this process is unknown, but it is assumed to follow chronic inflammation in and around glands. However, some authors believe that this entity is another complication of reflux esophagitis.

ESOPHAGITIS

A variety of inflammatory processes can involve the esophagus. These can be divided into peptic, infectious, and miscellaneous causes.

Peptic esophagitis is one of the most common abnormalities involving the UGI tract. Peptic changes are acute or chronic and are primarily the result of reflux as well as variants, such as Barrett esophagus, scleroderma, and those induced by prolonged insertion of a nasogastric (NG) tube, to mention a few. In acute esophagitis, vertically oriented linear ulcerations are

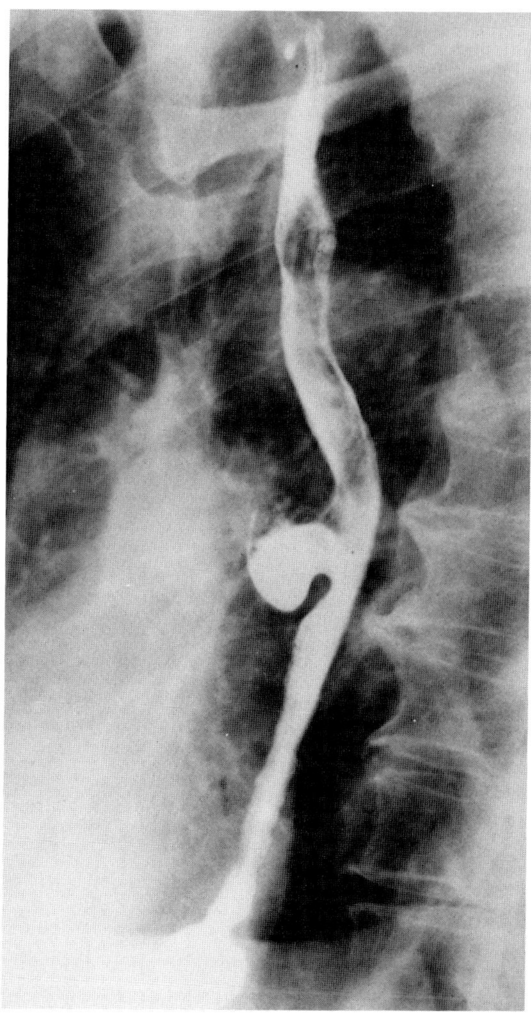

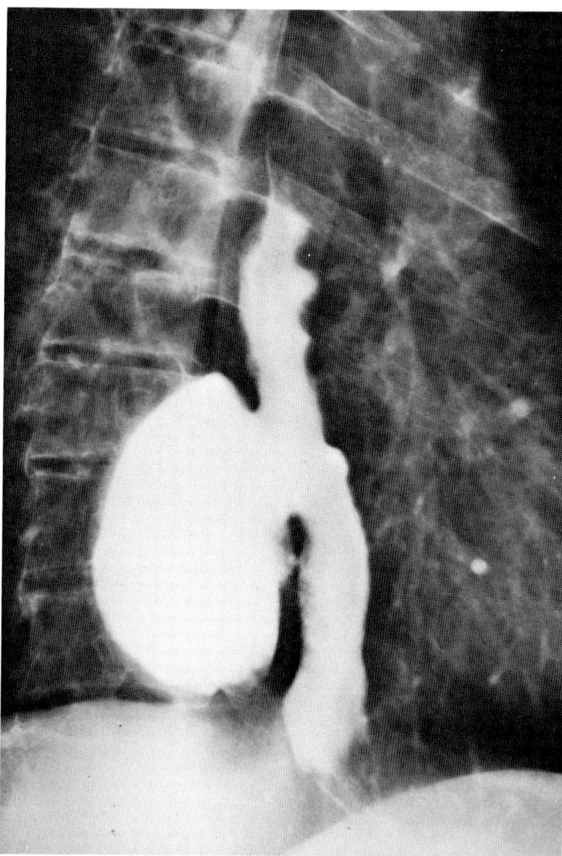

Fig. 1-22 Barium swallow, oblique view, in a patient with substernal discomfort. A large epiphrenic diverticulum is present. Note tertiary waves in esophagus.

Fig. 1-21 Oblique view of a barium swallow demonstrating a large traction diverticulum.

seen along with superficial erosions and deep ulcerations (Fig. 1-24). Thickening and nodularity of the longitudinal folds may also be present. In the chronic form, the most common manifestation is that of luminal narrowing with stricture.

The vast majority of esophageal infectious diseases occur in debilitated patients. The two most common organisms involved are the *Herpes simplex* virus and *Candida albicans.* With candidal infections, patients usually have abnormal motility. Using air-contrast techniques, plaquelike filling defects, representing colonies of fungus, are present. A shaggy mucosal contour secondary to pseudomembranes of necrotic exudate may be observed. Ulcerations can be extensive (Fig. 1-25). Herpetic esophagitis may be indistinguishable from candidiasis; however, discrete focal ulcers, with or without halos, strongly suggest herpetic involvement.

A variety of clinical problems and disease states can involve the esophagus. These include radiation changes, corrosive ingestion, Crohn disease, dermatologic problems, and a variety of medications. In radiation esophagitis, there is a history of thoracic radiation for primary or metastatic disease; the most common morphologic abnormality is a smooth stricture that often occurs months after the radiation.

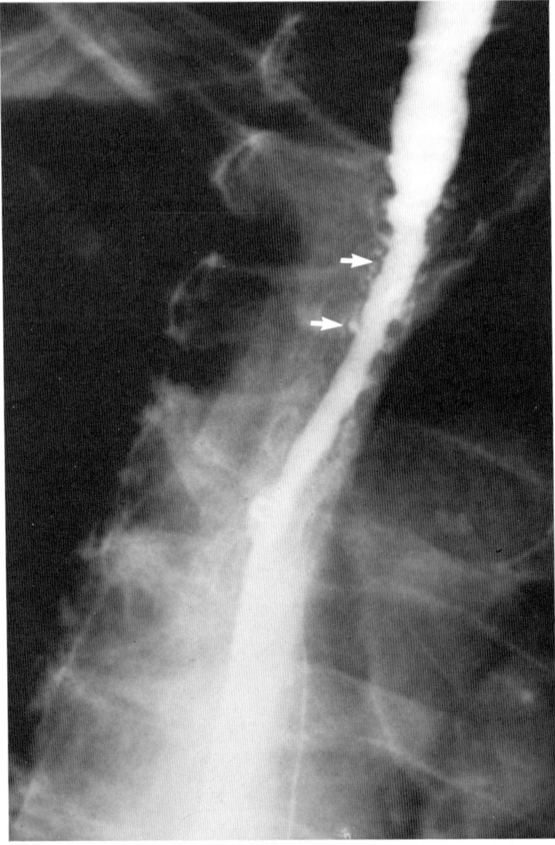

Fig. 1-23 Barium study of thoracic esophagus, demonstrating multiple, small saclike outpouching from intramural esophageal diverticulosis *(arrows)*.

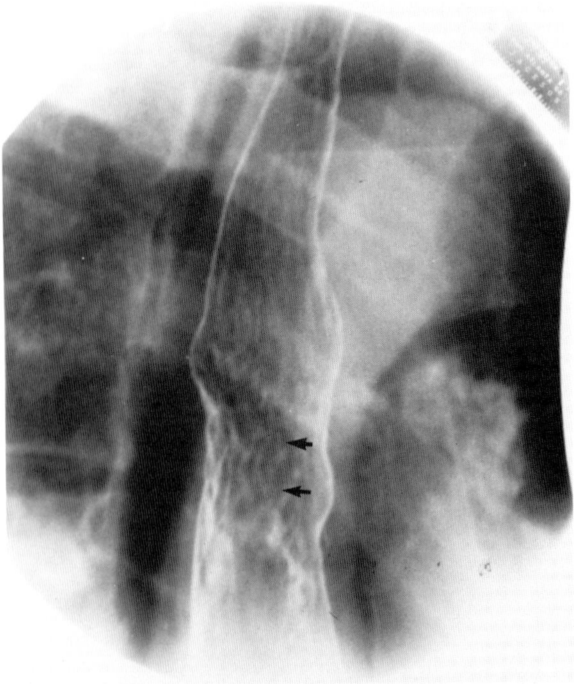

Fig. 1-24 Air-contrast view of thoracic esophagus showing nodularity and linear ulcerations *(arrows)* in a patient with esophagitis.

Ingestion of acids and alkali affect the esophagus in different ways. The ingestion of acid causes coagulation necrosis, a process that limits its further penetration. The squamous epithelium of the esophagus offers greater resistance to acid compounds; therefore, burns from acids usually cause more serious problems in the stomach. On the other hand, with alkali ingestion, tissue is dissolved and consequently, penetration is deeper; the mouth, pharynx, and esophagus are more commonly affected. In the acute stage, submucosal edema and hemorrhage give the esophageal wall a scalloped appearance. At this point, normal peristalsis is absent and painful contractions occur. With time, the esophagus becomes narrowed.

Some medications have been associated with esophageal inflammation. Tetracycline and its derivatives can cause focal ulceration — usually in the proximal or midesophagus — thought to result from the ingestion of medication immediately before retiring or to obstruction by a prominent aortic arch. Other medications, such as potassium chloride and quinidine, have also been implicated.

Dermatologic diseases, such as pemphigoid and epidermolysis bullosa, can produce esophageal inflammation that can progress to fibrosis and strictures.

Radiographically, the area involved is often the distal third of the esophagus, but the entire length can be affected. With air-contrast studies, the diagnosis of esophagitis has been simplified. Even minor morphologic changes of the mucosa are easily seen. Unfortunately, the changes are nonspecific and need to be correlated with endoscopy and clinical findings.

It is not unusual for patients with early changes of esophagitis to have a mild esophageal motility disturbance, often associated with mild prominence of the longitudinal folds. With progression of the disease, erosions and superficial ulcerations develop, and as

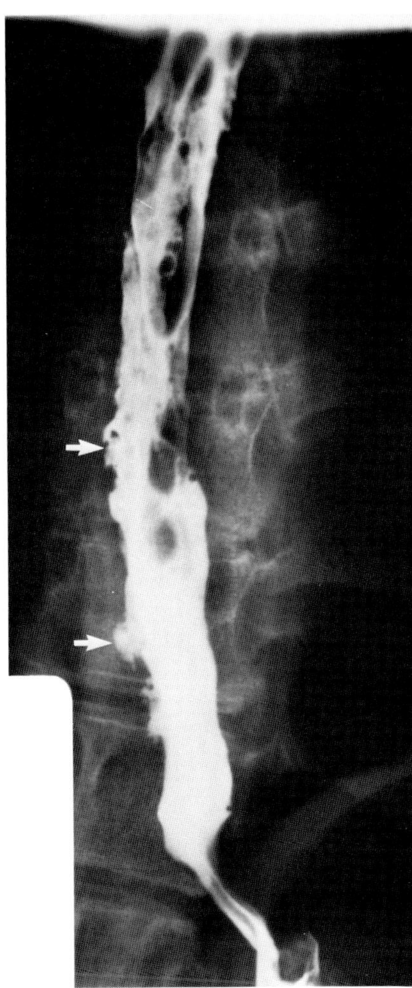

Fig. 1-25 Dysphagia in a 17-year-old with leukemia. Barium swallow demonstrates marked mucosal irregularity distally with ulceration *(arrows)* secondary to Monilia (Candida).

the process continues, fine, nodular filling defects are seen, especially in the distal esophagus. When the disease has persisted for a long period of time, inflammatory changes involve all layers of the esophagus. With subsequent healing, there is fibrosis with stricture formation.

VARICES

Esophageal varices are formed from venous dilatation in the subepithelial connective tissue of patients with portal hypertension. In the Western world, the most common cause of varices is hepatic cirrhosis, but they can be caused by other entities such as pyelophlebitis and portal vein thrombosis. Varices, most common in the esophagus, are easily demonstrated by either barium swallow, endoscopy, or angiography. Two types of varices, termed uphill and downhill varices, are seen. The uphill variety develops when blood attempts to ascend around an obstruction in the liver, toward the heart. In downhill varices, the cause is a blocked superior vena cava that leads to formation of venous collaterals as blood tries to descend toward the heart. Uphill and downhill varices can be seen on barium swallow. They begin as thickening and tortuosity of normally thin esophageal folds and end up as serpiginous or wormlike structures that produce marked distortion of the normal esophageal folds.

To evaluate a patient with suspected varices, a study should be performed in suspended respiration, using thick barium. The aim is a nondistended, barium-coated esophagus. Demonstration of varices is not constant during a barium study and depends on the alternate filling and collapsing of collateral veins (Figs. 1-26 and 1-27).

ESOPHAGEAL PERFORATION

Esophageal perforation, tears, or both can result from a variety of causes — esophagitis, peptic ulcer, neoplasm, instrumentation (Fig. 1-28), or trauma — and involve the mucosa only (Mallory-Weiss), the entire wall (Boerhaave syndrome), or the esophageal wall without actual rupture, but with submucosal dissection.

Esophageal tears are infrequent, and can result from prolonged vomiting after an alcoholic binge or from external trauma to the chest. In this syndrome, termed the Mallory-Weiss syndrome, there is an increase in intraluminal pressure. Most tears are gastric (76 percent); the remainder are gastroesophageal or esophageal. Approximately one-fourth of the patients have multiple tears, and the tears tend to be superficial and longitudinal. Often, they are difficult to demonstrate radiographically because they are shallow (Fig. 1-29).

Patient's with Boerhaave syndrome or complete rupture of the esophagus present with severe epigastric

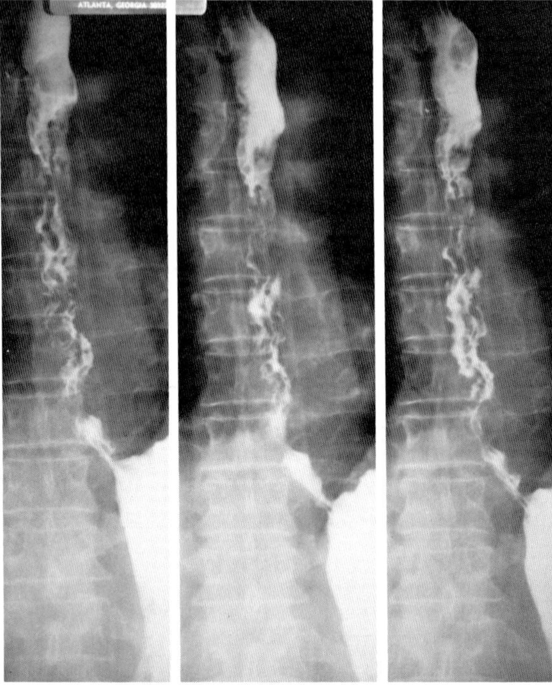

Fig. 1-26 AP view from barium swallow demonstrating serpiginous filling defects from varices.

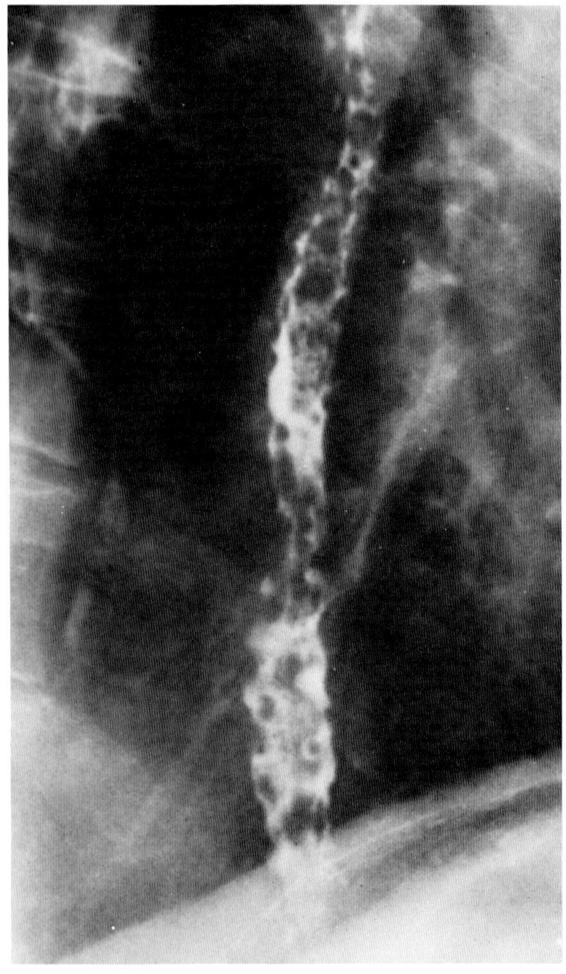

Fig. 1-27 Lateral view from barium swallow showing irregular filling defects from varices in a collapsed esophagus.

pain, symptoms that suggest ruptured abdominal viscera, myocardial infarction, or pancreatitis. Vomiting, although often seen, is not a necessary feature. Other causes include increased intraabdominal pressure from coughing, heavy lifting, blunt abdominal trauma, straining at stool, and external cardiac massage. Esophageal rupture involves the lower esophagus immediately above the diaphragm, usually on its left lateral aspect. Survival without therapy is rare.

Intramural rupture is the least common of the emetogenic injuries. Since it responds to conservative therapy, it needs to be separated from complete rupture. With laceration, an intramural hematoma forms, which can dissect up or down the esophagus. Radiographically, the mucosa is outlined on both sides by barium, the so-called mucosal stripe sign.

Radiographically, the signs of perforation are pneumomediastinum and extravasation of contrast outside the esophagus (Fig. 1-30). The association of gas in the upper mediastinum and/or cervical region, left-

sided pleural disease, and pneumothorax/hydropneumothorax are the classic radiographic findings in a perforated esophagus (Fig. 1-31). In the evaluation of patients with questionable perforation, 25 percent are missed when water-soluble contrast material is used. Barium, the contrast of choice, can also help guide the surgeon to the exact area to be explored at the time of thoracotomy.

POSTOPERATIVE ESOPHAGUS

Evaluation of the esophagus in the postoperative setting can be challenging. The esophagus is seen, in

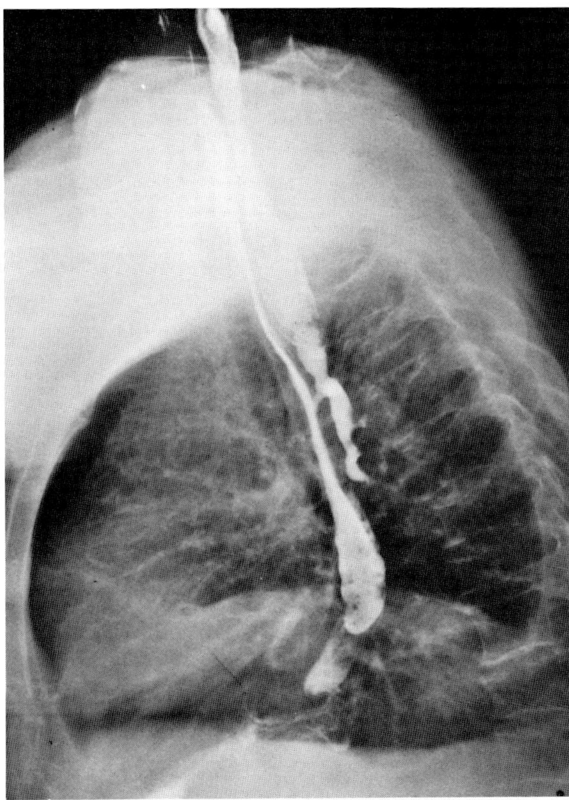

Fig. 1-28 Lateral view from barium swallow showing perforation in the midesophagus, secondary to instrumentation. Note barium tracking-up posteriorly to cervical area.

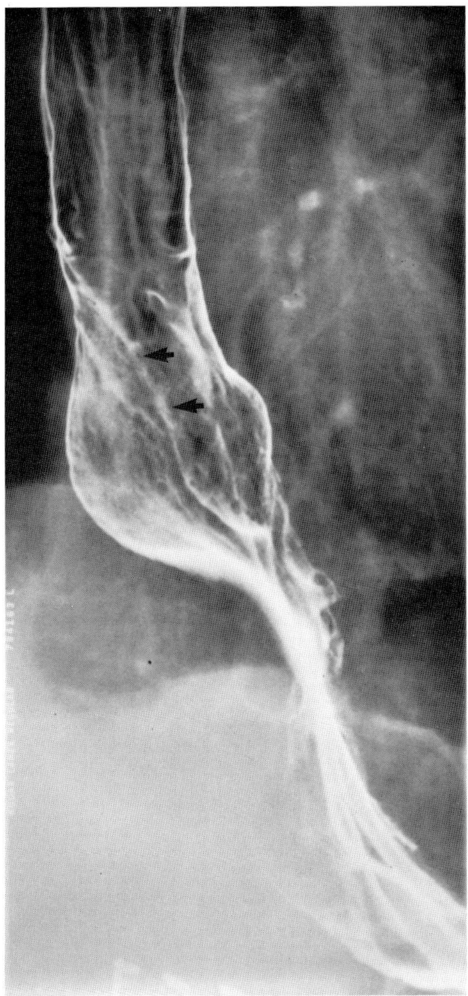

Fig. 1-29 View of gastroesophageal junction in alcoholic patient. Note oblique mucosal tears *(arrows)* secondary to Mallory-Weiss syndrome.

an unpredictable fashion, at a time when things are happening quickly, which can be a source of great confusion. Knowledge of the patient's prior surgery is essential, a fact not always provided by either the patient or the referring physician. With an understanding of the surgical anatomy and the expected postoperative appearance, the radiologist will know which study to perform and how to go about performing it. Postoperative patients may initially require different density barium as well as different positioning.

Immediately postoperative, an examination may be requested to look for evidence of early complications, such as obstruction or extravasation of contrast material. Early postoperative edema is usually present, and a barium tablet should not be given since its nonpassage has little meaning. Baseline postoperative exams are important because they are of value in the interpretation of subsequent radiographic studies. Late

postoperative patients are often studied to search for evidence of recurrent disease or stricture formation.

Surgery of the esophagus is performed for a variety of benign lesions such as diverticula, strictures, and hernias, as well as for malignant lesions. Resection of an esophageal diverticulum, for example, can be followed by a leak or stricture at the operative site. With a stricture, local resection with reanastomosis can be performed. In more severe cases, an esophageal bypass is done with either gastric pull-through or colon interposition. With malignant disease, the esophagus is

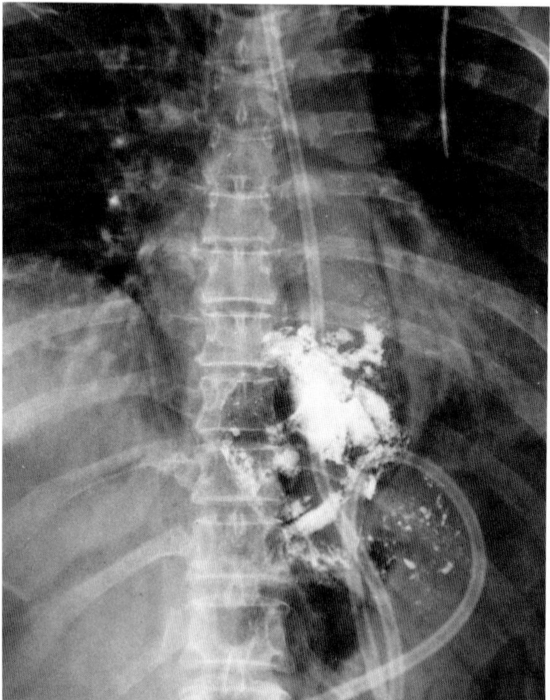

Fig. 1-30 AP view from contrast study in patient with suspected esophageal rupture. Note contrast outside lumen of esophagus. Air is seen paralleling the aorta.

either bypassed or the lesion is resected and the normal esophagus reanastomosed.

Surgery for repair of a hiatus hernia can be performed in a variety of ways (see Chapter 2). One of the most common operations is the Nissen fundoplication, in which the hernia is reduced and the fundus of the stomach wrapped around the now reduced esophagus to form an antireflux structure (Fig. 1-32). Following successful surgery, a pseudotumor is seen; this defect is caused by the gastric fundus wrapped around the esophagus. In the postoperative patient, a contrast-swallow study is performed to rule out anastomotic leakage or obstruction. Initial examinations in these patients are usually performed with a water-soluble contrast agent, unless there is the possibility of a tracheoesophageal fistula. If a leak is not identified, barium should be used to further evaluate the esophagus, since it provides better coating.

Reconstruction of the cervical esophagus, hypopharynx, and oral cavity following hypopharyngeal carci-

noma has been attempted in a variety of ways. A recent technique is the free transfer of jejunum. In this procedure, a proximal segment of jejunum on a vascular pedicle is isolated and removed (Fig. 1-33). The bowel is anastomosed to the hypopharynx and cervical esophagus as well as to adjacent vessels. The procedure has been associated with a very low incidence of complications and low morbidity.

Reconstruction of the thoracic esophagus has been attempted for a variety of reasons in adults, in benign conditions such as achalasia and scleroderma, and in severe strictures. However, the most common single indication is esophageal carcinoma.

The colon has long been used in reconstructing the esophagus, because of its inherent properties, such as a good marginal blood supply and some resistance to digestion by hydrochloric acid. In colonic interposition, the colon is mobilized—retaining its blood supply—and placed in the chest (Fig. 1-34). Many investigators believe that the colonic segment empties and fills by gravity and that little, if any peristalsis is seen.

Gastric interposition can also be used for esophageal replacement. In this technique, the stomach is pulled through the hiatus into the chest and anastomosed to the esophagus (Fig. 1-35).

FOREIGN BODIES

A variety of foreign bodies can become impacted in the esophagus, especially in the cervical esophagus at or just above the level of the thoracic inlet. Metallic, radiopaque objects are easily seen; objects of aluminum or other alloys may be impossible to detect radiographically. The object should be viewed in at least two planes to ascertain its true location. Nonopaque foreign bodies such as a food bolus, can only be demonstrated using contrast material (Fig. 1-36). Often, they become impacted in the distal esophagus, just above the hemidiaphragm, in association with a stricture.

STRICTURES

Although there are numerous causes of strictures, the most common etiologies are fibrosis secondary to

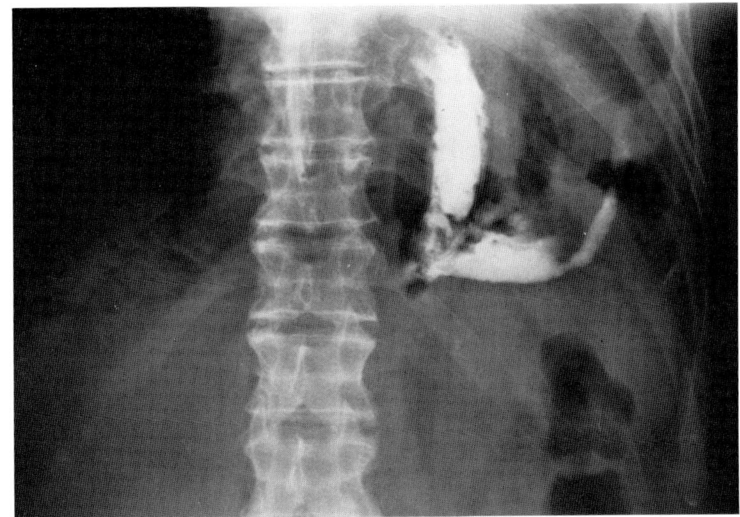

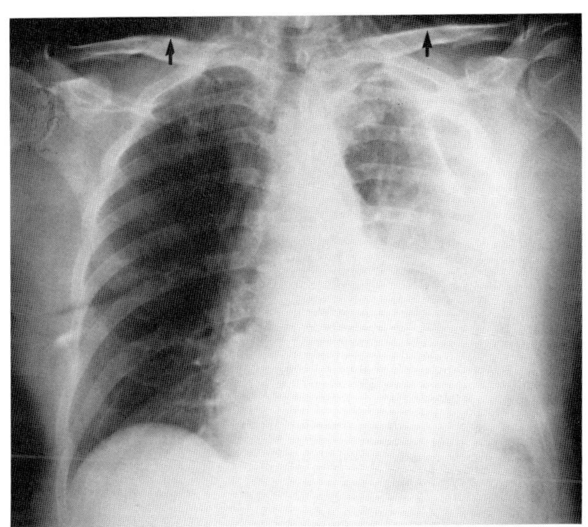

Fig. 1-31 **(A)** Complete rupture with contrast extending outside the esophagus. **(B)** AP chest radiograph showing a left effusion from a ruptured esophagus and subcutaneous gas in the neck *(arrows)*.

inflammation and neoplasia. Separating the benign from the malignant stricture is possible in most cases, but is not always easy. In general, benign strictures have a smooth, hourglass configuration and tapering margins that blend into the adjacent esophageal wall (Fig. 1-37). Malignant strictures, on the other hand, may have an irregular contour, often with ulcerations or tumor nodules. The narrowing is abrupt and often eccentric; the margins are undercut and end prior to the normal mucosa. Problems in diagnosis occur with inflamed strictures that can have ulcerations and irregular margins, which may simulate malignancy. Fibrosis can itself produce nodularity. Also, malignant strictures with fibrosis may appear to be benign. At times, radiographic differentiation is impossible and endoscopy, biopsy, or both may be necessary.

Differentiation from achalasia is also important. The presence of a measurable length of distal esophageal narrowing that does not change with increased hydrostatic pressure suggests the presence of a stricture, and not achalasia.

ESOPHAGEAL DUPLICATION

Esophageal duplication, a rare lesion, presents as a round or oval posterior mediastinal mass. The mass is

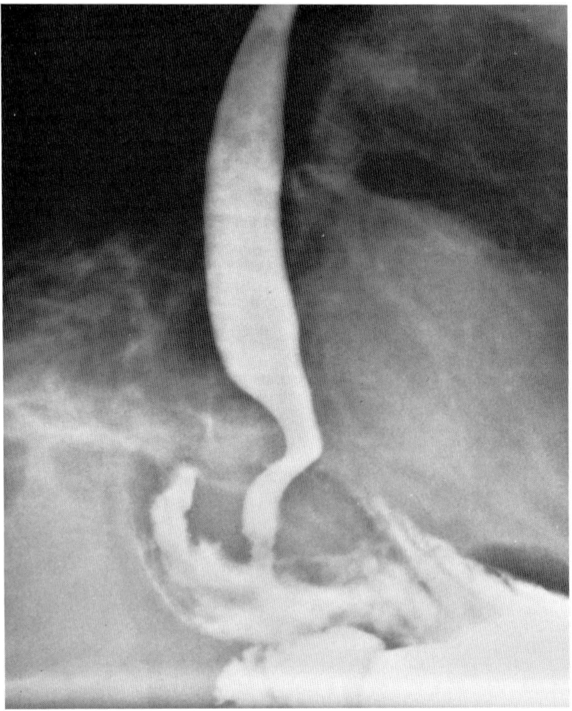

Fig. 1-32 View of the gastroesophageal junction demonstrating a pseudomass in a patient post–Belsey-Mark IV fundoplication.

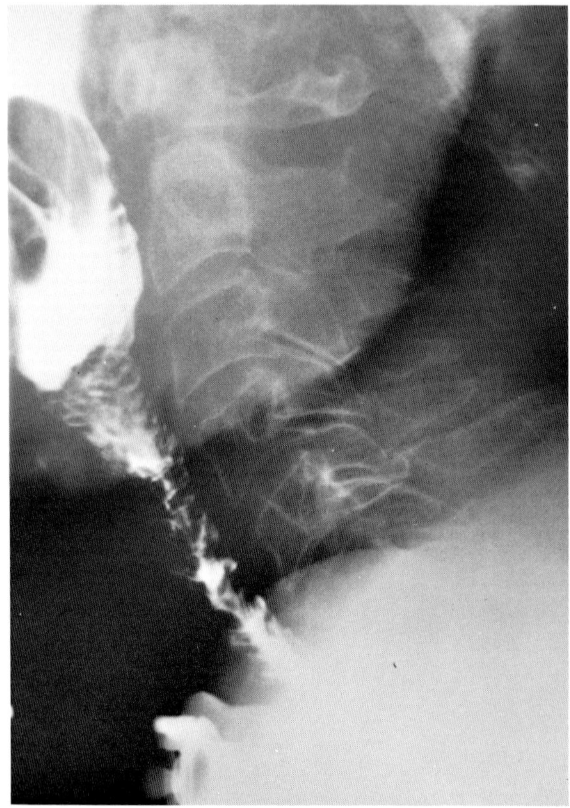

Fig. 1-33 Patient with en bloc resection of the trachea and cervical esophagus for carcinoma. A free jejunal flap is seen from hypopharynx to the thoracic esophagus.

often closely applied to and inseparable from the esophagus, at times causing deviation and compression. Two-thirds of these lesions are found in children; the remainder are found incidentally in adults. Most duplications are segmental, involving the lower posterior mediastinum; at times, the entire esophagus can be involved. Both spherical and tubular duplications can be seen. The spherical type does not usually communicate with the esophageal lumen, whereas tubular duplications often communicate with adjacent viscera. The content of duplications varies from mucosal lining, similar to that of adjacent bowel, to heterotopic; the latter can have bronchial or neural elements.

ESOPHAGEAL NEOPLASIA

Esophageal neoplasms, both benign and malignant, occur in a wide variety of locations within the esophagus and are among the least common types of gastrointestinal tumors. The vast majority of patients present with symptoms of dysphagia. The diagnosis is often made at the time of the initial barium swallow.

Differentiation of intraluminal or intrinsic lesions from extraluminal or extrinsic lesions is extremely important. Epithelial lesions, such as carcinoma, generally show some contour irregularity and when seen tangentially, they have acute shelflike margins. Submucosal tumors produce a symmetric moundlike lesion with smooth margins. Viewed in tangent, the margin tapers to form an obtuse angle with the normal esophageal wall. Esophageal defects produced by compression from an external mass are not usually as well defined as intramural submucosal lesions. At times, however, radiographic findings are such that differentiation is not possible.

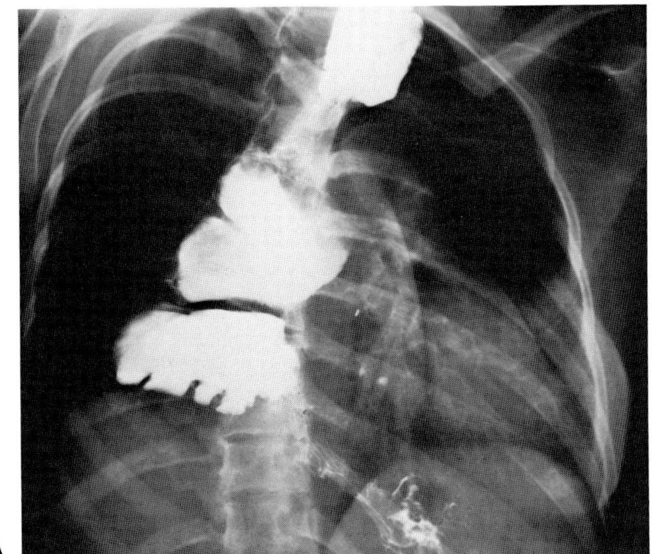

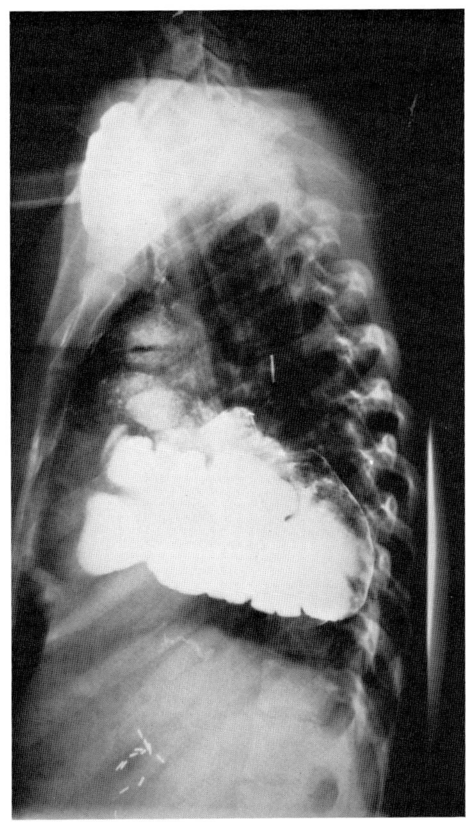

Fig. 1-34 **(A)** Oblique and **(B)** lateral views from a barium study, showing colon interposition in chest.

Benign tumors occur infrequently and are much less common than malignant tumors. The relative frequency of benign tumors has been reported as follows: leiomyoma and other myomas, 51 percent; polyp, 25 percent; cyst, 8 percent; papilloma, 3 percent; fibroma, 3 percent; and hemangioma, 2 percent. The remaining 8 percent is accounted for by extremely rare tumors, such as myofibroma, neurofibroma, adenoma, and others. There is no universally accepted pathologic classification for benign esophageal tumors. Esophageal tumors have been subdivided into two categories: (1) those having intraluminal origins and (2) those with intramural origins. Many, however, can have both intramural and intraluminal components.

Leiomyomas of the esophagus account for more than half of the benign tumors, often varying in size but with a smooth configuration. In the vast majority of cases, the lesion is only visible on a barium study (Fig. 1-38); occasionally it can be seen as it protrudes against the air-filled lung near the mediastinum.

Carcinoma of the esophagus, despite recent advances in surgery and radiation therapy, has a poor prognosis. The overall 5-year survival rate reported in the Western literature is in the 4 to 10 percent range. Risk factors include a history of smoking and heavy alcohol use. Furthermore, an increased incidence of squamous cell carcinoma is seen following chronic corrosive esophageal strictures and in longstanding achalasia.

Primary adenocarcinoma reported with Barrett esophagus (10 percent), accounts for approximately 20 percent of all adenocarcinomas involving the esophagus. Most adenocarcinomas are found in the distal esophagus, tend to involve the gastric cardia, and may be ultimately classified as gastric in origin. These tumors can produce an achalasia-like appear-

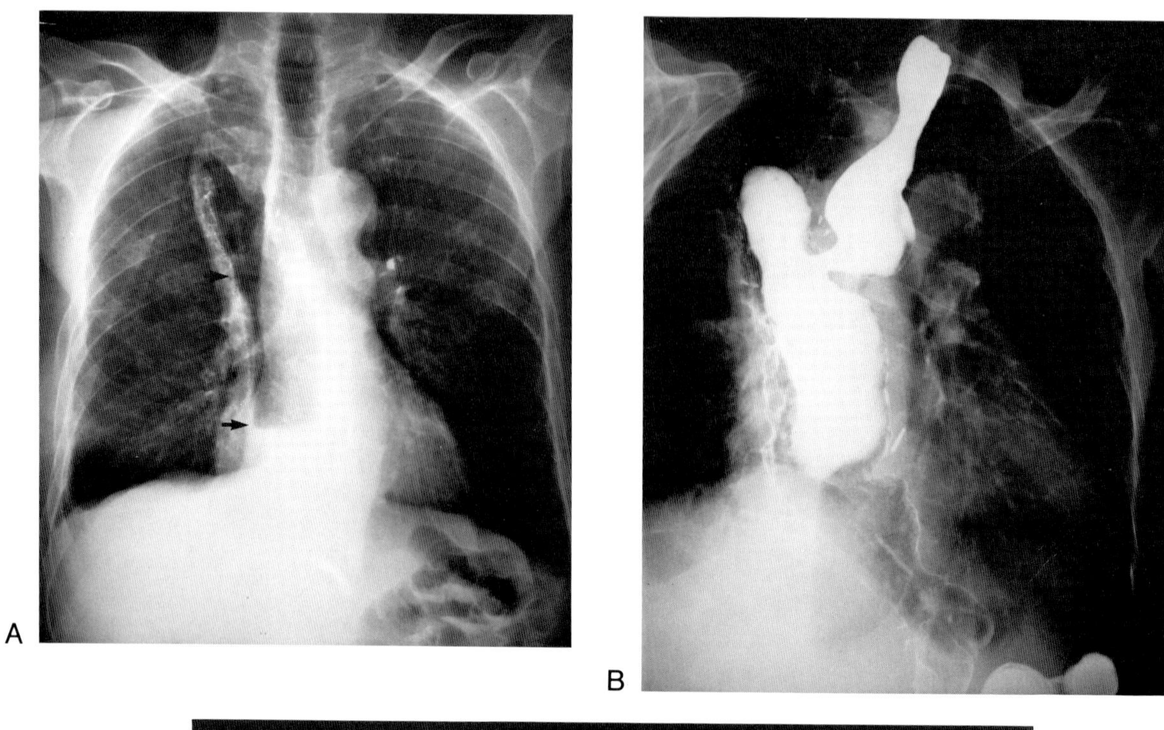

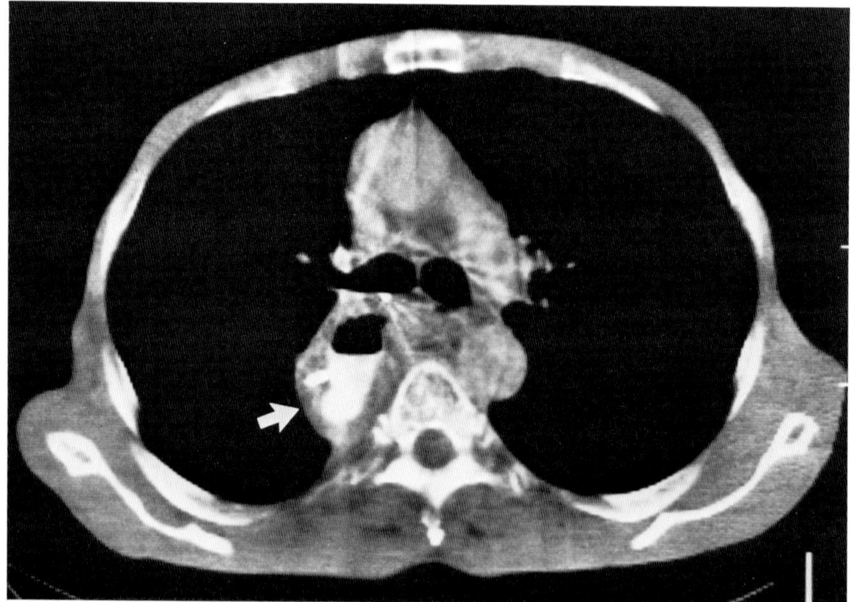

Fig. 1-35 (**A**) PA chest radiograph without contrast demonstrating a large air-containing structure *(arrows)* with a fluid level representing the gastric pull-through. (**B**) Oblique barium study showing the remaining esophagus and stomach. (**C**) CT scan with oral contrast, demonstrating the gastric pull-through.

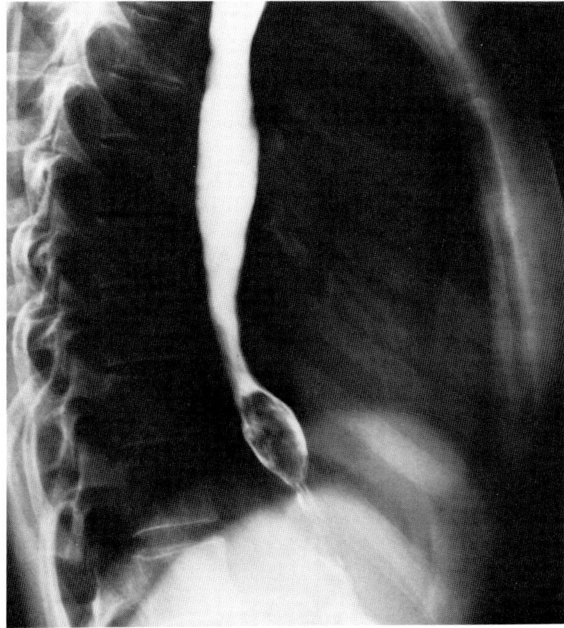

Fig. 1-36 Lateral barium swallow with large bolus of food partially obstructing the distal esophagus.

ance (see section on Strictures). The vast majority of esophageal malignancies are of the squamous cell variety (90 percent), with adenocarcinoma the next most frequent (6 percent), and other entities such as carcinosarcoma, lymphoma, and metastasis much less frequent. Carcinosarcoma, an unusual primary malignancy, contains components of both epithelial and connective tissue. Often the tumor, which has a bulky polypoid growth, expands the esophageal lumen. These tumors grow slowly, metastasizing late in the disease.

Although they rarely do so, any of the multiple histologic types of lymphoma can involve the esophagus. Radiologically, contiguous nodular involvement of both the distal esophagus and the stomach can be seen. However, a wide spectrum of radiologic appearances has been reported, since any part of the esophagus can be involved.

Carcinomas of the esophagus are usually superficially ulcerated, can be well-circumscribed, and can involve the entire circumference or only a portion of the esophagus. If severe stenosis is present, the esophagus proximal to the lesion can dilate. Often, submucosal

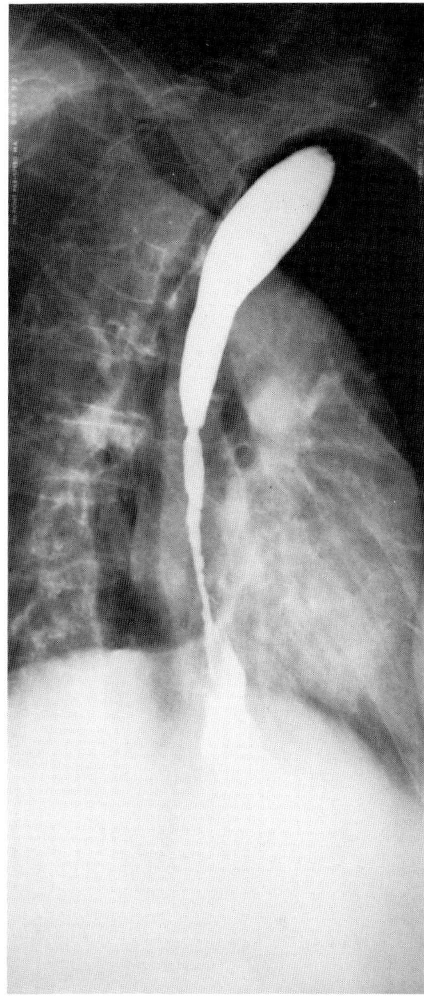

Fig. 1-37 View of the esophagus with marked narrowing secondary to a benign stricture.

invasion is present so that the lesion is more extensive than is seen radiographically.

The diagnosis of esophageal cancer, unfortunately, is rarely made before local invasion or distant metastasis has occurred. Plain radiographs of the chest generally show no abnormalities, but can reveal mediastinal widening, an esophageal air-fluid level, soft tissue mass with bowing of the trachea anteriorly, or widening of the azygoesophageal stripe.

Radiographically, the features of esophageal cancers can be classified into four categories: annular con-

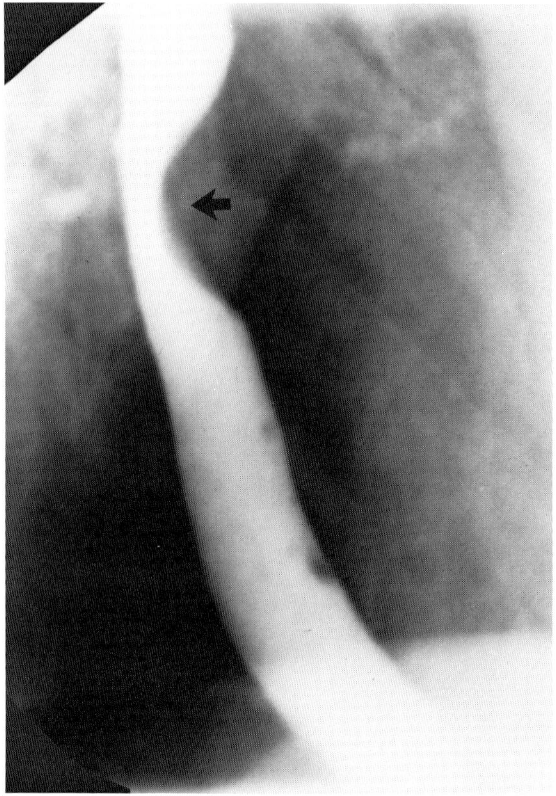

Fig. 1-38 Barium swallow radiograph showing a smooth mass involving distal esophagus secondary to a leiomyoma *(arrow)*.

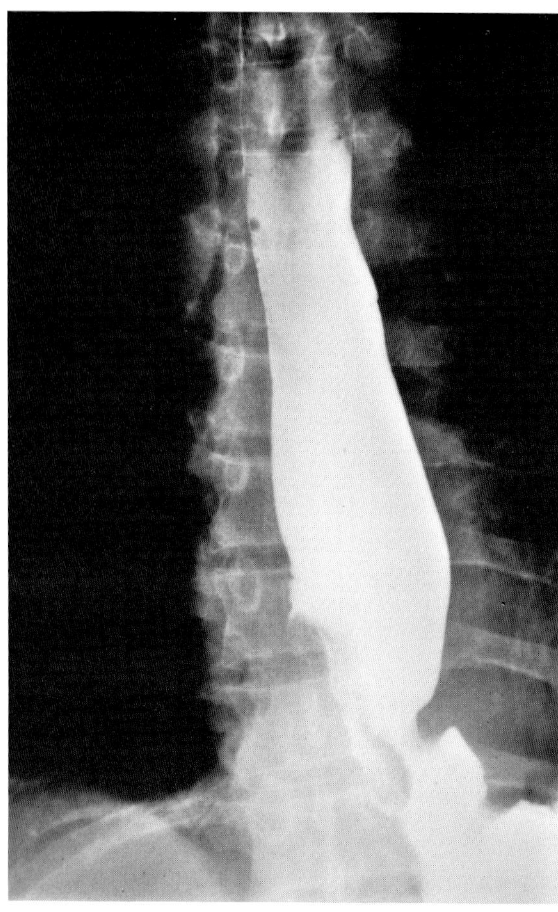

Fig. 1-39 AP barium swallow radiograph with irregular mass involving the distal esophagus secondary to adenocarcinoma.

stricting, polypoid, infiltrative or stenosing, and ulcerative. The most frequent type is the annular constricting lesion. Characteristically, in these lesions an overhanging shelf is seen proximally. The narrowed lumen is usually irregular and ulcerated, with destroyed mucosa (Fig. 1-39). The next most common type is the polypoid carcinoma. Early, the lesion can be seen extending from the esophageal wall. The neoplasm can eventually encircle the esophagus, producing an annular configuration or a bulky obstructing lesion. The infiltrative type can easily be confused with a benign stricture because the lesion is primarily submucosal (Fig. 1-40). Often, the mucosa is preserved and the margin of the tumor is tapered. The least common type of esophageal cancer is the ulcerative. Here, lesions are entirely ulcerated.

Early lesions begin as areas of focal mucosal irregularity, eventually develop into plaquelike structures on one wall of the esophagus (Fig. 1-41), then spread easily along the esophagus. Since there is no serosa surrounding the esophagus, cancer can easily spread through the muscularis to invade the mediastinum. Early symptoms are few. Dysphagia usually is not present until the lumen of the esophagus is surrounded by tumor. Since the lumen of the esophagus is distensible, it can accommodate a bolus of food even if a lesion involves one wall.

Early lesions can be demonstrated easily with an air-contrast technique. This technique helps to assess tumor boundaries by providing information about the distensibility of the esophageal wall and the mucosal surface of the esophagus.

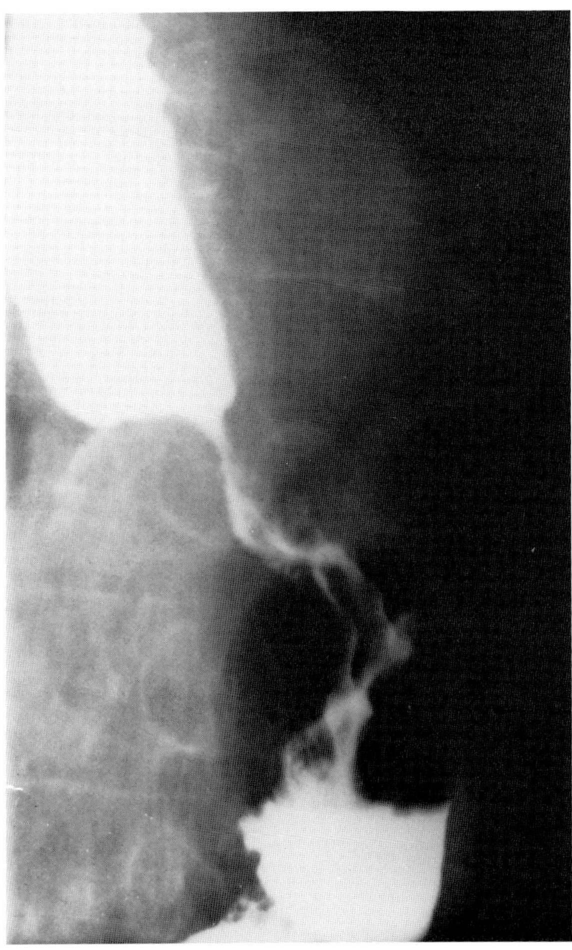

Fig. 1-40 View of the gastroesophageal junction shows marked irregularity of the mucosa involving the distal esophagus and gastric fundus. Patient had squamous cell carcinoma of the esophagus, invading the fundus.

In 1950 Barrett described a now controversial condition in which the lower esophagus is lined with columnar epithelium instead of the stratified squamous epithelium normally present. This process has been found to be associated with primary adenocarcinoma of the esophagus. Most believe that the abnormal columnar epithelium is acquired as the result of injury to the stratified squamous epithelium with metaplasia from chronic gastroesophageal reflux (See Fig. 1-18).

At times, a varicoid carcinoma of the esophagus can resemble esophageal varices. This variant of squamous cell carcinoma presents with nodular filling de-

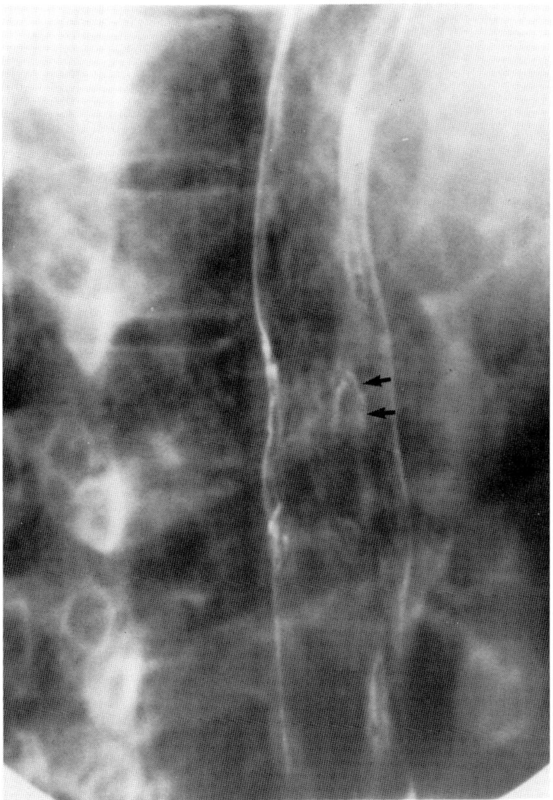

Fig. 1-41 Air-contrast view of the midesophagus demonstrating a placquelike lesion *(arrows)*.

fects and areas of rigidity that do not change in size or with peristalsis, as do true varices.

In recent studies, CT has been shown to be of great value in staging carcinoma of the esophagus. Until the advent of CT, there was no accurate method for the nonsurgical, pretreatment staging of patients with esophageal cancer. Currently, endoscopy and cytology can provide an unequivocal diagnosis of esophageal cancer.

CT can accurately display the anatomy of the esophagus and mediastinum and is also a rapid, noninvasive method of staging esophageal carcinoma. CT can provide necessary information about the length and diameter of the tumor, lymph node involvement, and metastatic disease to determine resectability and to plan radiation treatment. The most common abnormality found on CT is focal esophageal wall thickening by large masses that almost obliterate the lumen of

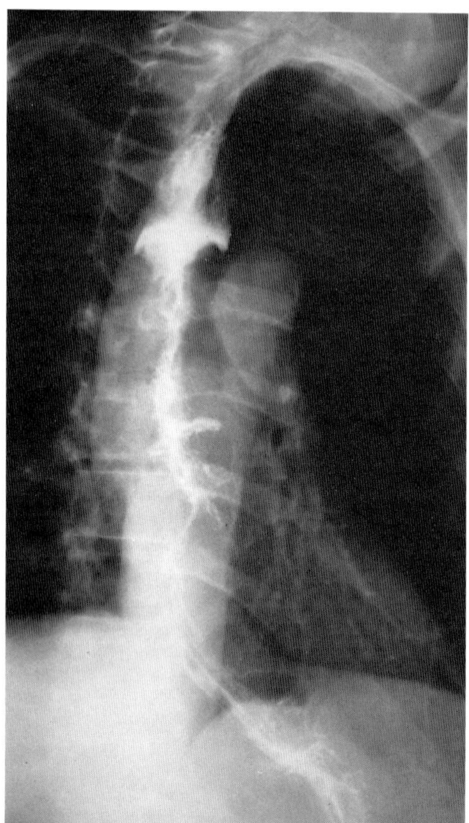

A

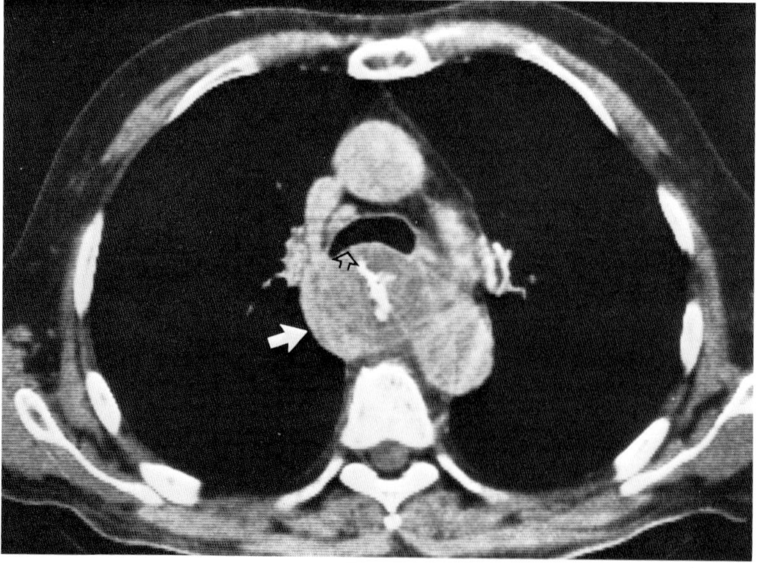

B

Fig. 1-42 **(A)** A barium-swallow radiograph demonstrating a large, irregular lesion involving the midesophagus, from an adenocarcinoma. **(B)** CT scan showing markedly thickened esophageal wall *(white arrow)* compressing adjacent trachea *(open black arrow)*.

the esophagus (Fig. 1-42). Esophageal cancer invading a variety of structures, including the trachea, bronchi, left atrium, aorta, and pulmonary arteries and veins can also be demonstrated by CT. Metastatic diseases of the mediastinum, abdominal lymph nodes, liver, and adrenals are also easily identified, thus, allowing precise preoperative staging. If radiography reveals a suspect lesion but the biopsy is negative, the results should not be accepted without question.

Primary and secondary malignant tumors that are submucosal in origin can yield negative mucosal biopsies. The differential diagnoses that should be considered include esophagitis (including Barrett esophagus), benign neoplasms, duplication cysts, large varices, and extrinsic masses.

SUGGESTED READINGS

Braver J: Iatrogenic disorders of the esophagus. p. 161. In Herman PG (ed): Iatrogenic Thoracic Complications. Springer-Verlag, New York, 1983

Calenoff L, Rogers LF: Esophageal complications of surgery and lifesaving procedures. p. 123. In Meyers MA, Ghahremani GG (eds): Iatrogenic Gastrointestinal Complications. Springer-Verlag, New York, 1981

Intrinsic diseases of the adult esophagus. Semin Roentgenol 16:168, 1981

Moss AA, Thoeni RF: Computed tomography of the gastrointestinal tract. p. 535. In Moss AA, Gamsue G, Genant HK (eds): Computed Tomography of the Body. WB Saunders, Philadelphia, 1983

Ott DJ, Gelfand DW, Wu WC, et al: Esophagogastric region and its rings. AJR 142:281, 1984

Spjut HJ, Dodds WJ, Anderson MF, et al: Esophagus and esophagogastric region. p. 491. In Margulis AR, Burhenne HJ (eds): Alimentary Tract Radiology. 3rd Ed. CV Mosby, St Louis, 1983.

Williford ME, Rice RP, Kelvin FM, et al: Revascularized jejunal graft replacing the cervical esophagus radiographic evaluation. AJR 145:533, 1985

Zboralske FF, Dodds WJ: Roentgenographic diagnosis of primary disorders of esophageal motility. RCNA 7:147, 1969

2
Radiology of the Stomach

R. Kristina Gedgaudas-McClees
Eric C. McClees

EXAMINATION OF THE STOMACH: TECHNICAL ASPECTS

Double-Contrast Technique

The formal double-contrast examination of the stomach is designed to produce optimal visualization of the gastric mucosa. This is achieved with gaseous distension and resultant effacement of the normal folds and use of an appropriate barium suspension to achieve good coating. Attention to rigorous technical detail is of paramount importance if the stomach is to be evaluated accurately.

Patient preparation includes an overnight fast. In addition, some examiners have insisted that their patients abstain from smoking the morning of the examination. Smoking has been implicated in excess mucus production, which theoretically can hinder optimal contrast coating of the gastric mucosa. Before the stomach is examined, all required materials (to be listed later in this chapter) should be ready for use. Various authors have advocated the routine administration of hypotonic agents. Pro-banthine has been used in the past but, because of its anticholinergic side effects, it has been replaced with glucagon. Glucagon has been used in intravenous doses ranging from 0.10 to 1.0 mg; however, it is generally felt that in examinations of the stomach a dose of 0.10 mg allows for adequate hypotonia in most patients and is effective for 3 to 5 minutes. If more time is required, 0.25 mg can be administered intravenously. (Intramuscular injections are not recommended as they require larger doses and take up to 15 minutes to take effect). Glucagon has essentially no side effects (although some patients may experience nausea) and is only contraindicated in patients with brittle diabetes mellitus, insulinoma, and pheochromocytoma.

Users of glucagon have little doubt that the hypotonic agent significantly improves the quality of the upper gastrointestinal (UGI) examination. Glucagon does, however, prolong the examination because it does not have a relaxing effect on the pylorus and subsequently delays emptying into the duodenum. This is not considered a significant problem in most patients. After the hypotonic effects have worn off, barium is free to empty into the small bowel so that subsequent small bowel follow-through examinations can be performed, if clinically indicated.

As mentioned, one of the key features of good technique is adequate distension of the stomach so that the normal rugal folds are totally effaced, facilitating visualization of small polypoid or ulcerated lesions that can readily be lost among tortuous folds. A variety of effervescent agents are currently in use. They contain sodium bicarbonate, which releases carbon dioxide when it is mixed with liquids. Also present is simethicone, which is important in dispersing the bubbles rapidly. Two popularly used effervescent agents are E-Z gas powder, made by the E-Z-EM company, and Baros effervescent granules manufactured by Mallinkrodt. Both are effective distending agents and are prepackaged in optimal single-dose packets.

The second feature of a satisfactory UGI double-contrast examination is adequate mucosal coating. The quality of coating depends on the specific properties of the barium suspension. The suspension has a gritty consistency that allows it to wash over the gastric mucosa, removing superficial gastric mucus. This allows the barium to spread in a thin adherent coat uniformly over all surfaces of the stomach as the patient is turned leftward through two 360-degree rotations. Several patient rotations generally provide adequate mucosal coating and, by turning the patient to the left, only a minimal amount of barium, if any, empties into the duodenum. If the radiologist considers the coating technically suboptimal prior to filming, additional patient turning may be necessary or more contrast material may have to be ingested at the discretion of the examiner.

Several so-called heavy barium products are on the market. Generally, E-Z HD (E-Z-EM Co) barium is preferred. It is currently prepackaged to dispense 4.5 oz of liquid when the powder is mixed with a specified measure of water. It produces a 250% W/V barium suspension, which has a moderate viscosity. (The fluoroscopist must be sure to mix the barium shortly before use, as it can precipitate when left standing for several hours.)

The presence of fluid in the stomach definitely interferes with the quality of mucosal coating. As mentioned, if the coating is suboptimal, additional barium can be administered. If the excess fluid continues to prevent adequate coating, the examiner should then switch to a conventional single-contrast examination of the stomach (to be discussed later), or the patient should return for reexamination after proper preparation.

A set pattern of patient maneuvers, which allow the entire stomach to be visualized in several projections, requires a combination of skill and relative speed. Because glucagon's effects on the stomach are limited, the examiner has 3 to 5 minutes in which barium can be retained in the stomach. Also, barium adequately coats the stomach for only a short period of time, about equal to the effect of glucagon. The examiner should, therefore, establish a good technique and begin filming immediately, making pertinent fluoroscopic observations simultaneously.

Filming with the 105 mm camera is extremely convenient for the radiologist. (The resolution of these films, however, is less than for conventional cassette films.) Spot films should be taken at 100 kVp, unless rare earth screens are being used, in which case the kVp can be lower. Density settings must be carefully lowered to prevent overpenetration of surface details. Although overhead films are a necessary adjunct to spot filming, the radiologist should not rely on them excessively and end the filming when the examination is felt to be complete and adequate.

The following is a list of specific maneuvers for the double-contrast UGI. For patients who are mobile, cooperative, and are not at risk for aspiration, the double-contrast examination should be used if mucosal disease is clinically suspect. All patients considered to be too ill, or in whom a nonmucosal condition is suspected (i.e., hiatal hernia, reflux, gastric outlet obstruction) should undergo a conventional single-contrast examination. (If gastric perforation is suspected, then water-soluble contrast agents *only* should be administered. Specific agents, such as Gastrografin or Gastrovue, contain diatrizoate meglumine and/or diatrizoate sodium solution with 37 percent bound iodine or 11 gr of iodine per ounce. If a nasogastric tube is present and the patient is not required to take the contrast agent orally, any water-soluble contrast can be used, provided its concentration is not greater than 40 percent iodine because subsequent hemorrhagic gastritis is an inherent danger.)

The various maneuvers listed can, of course, be modified for the individual patient, provided the end result yields several adequate views of each region of the stomach. Various manipulations and differing positions may be necessary, depending on the anatomy of the stomach.

DOUBLE CONTRAST UPPER GI SERIES (BIPHASIC)

Ingredients

4½ oz E-Z HD barium (250% W/V), E-Z-Paque (55% W/V)

E-Z gas powder or Baros effervescent granules

Glucagon 0.1 to 0.25 mg IV

Technique

1. In the erect position after receiving an injection of glucagon, the patient places the gas agent in his or her mouth, swallowing it down with 5 to 10 ml of water.* The patient then drinks a full cup of the high density barium as quickly as is comfortable. Film air-contrast views of the distal esophagus, with the patient turned slightly to the left to prevent the esophagus from projecting over the spine. (Warn the patient not to belch.)
2. The table is then placed in a horizontal position.
3. The patient rotates twice, 360 degrees toward the left. Having achieved good coating of the distended stomach, the distal half of the stomach is filmed with the patient in the supine position.
4. Next, film the distal half of the stomach with the patient LPO 30 degrees.
5. Film the fundus of the stomach with the patient in the right lateral position. (Additional upright views of the fundus can also be obtained.)
6. Film the upper body of the stomach with the patient in the RPO 30 degrees position (with the table horizontal).
7. The duodenal bulb and sweep, with barium-filled and air-contrast views, are examined using the prone oblique and supine positions, respectively. (Use compression of the duodenal bulb and distal stomach when the patient is in the prone oblique (GI) position.)
8. Finally, reexamine the esophagus for motility disorders or the presence of a hiatal hernia, with the patient prone and drinking the low density barium.
9. Conventional technique overhead films:
Esophagus (oblique)
Stomach prone
Stomach prone RAO
Stomach supine
Stomach lateral (optional)

---

*If Baros is used, the patient can swallow the granules with barium only.

Normal Appearance of the Stomach

In the normal stomach, a fine reticular or honeycomb pattern, extending from the fundus to the antrum (Fig. 2-1) should be identified. These are the areae gastricae, and they represent the micromucosal pattern of the stomach; the gastric rugae represent the macromucosal pattern. Any change in this reticular pattern in a technically adequate examination reflects pathology.

The gastric fundus is an extremely difficult area to examine because it offers an excellent hiding place for lesions; therefore adequate distension and coating is important in this region (Fig. 2-2). A normal, rounded radiolucency with radiating folds represents the cardia complex (the burnous), which can effectively be effaced with the Valsalva maneuver. Lesions in the cardia, however, can mimic this normal anatomic landmark. If respiratory maneuvers or the additional use of effervescent agents cannot efface or change this appearance, then pathology should be suspected (Fig. 2-3).

This leads us to the matter of interpreting the air-contrast examination of the stomach. In general, two types of lesions are diagnosed in the stomach — i.e., polypoid and depressed. Polypoid lesions are space-occupying masses that displace barium and are seen as negative filling defects. If the polypoid lesion is on the nondependent surface, the edge of the lesion will be

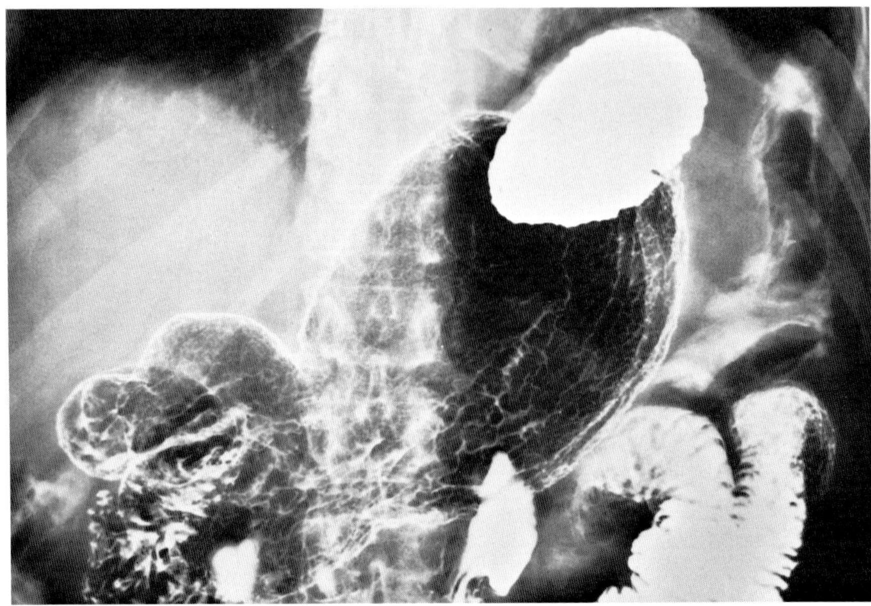

Fig. 2-1 The normal areae gastricae are well visualized throughout the entire stomach.

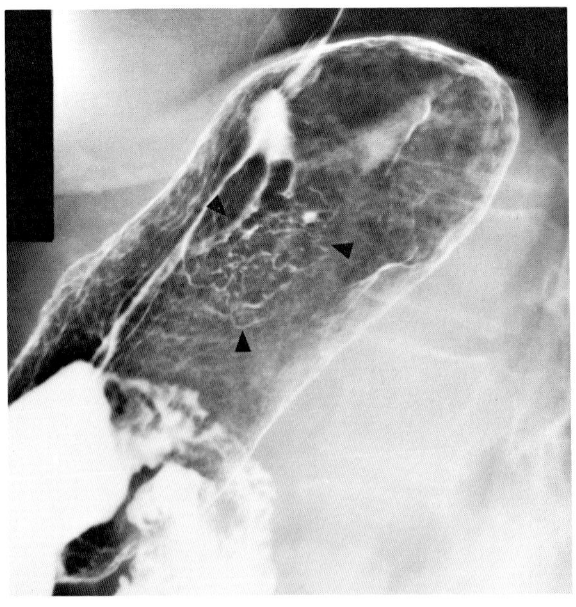

Fig. 2-2 Note the abnormal mucosal pattern just caudal to the burnous *(arrowheads)*. This represents a carcinoma in situ.

coated with barium. When the lesion is of mucosal origin, the areae gastricae pattern will be absent from its surface and its outline may be slightly irregular. Submucosal lesions, on the other hand, have a characteristically smooth surface, as if etched with a white pencil (Fig. 2-4). Polypoid lesions are best identified as such when seen in profile. In this view they can be seen as protruberant masses that project into the gastric lumen.

Depressed or ulcerating lesions have two distinctly different appearances depending on their location. When they are located on the dependent surface of the stomach, they collect barium to produce the typical ulcer niche. When the ulcer is on the nondependent surface, it will naturally be void of barium and will collect air. Generally, the edge of the ulceration coats with barium and, when seen en face, appears as a "ring shadow," a term coined by Laufer (1979) (Fig. 2-5). Partially coated, the ring may assume a crescentic or linear outline. Identified in profile, the ulcer is noted to project away from the lumen of the stomach and, therefore, can be distinguished from a polypoid lesion.

It is important that the reader not be confused with the stalactite phenomenon described by Op den Orth

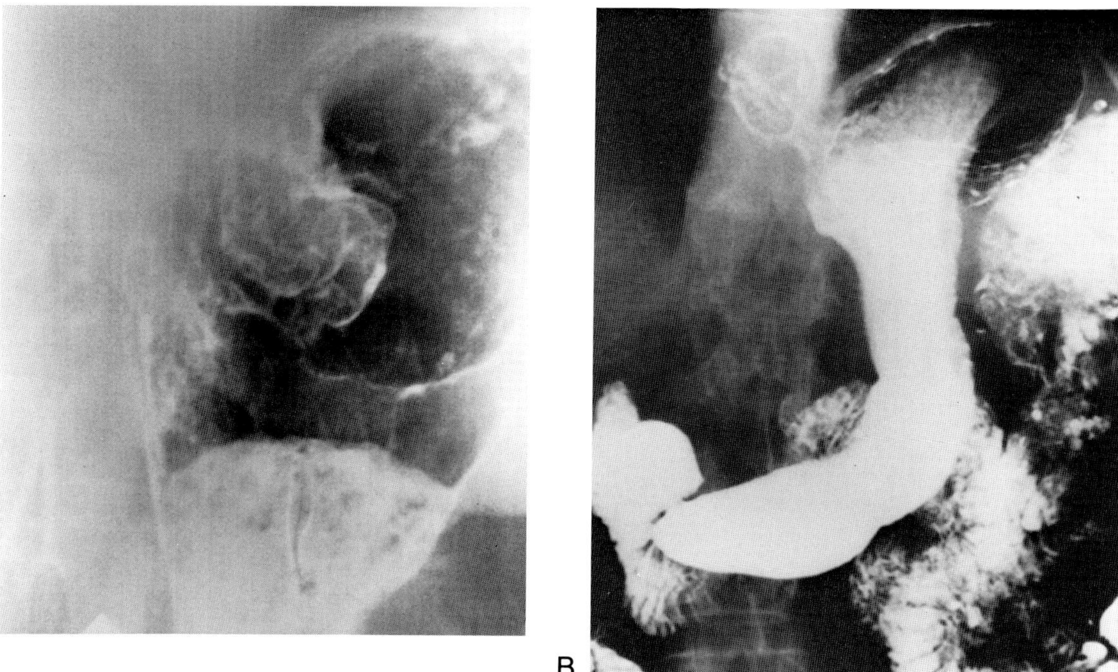

Fig. 2-3 (A) Mass effect is present at the cardia, mimicking a polypoid tumor. This represents a prolapsed hiatal hernia. **(B)** During the Valsalva manuever, the hernia is evident and the mass effect has disappeared.

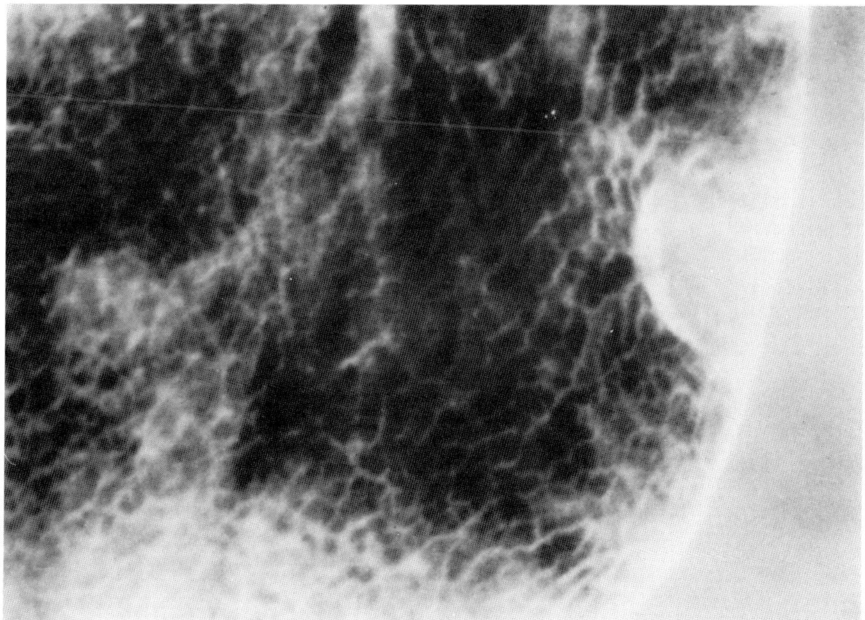

Fig. 2-4 A leiomyoma is apparent within the stomach. Note the normal mucosal pattern overlying it, and the smooth interface of the mass with the mucosa, confirming its submucosal origin.

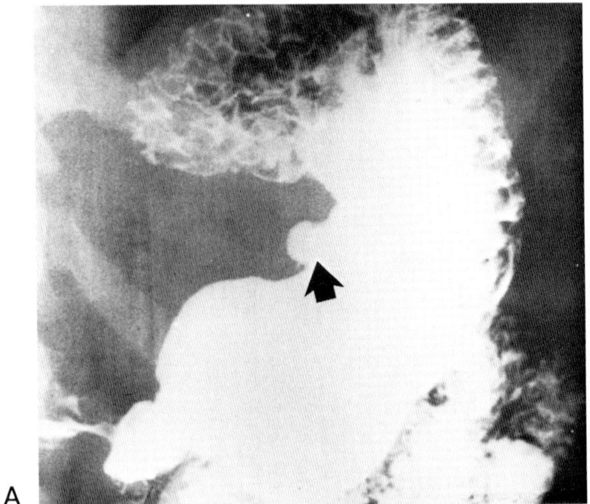

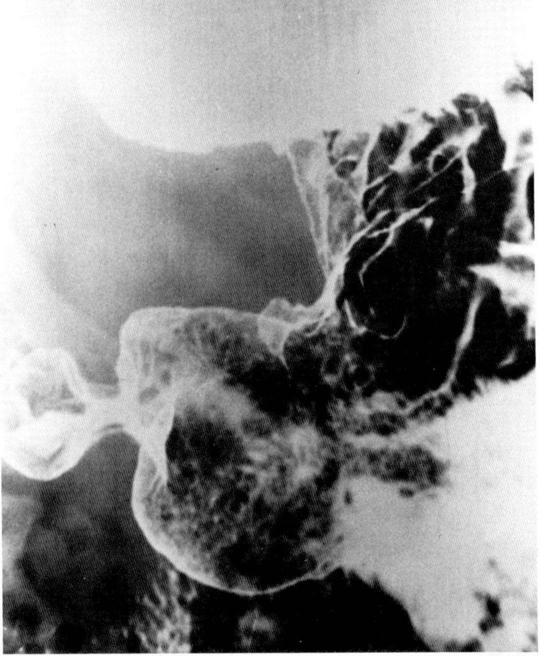

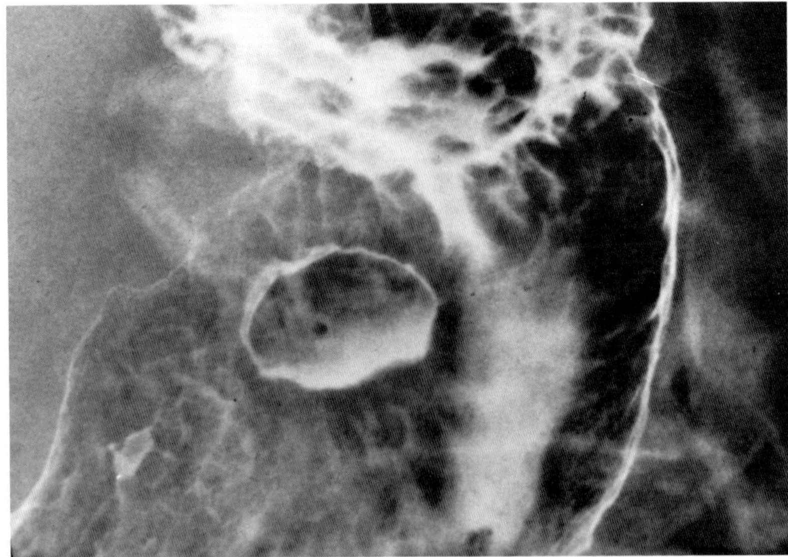

Fig. 2-5 (A) A barium-filled ulcer niche is present on the lesser curvature *(arrow)*. **(B)** Void of barium, the ulcer is identified in profile. **(C)** En face the air-filled ulcer has the appearance of a ring.

(1983), which represents a droplet of barium hanging from a protrusion on the nondependent surface of the stomach. Seen en face, it can be mistaken for an ulceration. With time, or on gentle palpation, the droplet falls to the dependent surface of the stomach and disappears (Fig 2-6).

Artifacts

Care should be taken not to mistake a variety of artifacts for pathology. Barium that has been mixed incorrectly can precipitate out in the stomach and appear as punctate collections. On quick inspection,

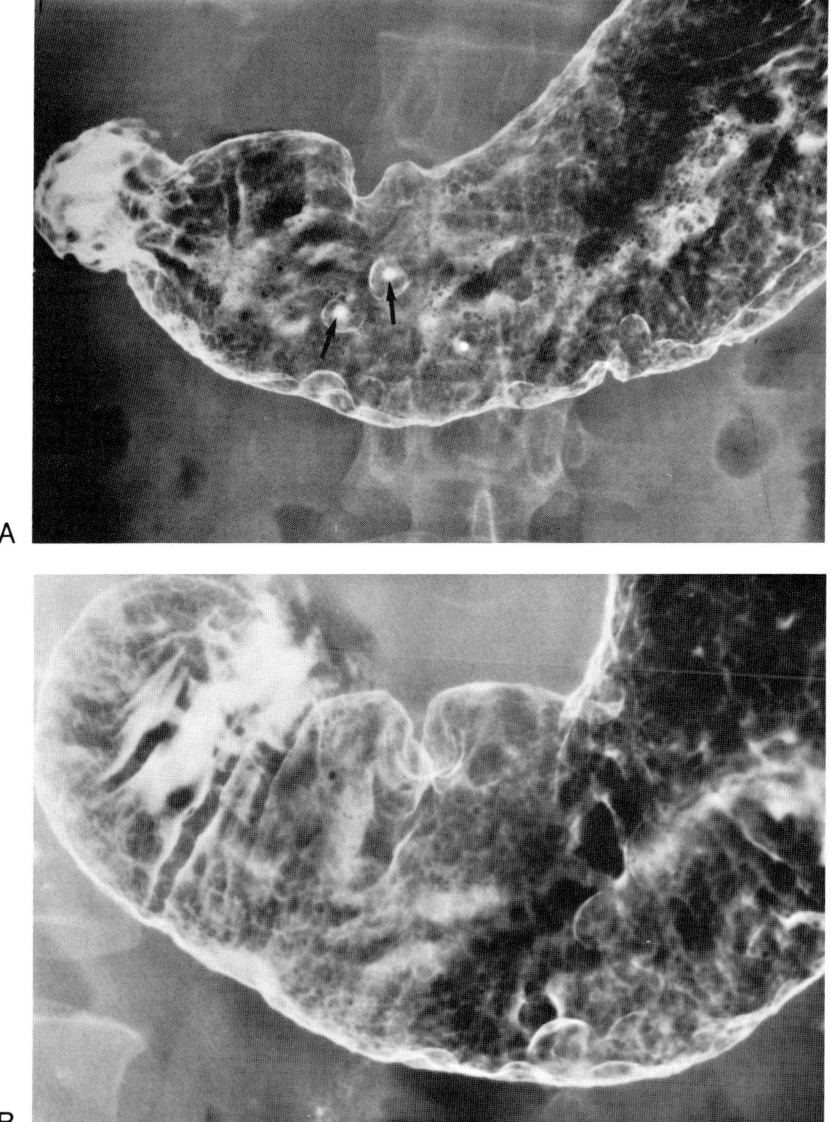

Fig. 2-6 (A) Droplets of barium *(arrows)* hang from inflammatory polyps on the nondependent surface of the stomach, creating a stalactite phenomenon. **(B)** Moments later the droplets have disappeared.

the barium collections look like aphthous lesions; however, differentiation is readily made since the precipitated barium is not surrounded by a well-defined halo of edema. Poorly dissolved effervescent granules can appear as tiny radiolucent defects that can be mistaken for tiny polyps. With time, and often with additional patient rotation, these filling defects disappear as the gas continues to defervesce.

The so-called kissing artifact mentioned by Laufer (1979) can mimic a mass lesion in the stomach. This artifact represents apposition of the anterior and posterior walls of the stomach as they are compressed, generally over the spine in asthenic patients. It can readily be altered by placing the patient in an oblique position, allowing air to separate the two surfaces of the stomach.

Finally, it is important to note that extragastric densities, such as the spine or projections from the small bowel, can be identified through the radiolucent stomach and be mistaken for polyps or ulcerations. This problem is generally obviated by filming the stomach in multiple projections.

Single-Contrast Technique

The single-contrast technique has received some criticism in the past by double-contrast advocates. However, it is a most important and useful radiologic examination. Even enthusiasts of the double-contrast technique rely on the single-contrast examination of the stomach in certain select patient populations. These are specifically patients immobilized by illness, those who are uncooperative, and patients with aspiration difficulties. Also, the single-contrast technique is indicated when mucosal disease is not suspected, as in patients with hiatal hernias, gastric outlet obstruction, and bezoars. Patients who have had recent gastric anastomoses of varying types may need only to be assessed for patency. Suspected malformations and malpositions, as well as motor disorders can be evaluated with the single-contrast technique.

Patient preparation includes an overnight fast. Hypotonic agents are not used. The patient swallows barium, of a thinner consistency than that used for the double-contrast examination. Barium preparations that can be used are Solopaque and E-Z-paque. After

the esophagus is examined, the stomach is filled and examined carefully, using manual compression. Graduated manual compression, applied carefully and systematically, allows the examiner to evaluate the entire stomach fluoroscopically, except for the fundus, which is located beneath the rib cage and, therefore, is not compressible. Spot radiographs are more selective than those taken with the double-contrast technique. However, the fluoroscopic impression is vital to the accurate evaluation of the stomach. The end result is a rapid and essentially accurate examination of potential organic lesions and functional disorders of the stomach.

In addition to anatomic abnormalities, functional disorders that affect gastric peristalsis can be evaluated by the single-contrast technique. The stomach can be examined completely in a maximum of 4 to 5 minutes using short repeated fluoroscopic flashes and four to six spot films. The following list is a guideline for single-contrast examination of the stomach.

SINGLE CONTRAST UPPER GI SERIES

Ingredients

E-Z-paque (55% W/V) or Solopaque

Technique

1. In the upright position, the patient drinks approximately ½ cup of barium as the examiner fluoroscopically observes the esophagus carefully, especially its distensibility and overall morphology.
2. Specific emphasis is placed on palpating and observing the body and antrum of the stomach to search for polypoid filling defects, ulcers, or contour irregularities.
3. If the bulb fills at this stage of the examination, spot films can be taken of the distended bulb.
4. With the table horizontal, the patient turns to the right lateral position, taking several swallows of barium so that the distended esophagus and the appearance of

the esophagogastric (EG) junction can be evaluated. When the EG junction appears entirely normal, a single spot film of this area is adequate in most patients. Esophageal peristalsis is then evaluated by observing the passage of a single swallow of barium down the length of the esophagus. Check for a hiatal hernia, using the Valsalva manuever when the distal esophagus is filled with barium.

5. With the patient in the right lateral position, the fundus is examined fluoroscopically and spotted. The stomach and duodenum are then evaluated for any anterior displacement.

6. The barium-filled stomach is fluoroscoped in the prone patient and appropriate spot films of the barium-filled bulb are obtained.

7. The patient is placed in the supine position and the barium-filled fundus as well as the body of the stomach are again evaluated with manual compression. The patient is then turned to the left posterior oblique position for air-contrast views of the duodenum.

8. The esophagus is observed for the presence of barium reflux.

9. Routine overhead films of the stomach are requested. If the patient has a very high transverse stomach, the tilt oblique view is requested, and if any abnormality is suggested fluoroscopically in the retrogastric position, a lateral view is also obtained.

GASTRITIS

Gastritis has been a topic of controversy for a number of years. Knowledge of gastritis is based on direct visualization and histologic examination of the gastric mucosa. In large part, diagnostic difficulties relate to differences in classification and terminology. The current trend is to classify gastritis based on etiologic and pathogenic features in addition to pure morphologic features.

TYPES OF GASTRITIS

Acute (erosive)
Chronic
    Superficial
    Atrophic
Granulomatous
Eosinophilic
Hypertrophic
    Menetrier disease
    Zollinger-Ellison syndrome
    Idiopathic
Miscellaneous types
    Radiation
    Phlegmonous
    Postoperative
    Corrosive

Acute Gastritis

Acute gastritis has been subtyped as erosive gastritis. It is occasionally asymptomatic in its milder forms but generally presents with varying degrees of epigastric pain and discomfort, often relieved by ingesting food or antacids. Occasionally the condition is persistent and may lead to chronic gastritis.

A variety of etiologies have been implicated, including reactions to stress; ingestion of gastric irritants such as alcohol, aspirin, acids, and alkali; as well as a variety of chemotherapeutic medications such as prednisone, adriamycin, methotrexate, cytoxan, and vinblastine, to name a few. Uremia and gastric radiation are common causes of gastric erosion and hemorrhage. A variety of infectious agents have been implicated, both bacterial (*Staphylococcus aureus, Escherichia coli, Clostridium welchii,* pneumococcus, *Proteus*); fungal (*Candida albicans* and *Candida tropicalis*); and viral (*Cytomegalovirus* and *Herpes*).

A number of radiographic criteria can be used in both the double contrast and the conventional techniques. Essentially five criteria can generally be used. These are (1) poor distensibility seen as flattening and incomplete distension along the lesser, greater, or both curvatures of the antrum; (2) crenulations (fine or coarse serrations) along the lesser, greater, or both curvatures of the antrum; (3) thickened or nodular folds; (4) spasm, evident as transient irritability of the stomach best appreciated on fluoroscopy; and (5) erosions characterized by pinpoint ulcers surrounded by a halo of edema (aphthoid ulcers) (Fig. 2-7). If any or a combination of these findings is present in the stomach, a presumptive diagnosis of gastritis can be made with a relatively high degree of accuracy. Naturally, the presence of erosions or aphthous ulcers is pathognomonic.

Chronic Gastritis

Essentially two forms of chronic gastritis are recognized—superficial and atrophic.

Superficial gastritis represents round-cell infiltration of the lamina propria with normal deeper zones of the mucosa and submucosa.

Atrophic gastritis is defined as round-cell infiltration with loss of normal glands. The mucosa, in fact, becomes atrophic and is thinner than normal. Of note is an entity called gastric atrophy, which demonstrates a complete loss of normal glands with little or no round-cell infiltration of the gastric mucosa. It is considered by some to be a morphologic entity separate from atrophic gastritis. This does not imply, however, that it is pathogenetically different from simple atrophic gastritis. Its progression is more rapid, but it generally develops through a stage of simple atrophic gastritis.

Gastritis shows a definite correlation with the function of gastric mucosa. The secretion of hydrochloric acid decreases linearly with the increasing severity of gastritis. Fasting serum gastrin levels are increased in the more severe cases, particularly in patients with gastric atrophy.

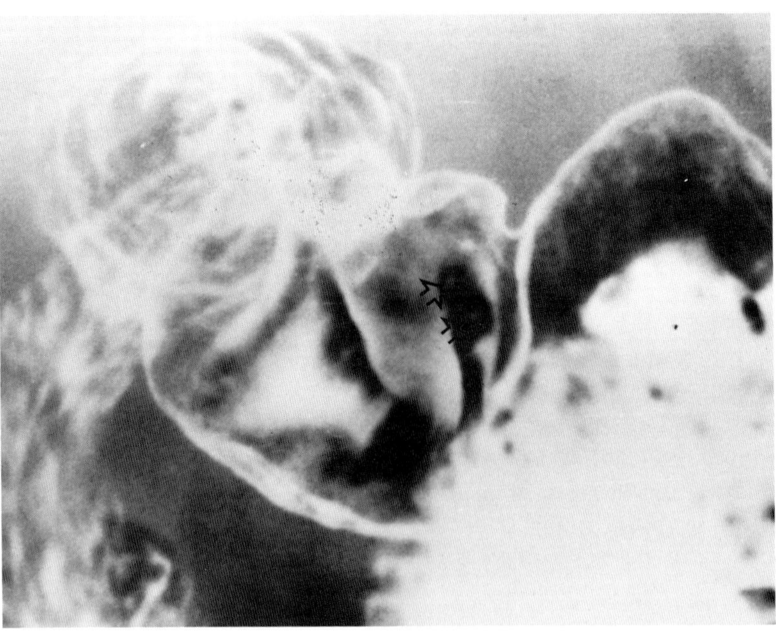

Fig. 2-7 Aphthous erosions *(arrows)* are surrounded by well-demarcated halos of edema in this patient with acute Crohn gastritis.

In general, two forms of atrophic gastritis are present: (1) that which occasionally is associated with achlorhydria, parietal cell antibodies, and high serum gastrin levels, forming a pattern characteristic of A-type or pernicious anemia type gastritis; and (2) B-type gastritis, which tends to be familial and is not associated with functional and immunologic alterations. It predominates in the antrum, sparing the parietal cells in the body of the stomach. Atrophic gastritis and gastric atrophy are associated with an increased risk of carcinoma of the stomach.

Radiographic findings of chronic gastritis are variable. Chronic superficial gastritis essentially cannot be diagnosed radiographically and is generally an endoscopic and histologic diagnosis. Atrophic gastritis reveals itself by thinning or absence of the folds in localized or generalized portions of the stomach. Generally, the contour of the stomach is smooth.

Granulomatous Gastritis

A variety of granulomatous gastritides have been diagnosed. These are specifically Crohn disease, syphilis, sarcoidosis, tuberculosis, histoplasmosis, and actinomycosis. Crohn disease is the most common of the granulomatous gastritides and is most often seen in conjunction with duodenal and ileal Crohn disease (Fig. 2-8). Of those patients with distal involvement, 20 percent will have gastric or gastroduodenal disease as well.

Radiographic findings depend on whether the disease is acute or chronic. Acutely, aphthous erosions or ulcerations may commonly be identified. Nodular thickening of the rugae, representing edema or submucosal granulomatous infiltration, can also be present. Generally, the various forms of granulomatous gastritis are indistinguishable from one another. In the more chronic stages of granulomatous gastritis the stomach generally — or focally in the antrum — becomes rigid and narrowed, with poor distensibility. A linitis plastica-like appearance is present. Scirrhous carcinoma cannot be differentiated from the more severe, chronic forms of gastritis (Fig. 2-9).

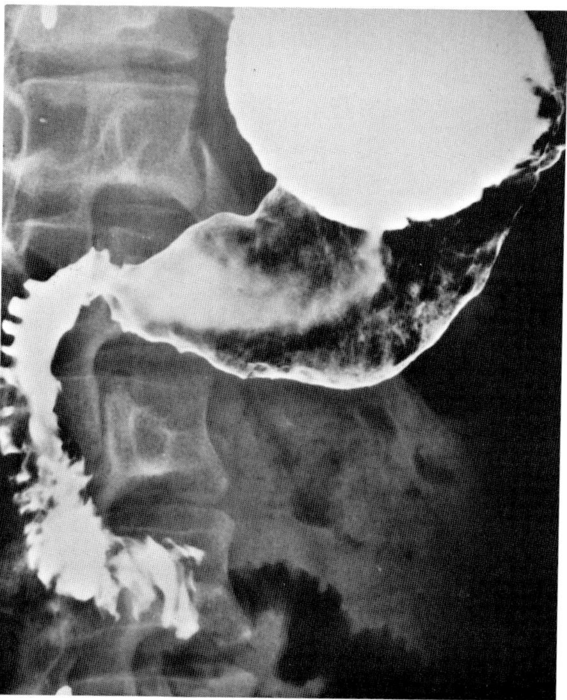

Fig. 2-8 Chronic Crohn involvement of the antrum and proximal duodenum revealed as nodularity, scarring, and effacement of the normal fold pattern.

Eosinophilic Gastritis

Eosinophilic gastritis is a disease known to affect all layers of the stomach and occasionally the small bowel as well. Gastric involvement occurs in 50 to 60 percent of cases and has a particular predilection for the antrum. Clinically, patients complain of abdominal pain and diarrhea, which occasionally are related to certain foods and reflect a hypersensitivity response. In other patients allergies cannot be demonstrated and dietary manipulations are ineffective. In general, approximately 60 percent of patients have a well-documented history of allergy with systemic as well as gastroenteric symptoms. A striking clinical feature that confirms the diagnosis is the presence of peripheral eosinophilia, again seen in 60 percent of patients.

Patients are generally young; the disease originates in the first and second decades of life. Hypoalbuminemia and hypogammaglobulinemia are particularly striking in these young individuals.

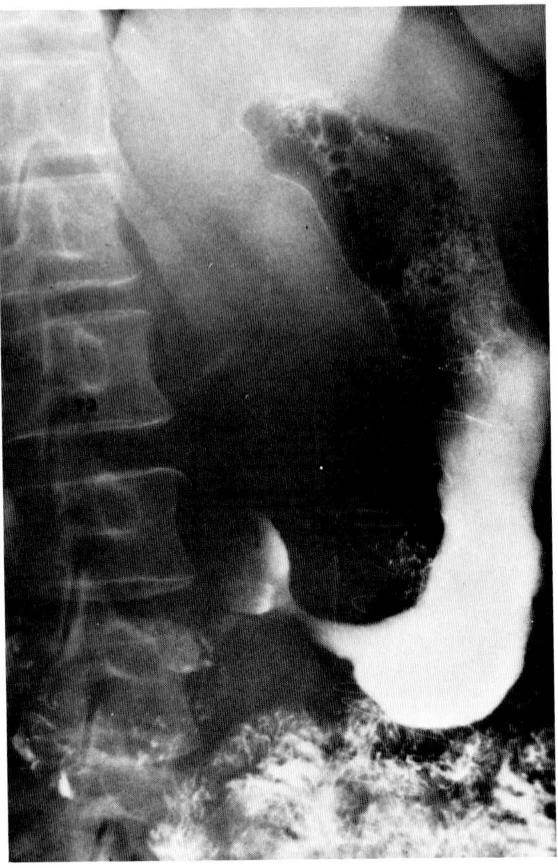

Fig. 2-9 Linitis plastica appearance of the entire stomach is generally caused by a diffusely infiltrative adenocarcinoma. This, however, represents a rare case of chronic gastric sarcoidosis.

Radiographically, the appearance of eosinophilic gastritis can vary. In its acute stages, folds become thickened and discrete polypoid lesions that arise in the submucosa eventually form. The polyps are composed of edema, fibroelastic tissue, and eosinophils. In the chronic phase of the disease the muscular involvement tends to narrow the antrum. Oftentimes it is indistinguishable from scirrhous carcinoma.

Hypertrophic Gastritis

Although the term hypertrophic gastritis is widely used in the literature, it is, in part, a misnomer because the disorder may lack the element of inflammation that warrants the term gastritis.

Histologically, there is marked thickening of the gastric mucosa with hyperplasia of the surface epithelium and enlargement of the glands. No inflammatory cells are usually identified. Endoscopically, the rugal folds are quite prominent, ranging widely from 5 to 30 mm in contrast to the normal 2 to 5 mm in diameter. They may often simulate the convolutions of the brain.

The disease, which may be detected at any age, is slightly more prevalent in males. Symptoms are nonspecific and include UGI bleeding, epigastric pain, nausea, and occasional diarrhea.

Therapy is optional and may not be required. Antacids and anticholinergics may produce mild relief. If symptoms are extreme, gastrectomy may be necessary. Otherwise, spontaneous remission is the usual outcome.

Several forms of hypertrophic gastritis are recognized. Menetrier disease is the classic example (Fig. 2-10). Clinically, protein loss with eventual hypo-

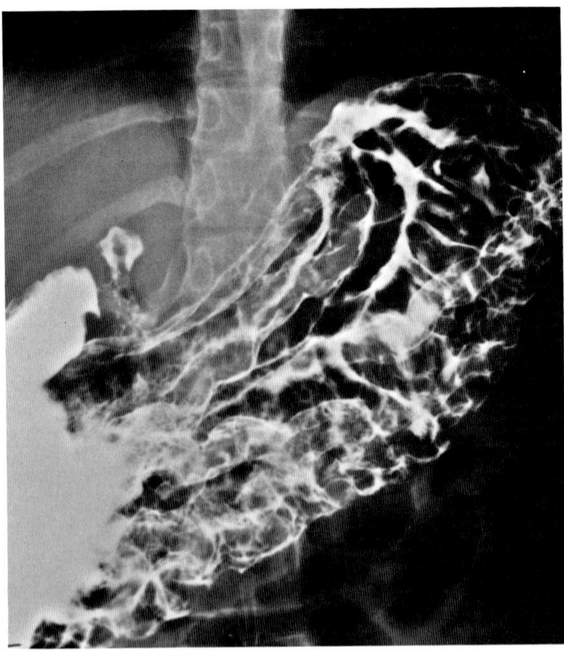

Fig. 2-10 Menetrier gastritis with giant rugal folds in the proximal half of the stomach.

proteinemia and edema are seen in patients with the disease. The patients may have achlorhydria, although a small percentage may actually hypersecrete acid.

Patients exhibit giant folds that primarily affect the fundus and body of the stomach, generally, but not always, sparing the antrum. The folds are soft and pliable and can be effaced on air-contrast examination. Prominent folds cannot always be distinguished from other forms of gastritis or, indeed, from lymphoma. In these cases biopsy is often required for a definitive diagnosis. When cystic changes of the glands are identified histologically, the diagnosis is certain.

There is some evidence to suggest that chronic metaplasia of the gastric mucosa in these patients may lead to an increased incidence of gastric carcinoma.

Another distinctive form of hypertrophic gastritis is Zollinger-Ellison syndrome. These patients have a non-beta, islet cell gastrin-secreting tumor, usually in the pancreas. A few of these tumors are located in the antrum, duodenal wall, or splenic hilus. Approximately 50 percent of the tumors are malignant and metastasize to the liver and adjacent lymph nodes. Ten percent of patients have a multiglandular syndrome involving other endocrine organs. Histologically, not only is there gastric mucosal hyperplasia but also an increase in parietal cell mass.

If the primary tumor is not removed immediately, a tendency toward aggressive peptic ulceration occurs. The ulcers not only form in the stomach but also in the duodenum and jejunum. The ulcers are often multiple and have a tendency to recur, even after adequate medical therapy.

Radiographically, the diagnosis can be suggested when severe gastric or proximal small bowel edema, or both are observed. Ulcers are identified often in extragastric locations, and hypersecretion is a common feature. When gastrin immunoassays are performed and confirm the suspicion, location of the tumor is best determined by angiography or computed tomographic angiography (CTA). Selective venous sampling can be carried out along the course of draining pancreatic and duodenal veins in a further

effort to localize the tumor. Evidence of metastases can also be evaluated by either CT or angiography. When longstanding disease is present, metastases have been known to calcify. (In patients with multiple endocrine adenomatosis resulting in hyperparathyroidism, nephrolithiasis has also been described.)

Therapy generally involves total gastrectomy. Subtotal gastrectomy and vagotomy is not completely effective, unless the tumor is also resected, at least partially. Total gastrectomy completely eliminates the danger of hyperacidity should resection of the primary tumor be incomplete. Occasionally metastases have been known to regress following total gastrectomy. Some surgeons, however, opt for subtotal gastrectomy with vagotomy because of the 5 to 10 percent mortality associated with total removal of the stomach. There is also some controversy regarding removal of the tumor, which tends to recur. Resection is optimally curative when tumors are located in the tail of the pancreas or in the duodenal wall.

Finally, an idiopathic form of hypertrophic gastritis, not surprisingly, has been described when no definite cause can be found and no clear histologic diagnosis can be made.

MISCELLANEOUS CAUSES OF GASTRITIS

Radiation-Induced Gastritis

When dose levels exceed 3,500 rads, radiation gastritis — manifested as mucosal edema and eventual fold loss — and gastric scarring can be observed. With higher doses, generally exceeding 4,000 rads, ulcers and eventual perforation may occur. Symptoms and radiographic evidence generally develop in an average of 6 months after radiation but can be seen as early as 1 or 2 months after therapy. Confusion with other causes of benign ulceration or malignancy is easy. Surgical intervention to prevent sudden exsanguination should be performed when perforation appears imminent.

Phlegmonous Gastritis

Phlegmonous gastritis is an acute, often fatal infection of the stomach that results in gastric necrosis and septicemia. In the vast majority of cases alpha-hemolytic streptococci are present; however, *Staphylococcus aureus, Escherichia coli, Clostridium welchii,* pneumococcus, and *Proteus* have also been identified. Endoscopically, the entire gastric wall is edematous, frequently without the presence of ulcerations. Although the inflammation generally involves the entire stomach, localized segments can be predominantly involved. Mortality is extremely high, decreasing with prompt gastrectomy and antibiotic therapy.

A common form of phlegmonous gastritis, when gas-forming organisms are identified in the wall of the stomach, is emphysematous gastritis (Fig. 2-11). In these patients *Escherichia coli* or *Clostridium welchii* are present, forming linear and small mottled collections of gas in the wall of the stomach. Other causes of emphysematous gastritis should also be considered. These include infarction, trauma, endoscopy, and erosive gastritis.

Radiographically, the diagnosis is generally made from plain films of the abdomen. To confirm the diagnosis of intramural pneumatosis, a left lateral decubitus film can be obtained to enhance the contrast between intramural air and intraluminal gastric fluid.

Postoperative Gastritis

Patients who have undergone partial gastrectomy with a patent gastroduodenostomy or, more commonly, a gastroenterostomy frequently have reflux of bile into the gastric remnant, resulting in bile-induced gastritis. (This subject is discussed in the section on The Postoperative Stomach.)

Corrosive Gastritis

Corrosive agents, represented by strong acids or alkalis, can have a devastating effect on the gastric mucosa. In general, alkalis commonly cause their greatest damage in the esophagus, sparing the gastric mucosa to a greater extent, whereas the reverse is true when acid is ingested.

Acutely, there is marked edema and swelling of the affected mucosa followed by rapid mucosal sloughing, erosion and ulcer formation, and eventual scarring of the mid- and distal portions of the stomach.

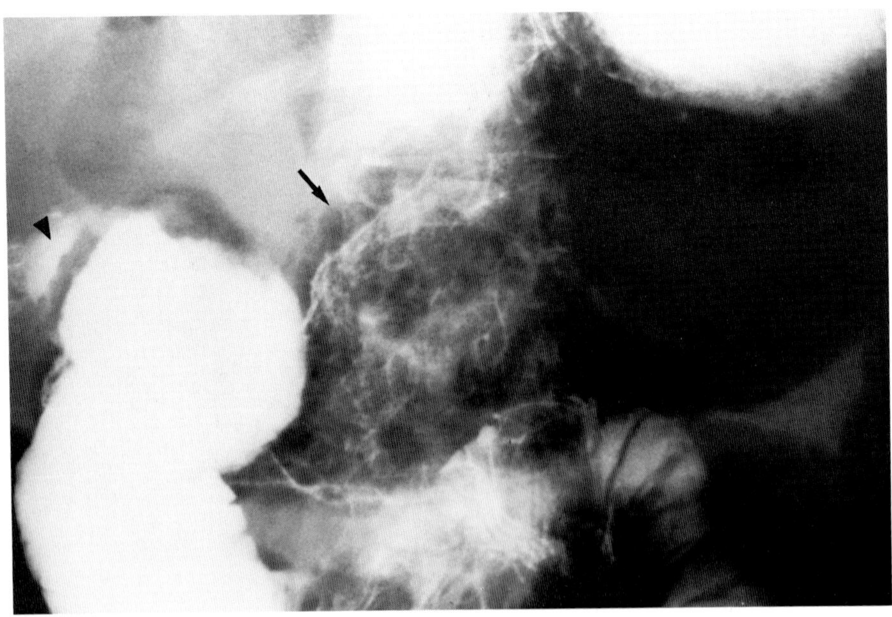

Fig. 2-11 Clostridium-induced gangrene of the stomach is the etiology of emphysematous gastritis in this case. Note the intramural air *(arrow)*, which dissected along the stomach to the duodenum, creating a localized perforation with extravasation of barium *(arrowhead)* and reflux of air in the common bile duct.

Because pylorospasm occurs in these patients, the duodenum is usually spared. Thus, gastric outlet obstruction can eventually occur 1 to 2 months later. Radiographically, these stomachs can eventually be indistinguishable from linitis plastica, the late manifestations of radiation-induced gastritis, eosinophilic gastritis, granulomatous gastritis, and metastatic disease (i.e., pancreas or breast).

GASTRIC CARCINOMA

Since the advent of the air-contrast technique, developed by the Japanese almost 20 years ago, it has been possible to diagnose gastric cancer in its early stages. The ability to diagnose early in situ gastric cancer is important because treated at this stage its prognosis is far better than that for gastric carcinoma in general; the 5-year postsurgical survival rate for early gastric cancer is greater than 90 percent.

Early gastric cancer, however, is an uncommon diagnosis in the United States; incidence rates are higher in Japan and South America. Epidemiologic studies have suggested that patients who move from high- to low-incidence regions adopt the risk of the new location. To date, however, data on environmental or dietary factors have not been convincing. Carcinoma of the stomach is slightly more common in males.

Several entities are known to be associated with an increased risk of gastric carcinoma. For example, adenomatous polyps occasionally undergo malignant change, whereas hyperplastic or inflammatory polyps rarely do so. Also, pernicious anemia is known to be associated with an increased incidence of carcinoma in the proximal stomach compared with the antrum, where gastric carcinoma is usually located. Furthermore, atrophic gastritis, a well-known precursor of gastric carcinoma, is commonly associated with pernicious anemia.

Classification

The macroscopic classification of early carcinoma, as proposed by the Japanese, has generally been used. The earlier classification suggested by Borrmann did not consider early changes in the mucosa and submucosa. The Japanese classification, which includes the macroscopic appearance of early gastric cancer, is used both by radiologists and endoscopists to establish a diagnosis.

Essentially, three types of early gastric carcinoma are recognized and classified (see box).

EARLY GASTRIC CARCINOMA*

I. Protruded type (polypoid lesion greater than 0.5 cm in diameter)
II. Superficial type
   A. Elevated (lesion less than 0.5 cm in diameter)
   B. Flat (no elevation of mucosa)
   C. Depressed (superficial ulcer)
III. Excavated type (prominent ulcer extending beneath the muscularis mucosae)

---

* Adapted from Laufer I: Double Contrast Gastrointestinal Radiology with Endoscopic Correlation. WB Saunders, Philadelphia, 1979.

PROTRUDED TYPE EARLY CARCINOMA (TYPE I)

Polypoid carcinomas are more commonly diagnosed in the antrum of the stomach, the incidence decreasing as one moves proximally toward the cardia (Fig. 2-12). Lesser curvature lesions are approximately twice as common as those in the greater curvature.

As stated, these lesions are at least 0.5 cm in diameter. Using the double-contrast technique, the surface pattern of the lesion is of paramount importance in determining whether the lesion is malignant or benign. The surface of a malignant lesion should have a coarse granular pattern similar to that of the surrounding normal areae gastricae as long as the lesion is superficial. As the lesion progressively invades the stomach wall, the surface pattern becomes increasingly distorted and generally ulcerates. The contour of the lesion should be slightly nodular. It is often difficult to differentiate a benign adenomatous polyp from a type I early gastric carcinoma. In general, however, lesions larger than 2.0 cm in diameter should be considered malignant since the incidence of malignant degeneration tends to increase with size. (Pedunculated adenomatous polyps less than 2 cm are almost always benign.)

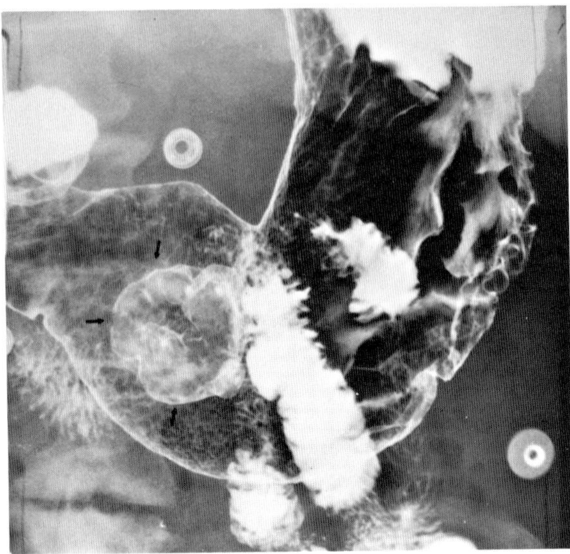

Fig. 2-12 A large polypoid type I carcinoma is readily identified in the body of the stomach *(arrows)*.

SUPERFICIAL TYPE EARLY GASTRIC CARCINOMA (TYPE II)

The type IIA or elevated superficial carcinomas are diagnosed using essentially the same criteria as for type I lesions, except for their size, which should be less than 0.5 cm in diameter (Figs. 2-13 and 2-14). Consequently, their size makes it very difficult to distinguish elevated superficial carcinomas from benign adenomatous polyps.

The flat, type IIB lesion is the most difficult to observe and diagnose (Fig. 2-15). Radiographically, the mucosa demonstrates focal irregularity. Subtle differences in coating from the surrounding normal mucosa should be looked at with a high degree of suspicion. These lesions are the least frequent of all early gastric carcinomas, both in the Japanese and the American experiences.

Depressed or type IIC carcinomas are the most frequently diagnosed gastric carcinomas and represent three-fourths of all early gastric carcinomas. The depression has sharp, spiculated, and irregular margins; is very shallow; and is generally surrounded by an irregular, nodular pattern of surrounding areae gastricae (Figs. 2-16 and 2-17).

"Converging folds" are often present and are extremely useful in the diagnosis of these early lesions. The folds are readily distinguished from benign folds

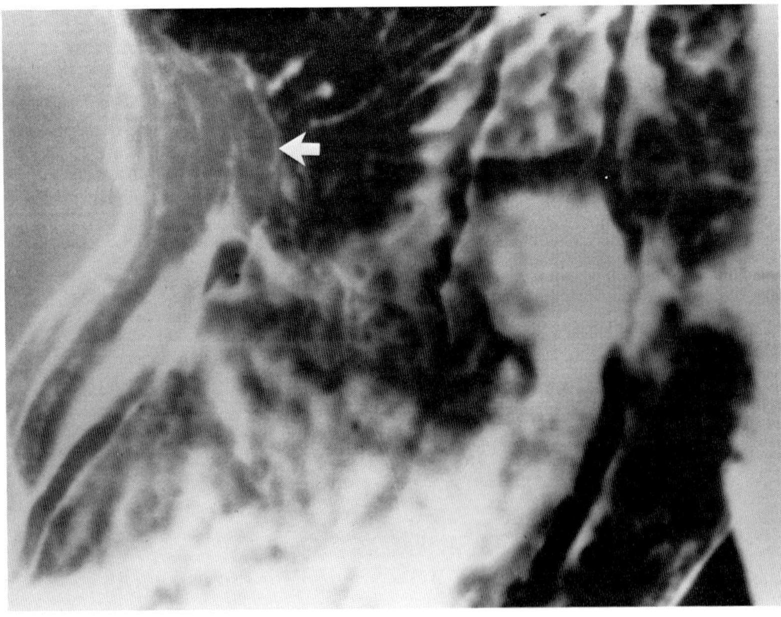

Fig. 2-13 A flat plaque-like type IIA carcinoma is identified along the lesser curvature *(arrow)*.
No peristalsis was present in this area at fluoroscopy.

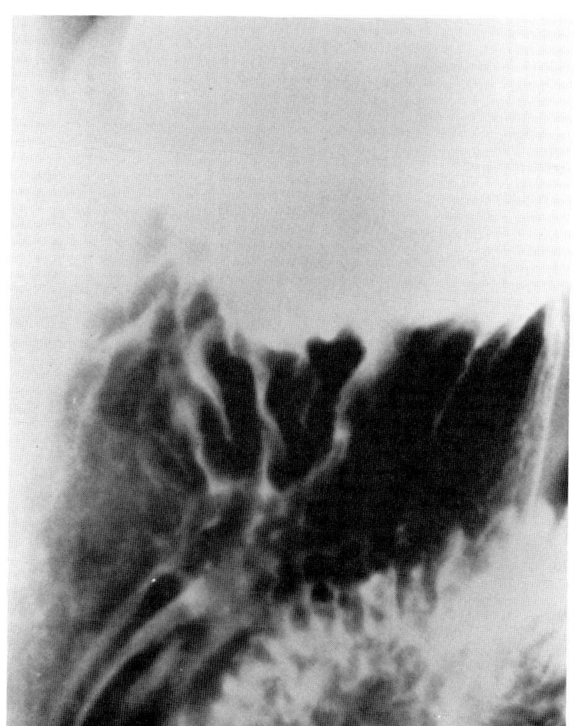

Fig. 2-14 Thickened, amputated folds, suggesting malignant infiltration, radiate toward a type IIA carcinoma in situ.

in that they tend to show tapering, clubbing, abrupt interruption, and fusion at the periphery of the depression. These changes are best identified en face and are virtually pathognomonic of malignancy (see Fig. 2-14).

Assessment of the depth to which early carcinoma has invaded underlying tissues largely depends on its size. In general, lesions greater than 2.0 cm in diameter histologically demonstrate submucosal invasion.

EXCAVATED TYPE EARLY GASTRIC CARCINOMA (TYPE III)

Type III early gastric carcinomas are differentiated from type IIC by the depth of the depression or ulceration. Both types of lesions are extremely common and the type III early carcinoma is particularly easy to diagnose radiographically. The location and radiographic characteristics are virtually identical (Fig. 2-18).

As the carcinoma progresses, becoming more invasive, the mass effect and size of the ulcer become increasingly pronounced. Fluoroscopically, all carci-

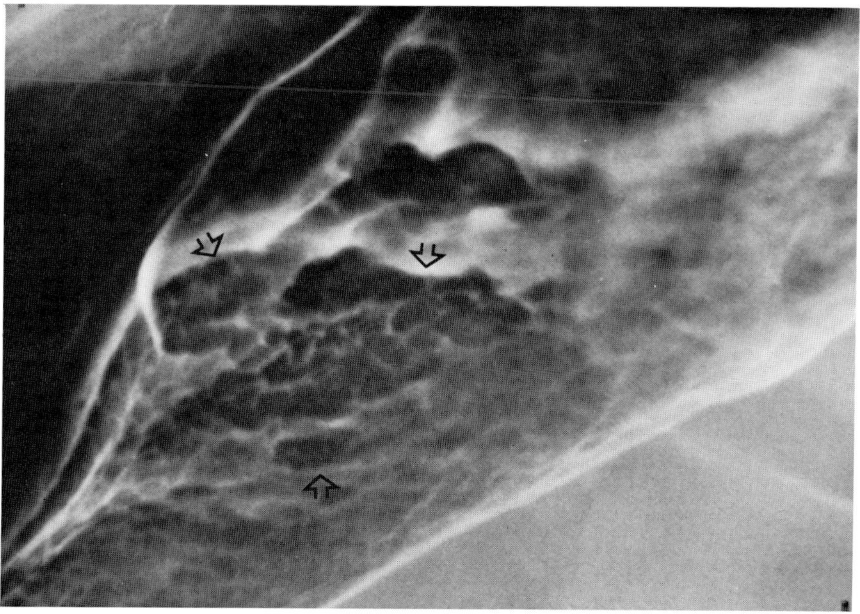

Fig. 2-15 A type IIB carcinoma is identified by focal alteration in the areae gastricae pattern *(arrows)*. The lesion was present in the fundus.

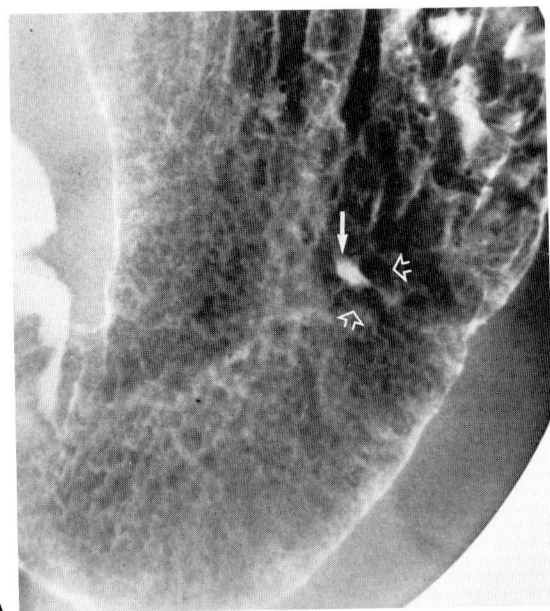

A

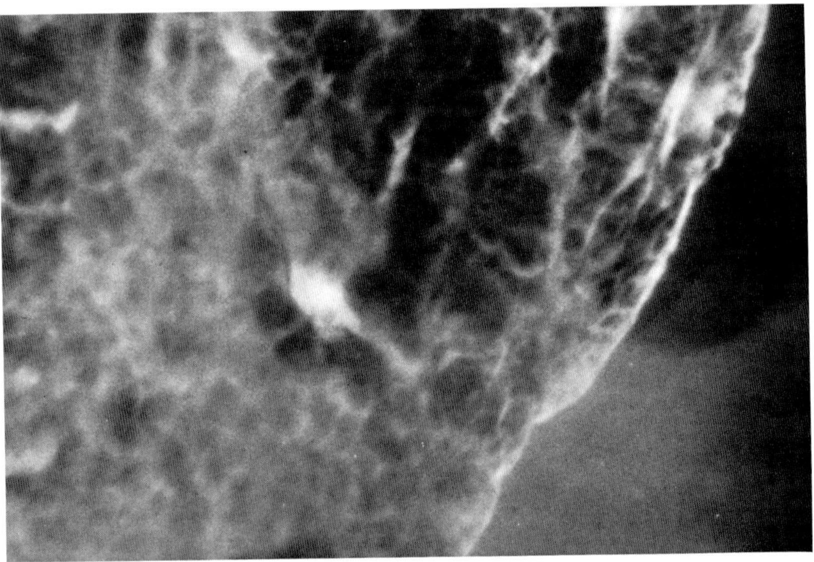

B

Fig. 2-16 (A) A 6 mm, shallow depression *(arrow)* is surrounded by an irregular, eccentric nodular mass *(open arrows)*. **(B)** Coned-down view of this type IIC carcinoma.

nomas show an absence of peristalsis when viewed in profile, with localized rigidity and flattening. The rigidity is most pronounced in the scirrhous type of carcinoma, when diffuse infiltration of the carcinoma leads to the ultimate progression of a shrunken and rigid stomach (linitis plastica). In these patients, the normal mucosal pattern is totally absent. The rugae are either completely absent or extremely disorgan-ized and nodular. However, a variety of benign disorders can radiographically simulate scirrhous carcinoma of the stomach. These disorders include the granulomatous, corrosive, radiation, and chronic eosinophilic gastritides. Diffuse metastatic disease, especially from the breast and Hodgkin lymphoma, can also give the appearance of a primary scirrhous carcinoma of the stomach.

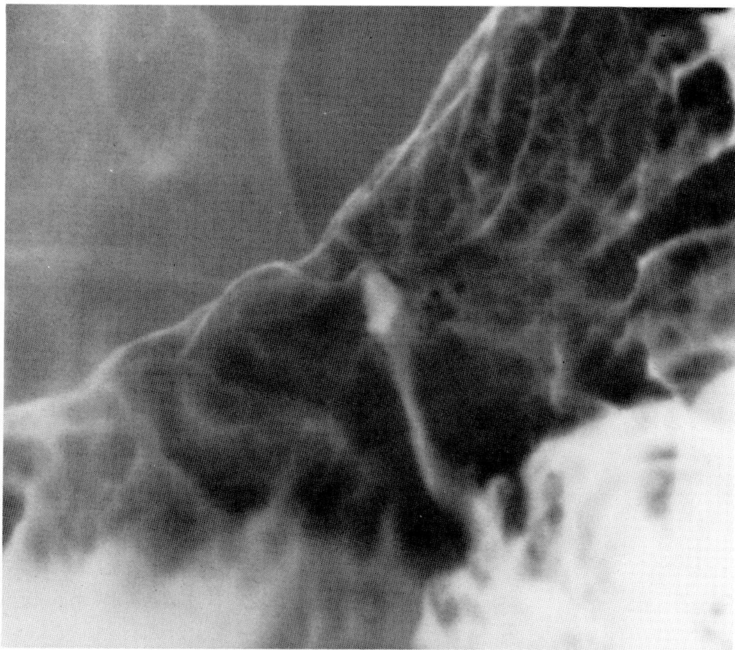

Fig. 2-17 A type IIC carcinoma reveals a nodular mass with a central shallow depression.

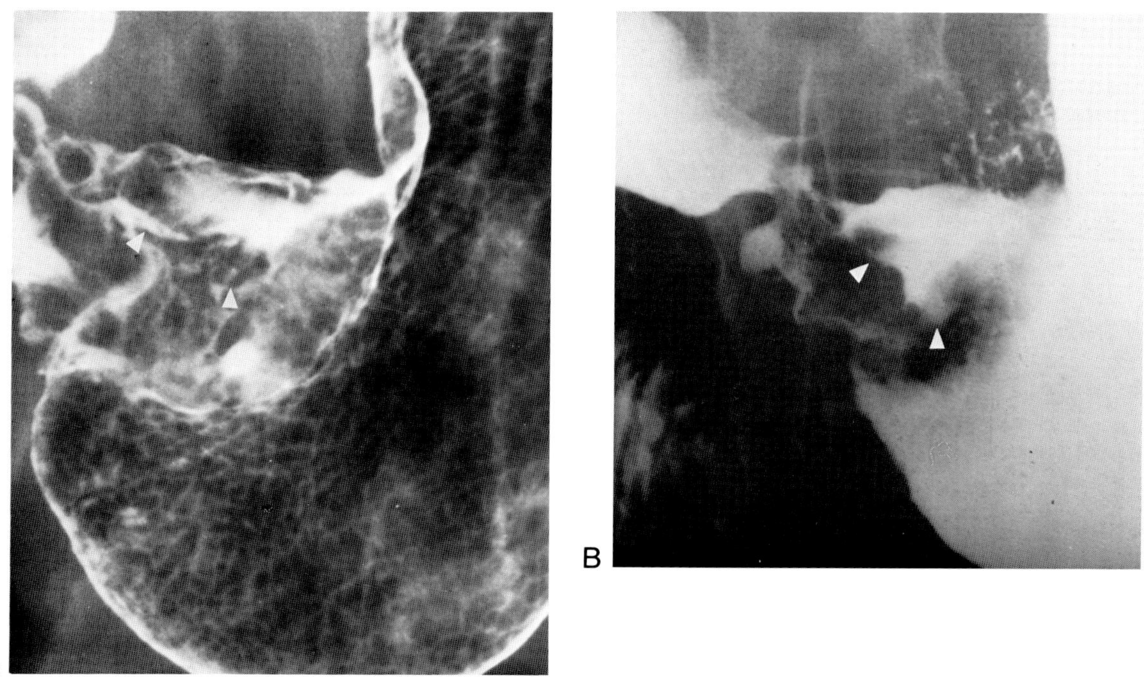

Fig. 2-18 (A) Air-contrast and **(B)** single-contrast views of a type III gastric carcinoma within the antrum. The malignant ulceration *(arrowheads)* produced a ring-sign on the air-contrast phase. Note the absent mucosal pattern within the mass.

Metastatic Carcinoma of the Stomach

Metastatic spread to the stomach can occur by either direct extension from adjacent organs or by a hematogenous route from distant sources.

The most common site of direct extension is from the pancreas into the posterior half of the body of the stomach. Another common source is the colon, where the metastasis spreads directly along the gastrocolic ligament to the greater curvature (Fig. 2-19). Left renal lesions that are extremely large can displace or invade the stomach as well.

Metastatic *bloodborne* metastases to the stomach are often manifested as submucosal lesions that can ulcerate, producing bull's-eye or target lesions. These are most commonly seen in metastatic melanoma and adenocarcinoma from the lung and kidney. Metastatic nodular lesions are difficult to differentiate from the lymphomatous nodules of non-Hodgkin lymhoma, or indeed from benign polyps (Fig. 2-20). Metastatic breast carcinoma, as previously mentioned, has a typi-

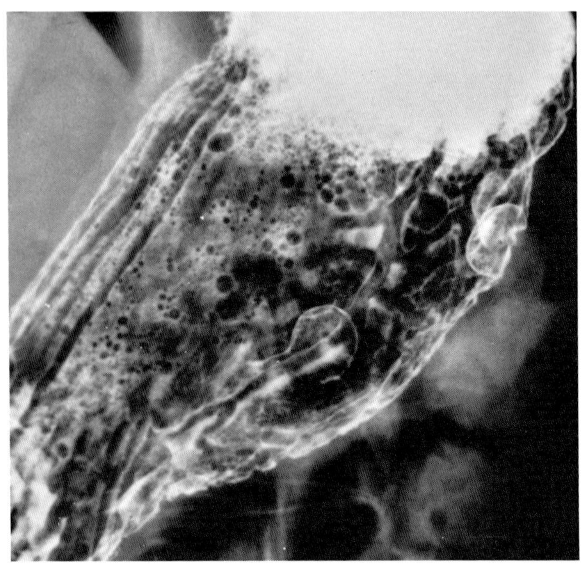

Fig. 2-20 Multiple nodules representing metastatic melanoma are identified in the body of the stomach.

cal scirrhous appearance that generally involves a large area of the stomach (Fig. 2-21).

When the carcinoma originates in the stomach, metastatic spread can be *lymphangitic* to the nodes along the lesser and greater curvatures, the celiac axis, porta hepatis, gastroduodenal, pancreaticoduodenal and paraaortic regions, and eventually to the lungs. It can also be *direct,* along the gastrocolic ligament to the superior border of the distal transvenous colon, or along the small bowel mesentery. In this case, the malignant cells cascade in the often-present ascitic fluid toward the ileocecal region, implanting along the medial border of the cecum and the intervening loops of small bowel. Gastric fundal carcinoma can spread directly toward the esophagus, as well. It may initially present as an irregular, often annular, distal esophageal mass that elicits symptoms of dysphagia. This secondary achalasia-like appearance may be impossible to differentiate from a primary esophageal carcinoma. Distal gastric carcinomas uncommonly (4 to 6 percent) spread across the pylorus to the duodenum, whereas lymphomas are far more likely to do so (95 percent) (Fig. 2-22). Other direct sites of spread include the gastrohepatic ligament, pancreas, diaphragm, jejunum, spleen, gastrosplenic ligament, infrahepatic surface of the liver, superior mesenteric and

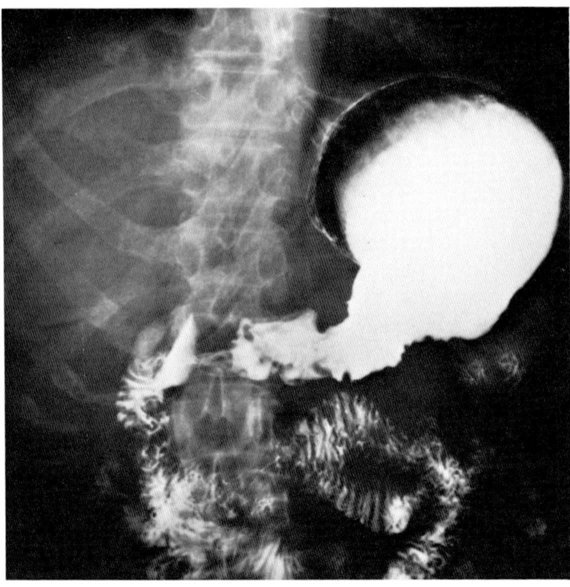

Fig. 2-19 Metastatic spread of transverse colon carcinoma along the gastrocolic ligament to the greater curvature, producing a focal irregular area of mass effect.

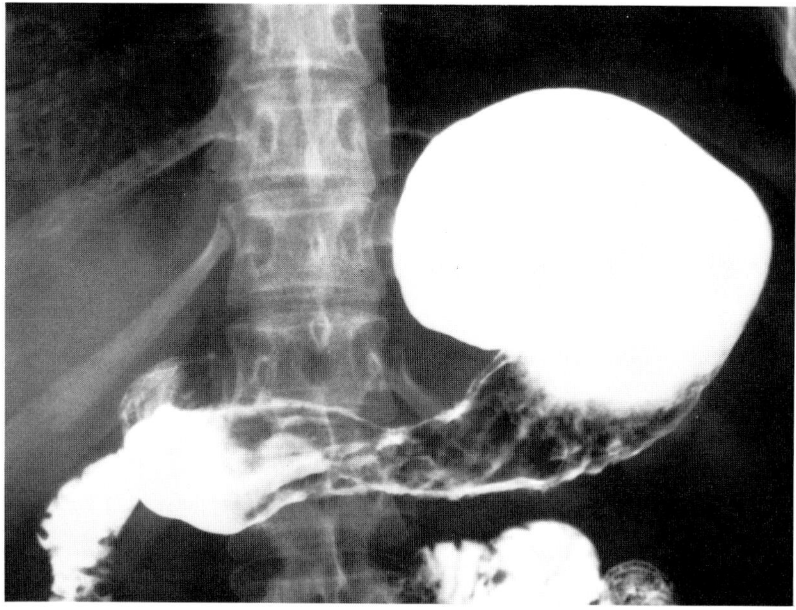

Fig. 2-21 Breast carcinoma metastatic to the stomach produces a rigid scirrhous appearance.

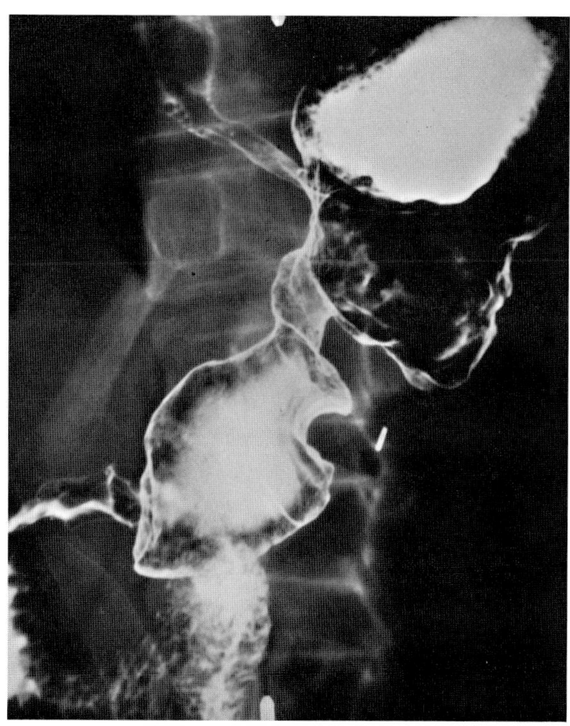

Fig. 2-22 Diffuse gastric lymphoma spreads across the pylorus into the base of the duodenal bulb.

celiac axis vessels, abdominal wall, and occasionally the left adrenal gland and kidney. *Intraperitoneal seeding* can occur in addition to the direct small bowel mesenteric spread. Commonly seeded sites are the pouch of Douglas, sigmoid mesocolon, and the right paracolic gutter. *Hematogenous spread* is primarily venous to the liver in about 30 percent of cases.

LYMPHOMA

Malignant lymphoma of the stomach may be primary or secondary. Primary lymphomas of the stomach constitute 3 percent of all gasric malignancies. Lymphomas of the stomach develop from the lymphatic tissue of the lamina propria mucosae. It has been stated that more than 70 percent of malignant lymphomas develop from both the mucosa and submucosa in the belief that the disease originates from the lymphoreticular cells therein.

Non-Hodgkin Lymphoma

Of all patients with non-Hodgkin lymphoma, primary gastric lymphoma can be found in approximately 25 percent. Secondary lymphoma is more commonly seen in patients with diffuse lymphoma. Clinically, males are more likely to be affected than females. Patients often present with nonspecific abdominal pain, anorexia, weight loss, nausea, and vomiting. Occult gastrointestinal bleeding is most often detected, whereas frank hematemesis and melena are not common.

The prognosis for primary gastric lymphoma is far better than that for intestinal lymphoma, perhaps related to earlier detection. Most patients are generally stage I or stage II when initially diagnosed and up to 66 percent are alive after 5 years.

Therapy includes subtotal or total gastrectomy followed by radiation therapy. Chemotherapy is used when systemic disease is present. Several classifications of non-Hodgkin lymphoma are currently being used by pathologists. The most common is the Rappaport classification of 1966, but the Lukes and Collins classification of 1974 is also used (Table 2-1).

The radiographic appearance of non-Hodgkin lymphoma can be somewhat variable. It can appear as a diffuse, infiltrating disease involving the distal stomach, where folds are thickened and nodular (Fig. 2-23). Peristalsis is decreased or absent but the stomach is generally more distensible than would be characteristic for carcinoma. Ulcerations of any size can occur.

Differentiation from severe gastritis (Menetrier) and, occasionally, carcinoma can be difficult. Lymphoma can also present locally in the stomach. When it does, it can appear as an ulcerating mass that grows to an enormous size at times and occasionally perforates, causing a grossly distorted configuration to that portion of the stomach (Fig. 2-24). At other times, smaller discrete polypoid masses can be present. These are generally multiple. Ulcerations may present in these lesions as well.

Hodgkin Disease

Hodgkin involvement of the stomach is extremely uncommon. Although primary Hodgkin disease rarely involves the stomach, approximately 15 to 20

Table 2-1 Classifications of Non-Hodgkin Lymphoma

Rapport	Lukes and Collins
Low grade	
Diffuse lymphocytic, well differentiated	Small lymphocytic and plasmatoid lymphocytic
Nodular, poorly differentiated lymphocytic	Small cleaved FCC[a], follicular only or follicular + diffuse
Nodular, mixed lymphocytic	Small cleaved FCC, follicular; large cleaved FCC, follicular
Intermediate grade Nodular histiocytic	Large cleaved or noncleaved FCC
Diffuse lymphocytic, poorly differentiated	Small cleaved FCC, diffuse
Diffuse mixed lymphocytic-histiocytic	Small cleaved, large cleaved or large noncleaved FCC, diffuse
Diffuse histiocytic	Large cleaved or noncleaved FCC, diffuse
High grade	
Diffuse histiocytic	Immunoblastic sarcoma, T or B cell
Lymphoblastic convoluted	Convoluted T cell
Undifferentiated, Burkitt + non-Burkett	Small noncleaved FCC

[a] FCC = follicular center cell

percent of all lymphomas that do so represent Hodgkin disease.

Hodgkin disease mimics scirrhous carcinoma because of its strong desmoplastic reaction. Occasionally, ulcerations may be noted in association with the narrowed stomach. It is uncommon for Hodgkin disease of the stomach to mimic non-Hodgkin involvement. However, when this occurs the differentiation is impossible.

The Rye modification of the Lukes-Butler classification, as used by pathologists, is as follows.

Lymphocyte predominance
Mixed cellularity
Lymphocyte depleted
Nodular sclerosing

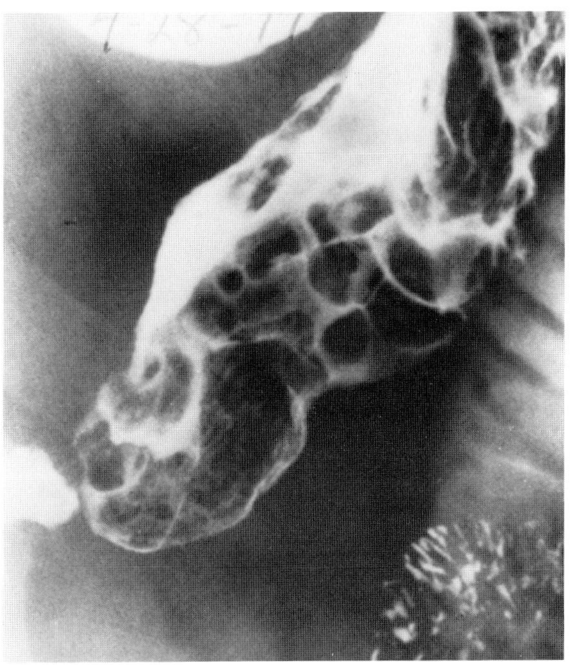

Fig. 2-23 Diffuse nodular thickening of the folds is a common presentation of non-Hodgkin lymphoma of the stomach.

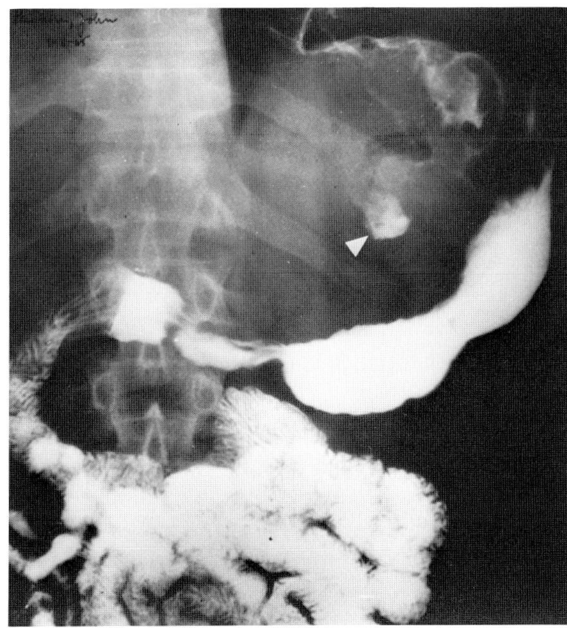

Fig. 2-24 Lymphomas can achieve enormous proportions. Large central areas of necrosis produce ulcerations, as indicated by the arrowhead.

Pseudolymphoma (Reactive Lymphoreticular Hyperplasia)

Focal diffuse proliferation of lymphoreticular tissue in the stomach has been recognized for the last four decades and is considered a form of gastritis often misdiagnosed as lymphoma. Reactive lymphoreticular hyperplasia demonstrates macroscopic findings that are easily confused with malignancy. The appearance is one of marked fold-thickening, often with ulceration (70 percent). It is felt to be a result of chronic inflammation and can be mistakenly diagnosed as lymphoma or even carcinoma, both radiographically and on frozen section. The final pathologic specimen, however, reveals a benign inflammatory response with lymphocytes, histiocytes, plasma cells, and fibroblasts.

Other Submucosal Tumors

The most common submucosal tumor of the stomach is by far the leiomyoma (See Fig. 2-4). It is impossible, however, to differentiate from many other submucosal tumors (see box). Leiomyomas, leiomyoblastomas, Kaposi sarcoma, plasmacytomas, ectopic pancreatic tissue, neurofibromas, lipomas, and carcinoids can ulcerate and appear as target or bull's-eye lesions. Carcinoid tumors occur rarely in the stomach and originate from the deeper portions of the mucosa and superficial submucosa. They often ulcerate. Malignate transformation takes place in approximately 20 percent.

SUBMUCOSAL LESIONS OF THE STOMACH

Spindle cell tumors
    Leiomyoma/leiomyosarcoma
      Neurogenic tumors
        Schwannoma (neurilemmoma)
        Neurofibroma
        Fibroma
Myomatous tumors
    Leiomyoblastoma/myosarcoma
Other mesenchymal tumors
    Lipoma/liposarcoma

(List continued)

Vascular tumors
    Hemangioma
    Lymphangioma
    Glomus tumor
    Kaposi sarcoma
    Hemangiopericytoma
Plasmacytoma
Carcinoid
Aberrant pancreas
Eosinophilic granuloma

GASTRIC POLYPS

Gastric polyps are less common than polyps found in the colon and are generally discovered incidentally during routine UGI examination. The overall incidence of gastric polyps is less than 1 percent.

The five classifications of gastric polyps are hyperplastic or inflammatory, adenomatous, hamartomatous, retention, and villous polyps.

Hyperplastic Polyps

Hyperplastic or inflammatory polyps are by far the most common and represent at least 90 percent of all gastric polyps. Histologically, the polyp consists of hyperplastic gastric glands with associated cystic and edematous changes. Inflammatory infiltrates may also be present. Hyperplastic polyps are associated with chronic gastritis and have rare malignant potential.

Radiographically, these polyps are generally less than 1 cm in diameter, they may be single or multiple, and they have a smooth contour. Occasionally these polyps may be pedunculated and can occur in any portion of the stomach, sometimes prolapsing into the duodenum. They infrequently ulcerate (see Fig. 2-6).

Adenomatous Polyps

Adenomatous polyps are the second most frequent type of gastric polyp. Unlike hyperplastic polyps, these are true neoplasms that histologically resemble adenomatous polyps of the colon. Papillary and villous patterns are occasionally seen histologically and gastric glands are generally not present. Adenomatous polyps often demonstrate growth, and malignant transformation (which increases with size) can occur with an incidence ranging from 40 to 50 percent. A coexistent carcinoma is three times more common in stomachs containing adenomatous polyps than in those with hyperplastic polyps. Radiographically, adenomatous polyps are generally 2 cm or greater in diameter. They may be single or multiple, are generally sessile, and commonly have irregular contours.

Adenomatous polyps of the stomach have been identified in approximately 5 percent of patients with familial polyposis coli (although hyperplastic and hamartomatous polyps have also been identified in this syndrome).

Hamartomatous Polyps

Hamartomatous polyps are rare. Histologically, they are composed of densely packed gastric glands. Radiographically, their appearance is similar to hyperplastic polyps in that they are generally small. They have been associated with Peutz-Jegher syndrome.

Retention Polyps

Retention polyps are also rare. Histologically, they represent focal cystic and edematous changes in the gastric glands. These polyps are associated with Canada-Cronkhite syndrome.

Villous Tumors

Villous polyps are similar to those found in the colon, both in their irregular cauliflower-like appearance and in their strong malignant potential. They are occasionally multiple, usually sessile but sometimes pedunculated, and can occasionally ulcerate.

As with all gastric neoplasms, endoscopy and biopsy are strongly recommended to establish the true histologic nature and malignant potential of the lesion.

GASTRIC ULCERS

The most common abnormality of the stomach that we, as radiologists, are asked to diagnose, is the ulcer. Improved techniques (described earlier) and knowledge of the various appearances of ulcers have increased our diagnostic ability. The task of differentiating between benign and malignant gastric ulcers is made easier when the anatomic basis for their different appearances is understood.

Good radiographic technique is of utmost importance in detecting gastric ulcers. Sloppy or inadequate air-contrast technique may lead to a false sense of normalcy. When an adequate double-contrast examination cannot be achieved, the radiologist should either examine the patient at a later date or utilize a good single-contrast compression technique, always assuming the presence of pathology.

Once a gastric ulcer is identified, it is vital to film it both in profile and en face so that criteria classifying it as benign or malignant can be applied accurately. Radiographic accuracy in differentiating benign from malignant ulcers has been the subject of some controversy, especially in the wake of skilled endoscopy. Japanese and American studies have shown that 1 to 3 percent of gastric ulcers, respectively, considered benign may actually be cancerous. Less than 1 percent of the gastric ulcers that exhibit complete healing on subsequent studies prove to be malignant. It is, therefore, safe to save endoscopy for patients with intractable or recurrent gastric ulcers, those in whom the radiographic diagnosis of benignancy is equivocal, and certainly for those in whom malignancy is considered a highly probable diagnosis. However, in most institutions nearly all gastric ulcers are endoscoped and biopsied.

Benign Gastric Ulcers

A number of radiographic criteria suggest the benign nature of a gastric ulcer. These have been enumerated by Nelson (1969). If two or more of the following signs are present, the ulcer is considered radiographically benign. The criteria are as follows:

1. Projection of the ulcer crater beyond or away from the gastric lumen
2. A smooth single mound of edematous tissue concentrically surrounding the ulcer crater
3. Undermining of the edematous mucosa at the base of the ulcer (the so-called Hampton line or ulcer collar)
4. Thin mucosal folds radiating to the base of the ulcer crater (Fig. 2-25)

Note that the number, location, and size of the ulcers are not useful criteria in distinguishing a benign from a malignant ulcer.

When the ulcer is identified in profile, it appears to project away from the gastric lumen because a benign ulcer originates in the mucosa and subsequently extends into the submucosa. Once the initial mucosal ulceration occurs, the submucosa can be further destroyed by acid and pepsin. Undermining of the mucosa creates a lip of edematous tissue which, when viewed in profile, creates a lucent band approximately 1 mm in diameter—known as Hampton's line—at the base of the ulcer crater. When seen, this is considered by some to be pathognomonic of a benign ulcer.

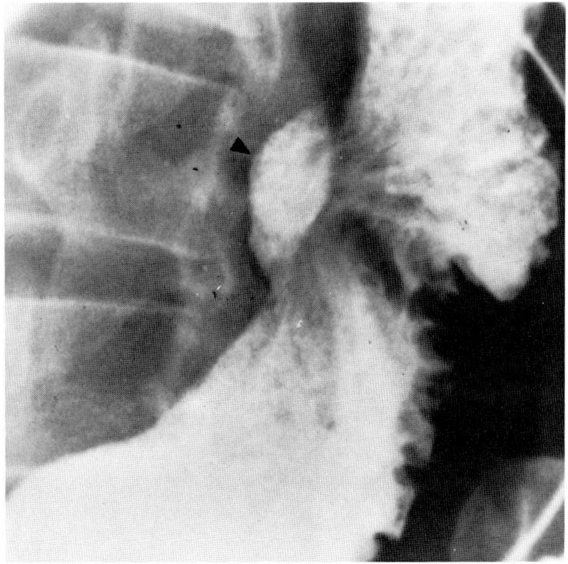

Fig. 2-25 A benign ulcer *(arrowhead)* projects beyond the gastric lumen into the wall. Thin folds radiate toward the crater.

In addition, a mound of edema is occasionally seen to surround the ulcer crater. The edema should be concentric with the ulcer crater because it is, in fact, secondary to the inflammatory ulcerogenic process. This is an important point because eccentricity generally suggests malignancy. If the ulcer is actively bleeding, blood clots may be noted at the base of the benign ulcer crater. When present, the clots can often create a somewhat nodular appearance within the crater. Viewed en face, the mucosal folds radiating to the benign ulcer crater are generally thin and extend directly to the base of the crater.

As stated in the section on early gastric carcinoma, the appearance of radiating folds is extremely important in differentiating benign from malignant lesions. If the folds are thickened and blunted or they do not extend beyond the surrounding mound of tissue, malignancy should be suspected (see Fig. 2-14). The areae gastricae immediately adjacent to the crater should be intact. Any irregularity in the micromucosal pattern should again suggest malignancy (see Fig. 2-18).

Diagnostic difficulties occur when the ulcers are either in the antrum or along the greater curvature. Benign ulcers in these areas may appear to be intraluminal rather than extend beyond the gastric lumen; therefore, all ancillary signs should be evaluated carefully when benignancy versus malignancy is being determined.

Malignant Gastric Ulcers

Several of the signs of malignancy have been covered in the section on gastric carcinoma. In general, the features suggesting malignant ulceration are as follows.

1. Carman meniscus sign
2. Eccentric mass effect surrounding the ulcer crater
3. Nodularity and irregularity of tissue surrounding the ulcer crater
4. Abnormal areae gastricae surrounding the ulcer
5. Abnormally thickened or amputated folds radiating to the mass but not extending to the orifice of the ulcer

The Carman meniscus sign results from the apposition of rolled halves of the tumor margin forming the periphery of the ulcerated carcinoma. The Carman sign is present when the ulcer is located along the lesser curvature aspect of the stomach (Fig. 2-26). The semilunar configuration of the barium within the ulcer creates the appearance of a meniscus. The eccentricity of the ulcer relative to the surrounding mass is easily explained. Tumors generally grow exophytically and the necrosis that occurs within them is oftentimes eccentric, occurring toward the edge of the mass. Eccentricity should be evaluated with the ulcer seen en face and in profile. Irregularity of the ulcer is usually, but not always, present. The mass, however, is almost always irregular and nodular in outline and, therefore, can be readily distinguished from pure edema.

Malignant ulcers rarely heal completely. Follow-up examination, therefore, is crucial to the evaluation of an ulcer. A residual scar may be present, which occasionally can retain barium. If a malignant ulcer heals, it will recur.

Double Pylorus

The double pylorus develops when a prepyloric benign ulcer erodes into the duodenal bulb, creating a gastroduodenal fistula. The fistula parallels the normal pyloric channel and is generally superior to the pyloric channel, because the ulcer creating the fistula is almost invariably located along the lesser curvature. The ulceration may not be evident at the time of examination, depending on the chronicity and duration of peptic disease. Accessory pyloric channels have been described in the literature and have been considered congenital anomalies. These are located along the greater curvature aspect of the stomach, revealing no evidence of prior peptic disease.

Pyloric Channel Ulcers

Pyloric channel ulcers are generally felt to originate in the distal antrum, although some feel they should be grouped as duodenal ulcers. They are generally located along the lesser curvature aspect of the pyloric channel and are usually less than 1 cm in diameter. Edema and spasm are often present. Acutely, gastric outlet obstruction is uncommon; however, with sub-

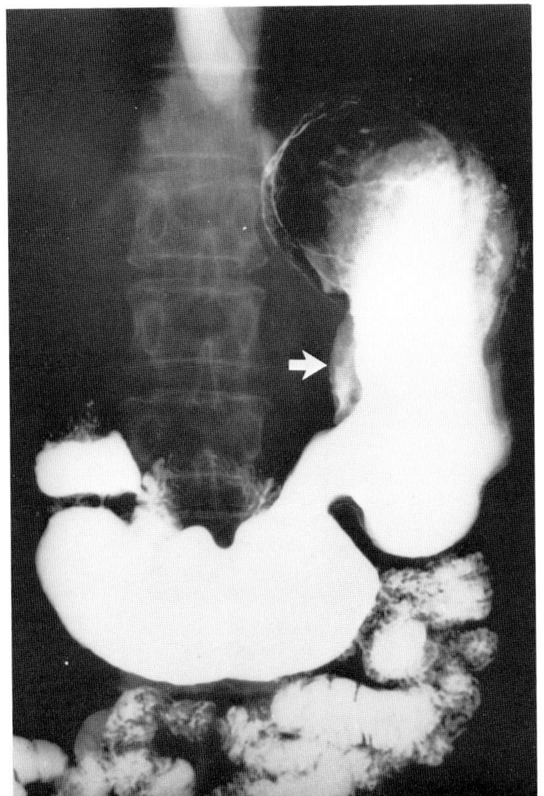 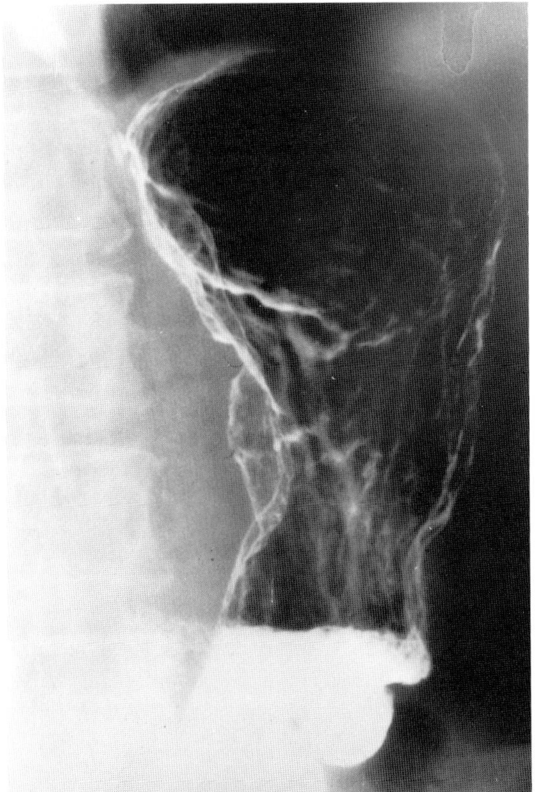

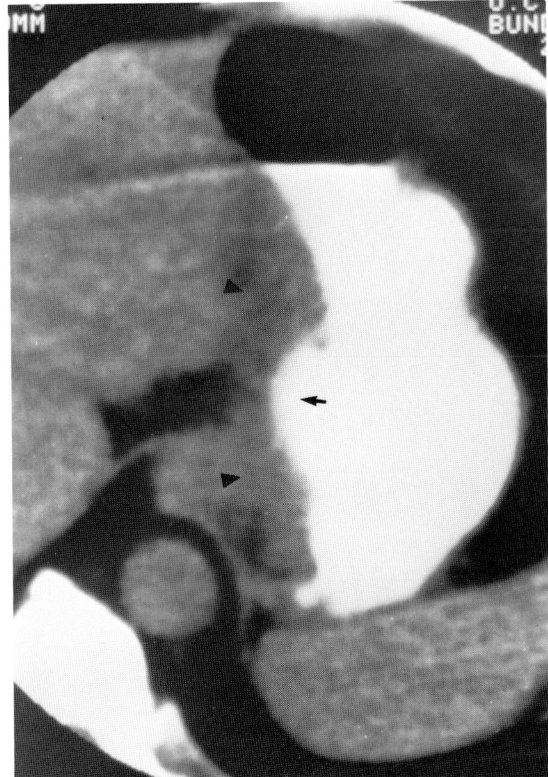

Fig. 2-26 (A) A single-contrast exam reveals the Carman sign of a malignant ulcer present along the lesser curvature *(arrow)*. **(B)** Same case, air-contrast exam of the Carman sign. **(C)** A CT scan (magnification) illustrates the Carman sign *(arrow)*, with barium filling a necrotic portion of the carcinoma. Note the mass effect *(arrowheads)*. CT can often identify thickening of the wall in patients with gastric malignancies.

sequent scarring, narrowing of the pylorus can lead to delayed emptying and even to total obstruction of the gastric outlet.

Hypertrophic Pyloric Stenosis

Two distinct forms of hypertrophic pyloric stenosis have been described. The first is primary or idiopathic hypertrophic stenosis which resembles the congenital pyloric hypertrophy of infants. It represents simple hypertrophy of the pyloric musculature not associated with significant pathologic lesions at or near the pylorus. This lesion may be focal, involving only the pylorus (torus hyperplasia), the prepyloric area, or both. (The torus represents the point at which the two loops of circular muscle fibers of the pyloric canal converge.)

The second form is known as secondary hypertrophic stenosis caused either by benign (inflammation, ulceration, mucosal adenomatosis, eosinophilic infiltration, fibrosis) or malignant (carcinoma) disease. Radiographically, pyloric stenosis is characterized by narrowing and elongation of the pyloric canal. A common finding is a barium-filled pyloric cleft within the torus defect (Twining's sign). This cleft is diamond shaped and can occasionally be confused with an ulceration (Fig. 2-27). Delayed gastric emptying is usually present. Generally, malignancy can be differentiated from benign or congenital disease when irregularity, fine crenulations, or abrupt shouldering between the antrum and pylorus are present. In contrast, the benign form reveals a smooth tapered contour. Surgical treatment includes simple myotomy, resection, or outlet bypass procedures.

POSTOPERATIVE STOMACH

In the immediate postoperative period the radiographic examination is performed either to determine whether complications have occurred or as a routine check before reinstituting oral feedings. Immediate postoperative complications include leakage at the anastomotic site, with the potential for abscess formation; the development of a fistula; and obstruction. In these patients, a water-soluble contrast is advised during radiographic examination in the event a leak may occur. At a later postoperation date barium can, of course, be used for follow-up exams. The technique in

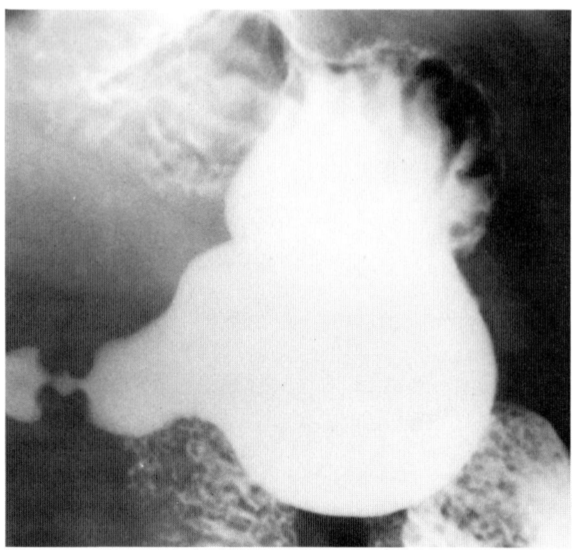

Fig. 2-27 Pyloric stenosis is characterized by an elongation of the pyloric canal, with the central cleft in the torus defect filling with barium. (Marshak RH, Lindner, AE, Maklansky D: Radiology of the Stomach. WB Saunders, Philadelphia, 1983.)

the former situation is not unlike the routine single-contrast UGI study, bearing in mind specific areas of interest in the region of surgery and limitations placed by the patient's diminished mobility. The barium examination, however, should be performed so that optimal mucosal definition is achieved. Using the double-contrast technique described earlier, marginal ulcerations and recurrent mucosal neoplasms, for example, are optimally detected.

Hiatus Hernia Repair

Surgical correction for chronic gastroesophageal reflux remains a common procedure, involving reduction of the hernia and narrowing of the gastroesophageal junction. However, several procedures are available to the surgeon. The following are the most popular, current methods used to reduce gastroesophageal reflux.

NISSEN FUNDOPLICATION

After the hernia is successfully reduced, the gastric fundus is freed from several of its attachments to the short gastric branches of the splenic artery. The posterior aspect of the fundus is then mobilized — via an abdominal approach — behind the abdominal portion of the esophagus. It is wrapped circumferentially about the distal esophagus and sutured anteriorly to form a 4- to 5-cm cuff or antireflux valve. Additional posterior diaphragmatic sutures are frequently placed to fix the stomach to the inferior surface of the diaphragm.

The radiologic examination following this procedure demonstrates narrowing of the wrapped intraabdominal portion of the esophagus and "mass effect" along the visualized fundus of the stomach, representing the plication.

Complications of the Nissen procedure include obstruction at the gastroesophageal junction, loosening of the sutures at the site of plication, and reappearance of the hiatus hernia.

BELSEY-MARK IV

This procedure is performed much like the Nissen fundoplication, mobilizing the lower esophagus and fundus and plicating the fundus to the esophagus in a 270-degree fashion, sparing the region of the vagus nerves. This creates an acute esophagogastric angle or radiographic dog-leg appearance characteristic of the procedure. The pseudotumor defect along the fundus decreases approximately one month after surgery (see Fig. 1-31).

ANGELCHIK PROCEDURE

A relatively recent innovation has been a silicone ring prosthesis placed above the esophagogastric junction below the diaphragm. This is a technically easier procedure that does not require sutures. The ring is rendered radiopaque by tantalum markers and measures 2½ cm in width. However, the ring is not without its complications, slipping distally over the body of the stomach or becoming completely dislodged. Consequently, its utility has been questioned.

OTHER PROCEDURES

Numerous gastric procedures are performed for peptic disease or neoplasia. These can be separated into those that do not require gastric resection and those that require partial or total gastrectomy.

PROCEDURES FOR NONRESECTION AND FOR GASTRECTOMY

Nonresection Procedures

Pyloroplasty
  Widening of the pyloric canal either by transverse suturing of a sectioned pyloric sphincter (Heineke-Mikulicz) or by a U-shaped incision for antroduodenal anastomosis (Finney)

Beck procedure
  Longitudinal transsection of the stomach for intrathoracic interposition following partial esophagectomy

Simple closure/excision
  Oversewing perforating uclers

Gastroduodenostomy
  Gastroduodenal anastomosis for distal gastric outlet obstruction

Gastroenterostomy
  Gastrojejunal anastomosis for distal gastric obstruction or ulcers

Gastrectomy

Partial
Generally accompanies truncal/selective vagotomy

1. Distal two-third gastrectomy and gastroduodenostomy
   End-to-end (Péan-Billroth I)
   End-to-side (Finsterer-Billroth I)

2. Distal two-third gastrectomy and gastrojejunostomy
   End-to-side (Polya-Billroth II) afferent loop retrocolic or (Finsterer [Hofmeister]-Billroth II) antecolic (Fig. 2-28)
   End-to-side Roux-en-Y (jejunojejunostomy distal to the gastrojejunostomy site)
   Whipple procedure (distal gastrectomy with gastrojejunostomy, choledochojejunostomy, and partial pancreatectomy)

(List continued)

(Note: generally all gastroduodenostomy procedures are termed Billroth I and gastrojejunostomy procedures [with the exception of the Roux-en-Y and Whipple's procedures] are Billroth II).

Total
1. Esophagojejunostomy
   End-to-end
   End-to-side
2. Interpositions
   Small bowel
   Colon

RATIONALE FOR DISTAL GASTRECTOMY

Generally, the distal two-thirds of the stomach are resected, including the pylorus and duodenal bulb, and the gastric remnant is anastomosed to either the duodenum or jejunum. These procedures have been used to treat gastric and duodenal ulcers as well as gastric carcinomas.

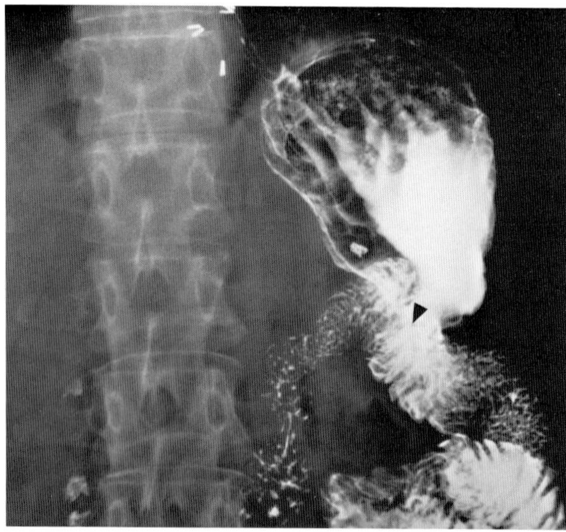

Fig. 2-28 The normal appearance of a Billroth II, gastrojejunostomy procedure with vagotomy clips present. Note preferential emptying into the efferent loop *(arrowhead)*.

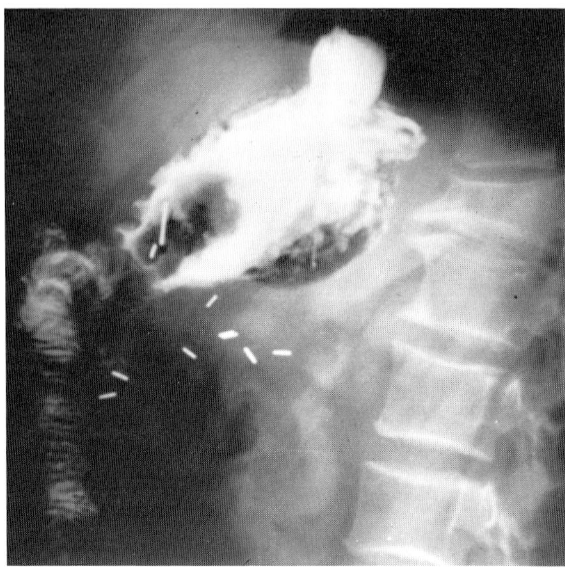

Fig. 2-29 A filling defect in the barium pool represents intussusception of the jejunum into the gastric remnant in a patient post–Billroth II surgery.

Duodenal Ulcer Disease

A decrease in the secretion of gastric acid (HCl) diminishes the corrosiveness of gastric juices entering the duodenum, thereby promoting healing. By eliminating the distal stomach, most of the chief and oxyntic cells are removed. By removing the antrum, the source of gastrin — the stimulus for the production of acid by oxyntic cells and of pepsinogen by the chief cells — is also removed.

Gastric Ulcer Disease

The rationale for distal gastrectomy is similar to that for duodenal ulcer disease, with the additional benefit of rapid gastric emptying which reduces the time the gastric juices are in contact with the gastric mucosa.

Complications of Gastric Resective Surgery

A number of complications can occur following gastric surgery. These are anastomotic leaks, abscess formation, fistulization to the skin or abdominal contents; hemorrhage; obstruction; bezoar formation; esophagitis, gastritis, or both, generally secondary to bile reflux but also occasionally caused by stasis; recurrent ulcer disease on either side of or at the anastomosis, more common distally; gastrojejunal intussusception, (antegrade or retrograde) (Fig. 2-29); afferent loop syndrome — undue distension of the proximal limb generally caused by obstruction distal to the gastrojejunal anastomosis or to unphysiologic construction of the anastomosis with preferential filling of the afferent loop; retained antrum with continued acid secretion from parietal cells in response to gastrin secretion by the antrum; and postgastrectomy syndrome — i.e., mechanical dumping caused by rapid gastric emptying.

Another complication that has been debated in the recent medical literature is the development of gastric carcinoma 10 to 15 years after partial gastrectomy for peptic disease thought to be secondary to chronic bile reflux gastritis. An incidence of 5 percent has been reported. The carcinoma occurs in the gastric remnant rather than distal to the anastomosis (Figs. 2-30 and 2-31).

CONGENITAL ANOMALIES

Congenital anomalies of the stomach are relatively rare, often seen as incidental findings, occasionally explaining vague symptomatology.

The complex embryologic development of the gut is not discussed in detail in this chapter (see the recommended reading list). More commonly encountered entities are briefly described.

Gastric Volvulus

Volvulus is an uncommon condition in which there is an abnormal rotation or torsion of one part of the stomach upon another part. It can occur at any age and is due to laxity of the suspensory gastric ligaments. That condition in which the greater curvature points upward in the chest, the so-called upside-down stomach, is not considered *true* volvulus because no obstruction is present. Generally, greater than 180 degrees of twist about an axis are required to produce

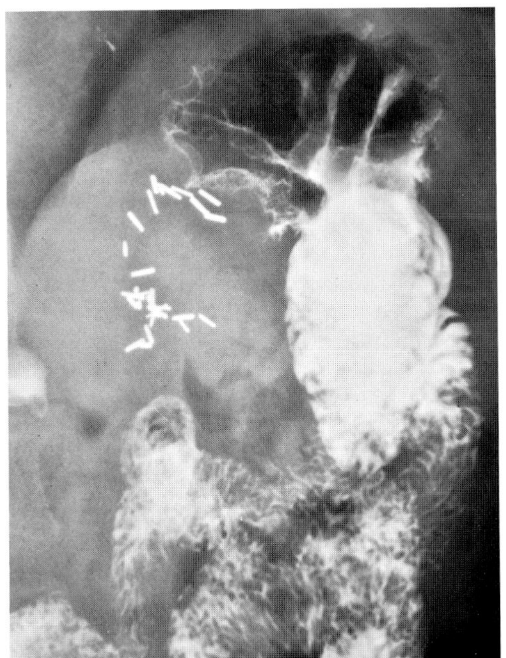

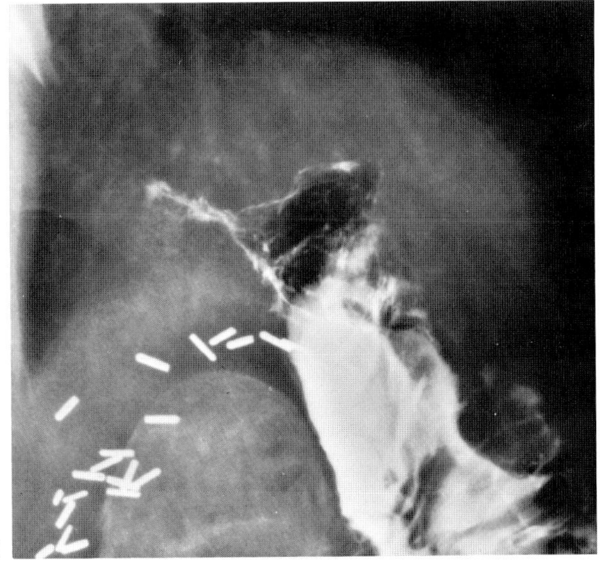

Fig. 2-30 (A) Several years following Billroth II procedure, folds of the gastric remnant are thickened secondary to bile reflux gastritis. **(B)** Malignant degeneration has produced a shrunken, narrowed gastric remnant 10 years later.

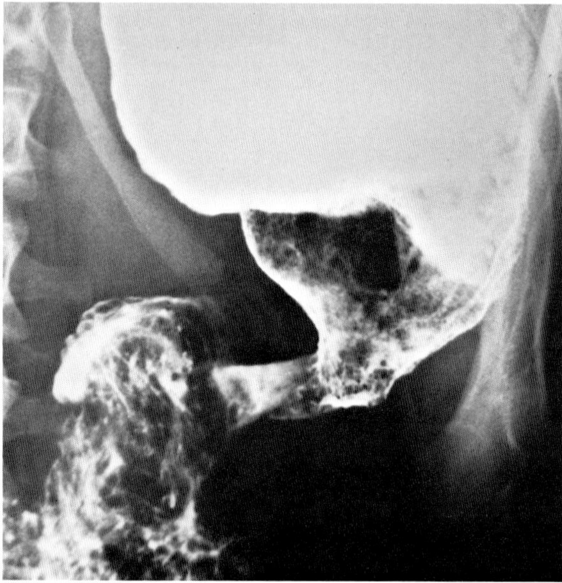

Fig. 2-31 Scirrhous narrowing of the distal gastric remnant provides evidence for an infiltrative adenocarcinoma following partial gastrectomy in this patient.

complete obstruction and vascular compromise with subsequent necrosis. Clinically, this produces an acute abdomen with a triad of pain, unsuccessful attemps at vomiting, and the inability to pass a nasogastric tube (triad of Borchardt).

Radiographically, plain films show a massively distended stomach. Its location is high, and there is a paucity of gas distally. Occasionally, intramural emphysematous gastritis is present when necrosis has occurred. Barium examinations reveal complete obstruction and malposition of the stomach, the appearance of the latter depending on the type of volvulus present. The two possible types of gastric volvulus are organoaxial and mesenteroaxial volvulus.

Organoaxial Volvulus

The stomach rotates along its long axis, along a line drawn from the fundus to the antrum. The stomach twists 180 degrees anteriorly or posteriorly so that the position of the greater curvature is cranial and that of the lesser curvature is caudal. Organoaxial volvulus is

generally seen in elderly patients with a history of hernias (particularly the paraesophageal type).

Mesenteroaxial Volvulus

The stomach rotates on its short axis along a line drawn perpendicular to the lesser and greater curvatures. The distal stomach rotates 180 degrees anteriorly and superiorly so that the fundus is caudal to the antrum. This type of volvulus is seen primarily in children and is commonly associated with traumatic diaphragmatic hernias (Fig. 2-32).

Gastric Duplications and Cysts

Duplications — also referred to as gastric cysts, enterogenous cysts, embryonal cysts, supernumerary or accessory stomachs — are extremely rare. About 4 percent of all gastrointestinal duplications are gastric in origin. The cyst is contiguous with the gastric wall and is lined with alimentary epithelium — gastric and occasionally, ectopic intestinal, respiratory, and pancreatic epithelium. The size of the duplication ranges from several centimeters to greater than 12 cm. It generally does not communicate with the true gastric lumen and, therefore, presents radiographically as smooth intramural masses with cystic or tubular configurations that have a slight preference for the greater curvature (Fig. 2-33). In one-third of cases, gastric duplications have been associated with other anomalies such as other enteric duplications, annular or ectopic pancreas, and vertebral anomalies.

Duplication cysts can be surgically excised when symptomatic.

Antral Diaphragm/Web

Mucosal diaphragm membranes, or webs, are located in the antrum. They are composed of two layers of mucosa separated by an inner layer of submucosa. These webs measure 2 to 3 mm in width, are circumferential, and are located perpendicular to the curvatures of the stomach. Apertures in the webs permit barium to pass (Fig. 2-34). The smaller the aperture, the more symptomatic the patient.

Webs are commonly associated with gastritis and gastric ulcers in as many as 50 percent of cases. In these patients the webs are quite likely acquired secondary to scarring and fibrosis. The fact that webs can also be seen in children, or in the absence of inflammation, indicates that a congenital origin is a definite possibility.

Aberrant Pancreas

Also known as an ectopic pancreatic rest, these islands of pancreatic tissue are not uncommon. They can be found anywhere in the stomach or duodenum as well as within the jejunum, Meckel diverticula, gallbladder, liver, spleen, mesentery, and even the mediastinum. The most common location is the gastric antrum, as a solitary, smooth, submucosal nodule (0.5 to 2.0 cm) with a central umbilication representing a pancreatic duct remnant. The nodule itself consists of true pancreatic tissue that can grow during life (Fig. 2-35).

Hypertrophic Pyloric Stenosis

There are two forms of hypertrophic pyloric stenosis — that found in the newborn and the adult type. In the neonate, it represents hypertrophy and hyperplasia of circular smooth muscle with resultant elongation of the pylorus. The infants present with large air-filled stomachs caused by the distal obstructing lesion, which is readily palpated.

Adult hypertrophic pyloric stenosis is a rare lesion that represents either an idiopathic or a secondary postinflammatory lesion. Anatomically, the specimen is similar to that seen in the infant. It is composed of hyperplastic and hypertrophic muscular tissue that extends into the antrum, thus creating an elongation of the pyloric canal. A central triangular outpouching of the pylorus is caused by barium trapped in mucosal clefts between the hypertrophied circular or torus muscle (see Fig. 2-27).

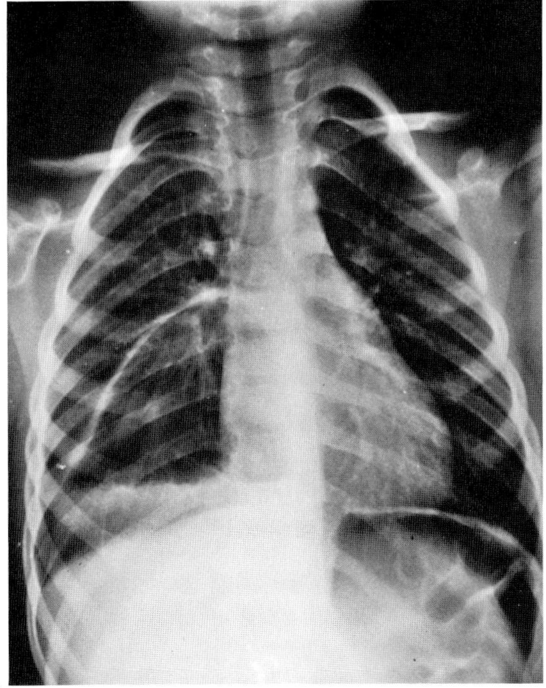

A

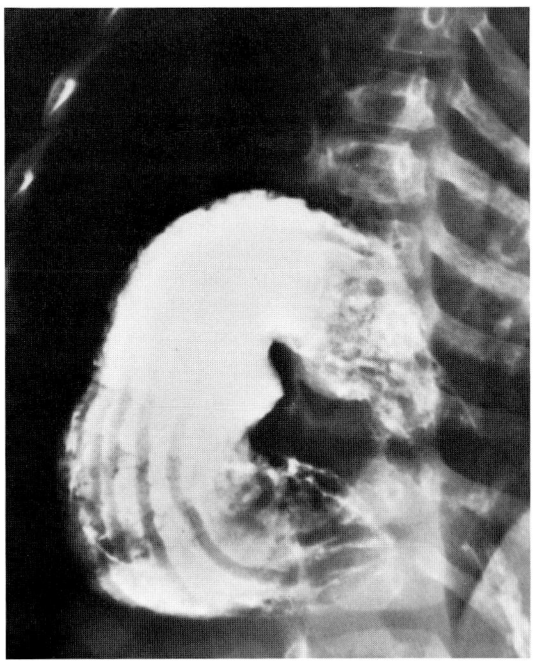

B

Fig. 2-32 (A) Admission chest radiograph of a young child with a mesenteroaxial volvulus of the stomach and a coincidental traumatic diaphragmatic hernia. The stomach is identified in the right hemithorax. **(B)** An upper GI exam showed complete gastric outlet obstruction of the malpositioned stomach.

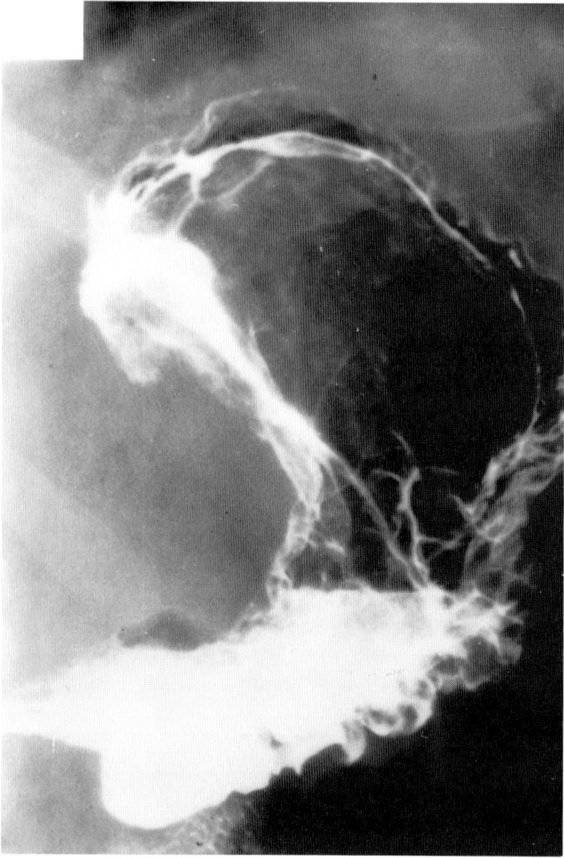

Fig. 2-33 A posterior wall gastric duplication presents with extrinsic mass effect on the stomach.

Patients present with symptoms of obstruction, which may be longstanding. The lesion must be differentiated from an annular carcinoma that generally demonstrates more mucosal irregularity radiographically. Therapy varies from dilatation attempts to surgical pyloromyotomy and resection. The latter procedure is optimal in that the specimen can be thoroughly inspected for evidence of carcinoma.

GASTRIC VARICES

Venous drainage along the stomach is accomplished through short gastric veins that drain the fundus of the stomach and enter the splenic vein posteriorly, the gastroepiploic vein along the greater curvature, and the coronary vein along the lesser curvature of the stomach. The latter two veins drain directly into the portal vein, whereas the splenic vein merges with the superior mesenteric vein to form the portal venous confluence. Esophageal veins drain into the coronary and azygos veins.

Gastric varices are caused by either portal venous hypertension or splenic vein thrombosis. In portal venous hypertension, elevated pressures generated along the coronary and splenic veins increase the blood flow to these vessels, with resultant gastric and uphill esophageal varices. In general, the varices occur simultaneously with preference for the former over the latter, although radiographically gastric varices are more difficult to demonstrate by techniques other than angiography.

Gastric varices in the absence of esophageal varices can be attributed to the second cause of varices — i.e., splenic vein thrombosis. In this situation, venous blood flow is reversed between the fundus and the spleen so that blood is diverted from the spleen through the short gastric veins to the coronary vein, thus bypassing the esophageal collaterals. The most common cause of splenic vein thrombosis is pancreatitis. Other causes include pancreatic neoplasms, adenopathy, retroperitoneal neoplasm (sarcoma, hypernephroma), and trauma.

Radiographic evaluation of the stomach by double-contrast UGI examination can demonstrate varices because the gaseous distension achieved eliminates a false-negative evaluation caused by prominent rugae that can readily mask varices on routine single-contrast studies. Varices can be identified in the fundus and along the distal body and antrum, appearing as serpiginous filling defects or large polypoid mass(es) (Figs. 2-36 and 2-37). A large fundal mass may represent a number of entities, in addition to varices, such as a neoplasm (carcinoma, lymphoma, metastases, leiomyoma, carcinoid, and others), a postsurgical defect from the fundoplication procedure, or a slightly prolapsed esophagus in a patient with a hiatal hernia (See Fig. 2-3). Unlike the evaluation of esophageal varices, the Valsalva maneuver is not helpful in distending gastric varices; however, this maneuver is particularly helpful in ruling out the more common entity of a

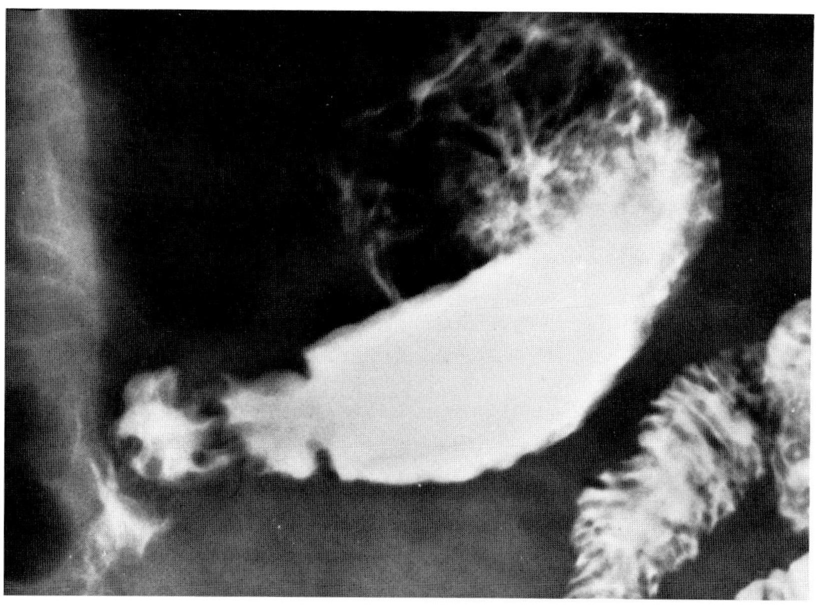

Fig. 2-34 A nonobstructing antral web (diaphragm) was diagnosed in this asymptomatic patient.

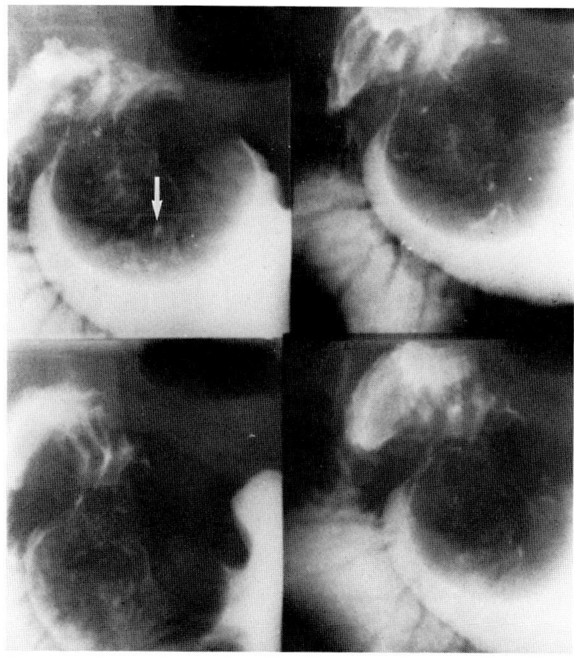

Fig. 2-35 A central umbilication representing the pancreatic duct remnant *(arrow)* is located in this pancreatic rest.

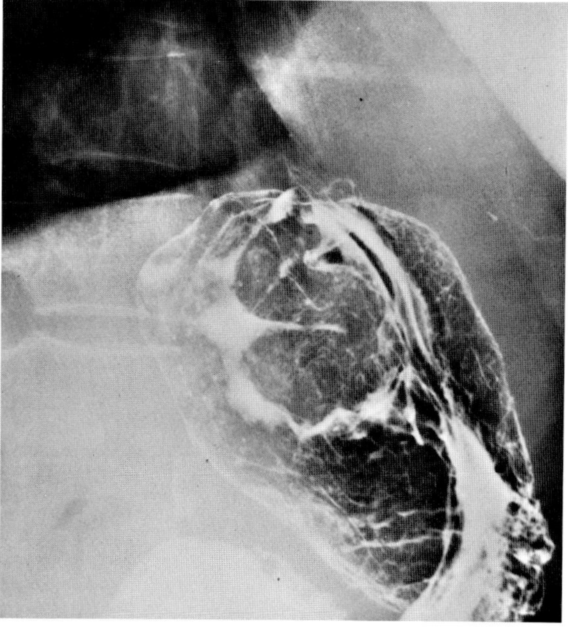

Fig. 2-36 A large serpiginous filling defect in the fundus represents a dilated collateral vein in a patient with portal hypertension.

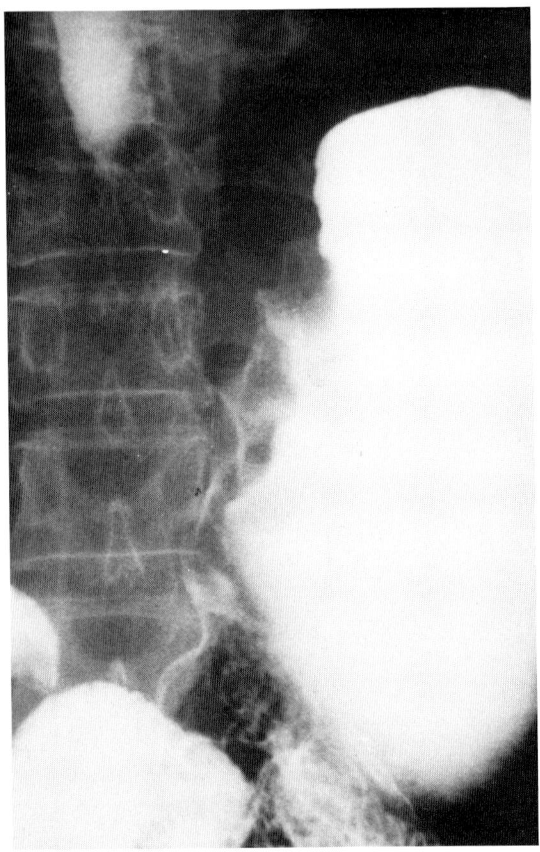

Fig. 2-37 Gastric varices can mimic fundal tumors.

prolapsed hiatal hernia. Angiography is the examination of choice in evaluating for varices as well as their causes. CT and recently MRI scanning have been shown to also demonstrate prominent collateral veins.

SUGGESTED READINGS

Callihan TR, Berard CW: Classification and pathology. p. 1. In Felson B (ed): Roentgenology of the Lymphomas and Leukemias. Grune & Stratton, New York, 1980

Kressel HY: Peptic disease of the stomach and duodenum. p. 716. In Margulis AR (ed): Alimentary Tract Radiology. CV Mosby, St Louis, 1983

Kressel HY, Laufer I: Principles of double contrast diagnosis. p. 11. In Laufer I (ed): Double Contrast Gastrointestinal Radiology with Endoscopic Correlation. WB Saunders, Philadelphia, 1983

Laufer I: Stomach. p. 155. In Laufer I (ed): Double Contrast Gastrointestinal Radiology with Endoscopic Correlation. WB Saunders, Philadelphia, 1979

Marshak RH, Lindner AE, Maklansky D: Radiology of the Stomach. WB Saunders, St Louis, 1983

Maruyama M: Early gastric cancer. p. 241. In Laufer I (ed): Double Contrast Gastrointestinal Radiology with Endoscopic Correlation. WB Saunders, Philadelphia, 1983

Nahum H, Fekete F, Margulis AR: Radiology of the Postoperative Digestive Tract. Masson Publishing, New York 1979

Nelson SE: The discovery of gastric ulcers and the differential diagnosis between benignancy and malignancy. Radiol Clin North Am 7:5, 1969

Op den Orth JO: The postoperative stomach. p. 289. In Laufer I (ed): Double Contrast Gastrointestinal Radiology with Endoscopic Correlation. WB Saunders, Philadelphia, 1983

Seaman WB: Non-neoplastic lesions. p. 688. In Margulis AR (ed): Alimentary Tract Radiology. 3rd Ed. Vol 1. CV Mosby, St Louis, 1983

3

Radiology of the Small Bowel

Peter Feczko
Robert Halpert
R. Kristina Gedgaudas-McClees

Despite considerable advances in gastrointestinal diagnostic techniques in the last several decades, the small bowel continues to represent an area where barium examination remains the primary diagnostic tool. Being largely inaccessible by endoscopic methods, various barium techniques continue to be utilized as front line diagnostic modalities for this "hinterland" of the alimentary tract. Other imaging techniques such as ultrasound, computed tomography, or magnetic resonance imaging do not approach the barium study for diagnostic detail of processes involving the bowel.

Despite this, barium examination of the small bowel has suffered from a reputation as being insensitive to everything but the most grossly obvious diseases. The expected usefulness and sensitivity of any imaging modality is directly proportional to the care, detail, and expertise the investigator brings to the process. The small bowel examination is no exception. Quite often, the exam proceeds without diligent monitoring; hence, diagnostic evaluation occurs after the fact rather than during the course of the study. The efficacy of the small bowel series also depends on the reason for which it is performed. Based on the clinical

evaluation or laboratory data, the small bowel series is indicated for the following reasons.*

1. Small bowel fistula
2. Metastasis
3. Abdominal trauma
4. Small bowel obstruction
5. Systemic disease with small bowel involvement
6. Inflammatory bowel disease
7. Primary small bowel tumor
8. Malabsorption

Various technical advances have been introduced to maximize diagnostic accuracy. However, changes in attitude are perhaps as significant to the success of small bowel barium imaging as are changes in technique. Delegation of the small bowel examination to a "poor cousin" status doomed to futility at the start should be replaced by a determination to extract maximum information whenever possible.

---

* List adapted from Rabe FE, et al: Radiology 140:47, 1981.

TECHNIQUES OF EXAMINATION

The types of radiologic examinations of the small bowel include the following.

1. The small bowel follow-through (SBFT)/small bowel series.
2. The dedicated small bowel examination/small bowel meal (SBM).
3. Small bowel enteroclysis/small bowel enema (SBE).
4. Peroral pneumocolon (PPC).
5. Water-soluble examination of the small bowel.

Small Bowel Follow-Through (SBFT)

The small bowel follow-through examination is the most commonly performed radiographic procedure for detecting abnormalities of the small bowel.

Following evaluation of the stomach and duodenum, additional amounts of low weight barium (20% to 40% W/V) are administered. It is recommended that 16 to 20 ounces (480 to 600 ml) of barium be ingested by the patient in order to visualize and distend the entire small bowel. The patient should drink this amount at one time to minimize inadequate delineation of segments of small bowel.

It is common to obtain 14″ × 17″ overhead radiographs 15 and 30 minutes following the start of the exam. Additional films are taken at 30- to 60-minute intervals, until contrast is identified in the right colon. Normally, this occurs within 45 to 90 minutes. Fluoroscopy and compression filming of the terminal ileum are routinely performed at this time in most departments. In fact, a criticism of this technique has been made by several authors indicating an overreliance on the overhead films to indicate pathology in areas proximal to the terminal ileum. In addition to careful monitoring by the radiologist of routine overhead radiographs, additional fluoroscopic evaluation of all individual segments of the small bowel with manual compression decreases technical and perceptive errors when lesions are hidden in overlapping loops of bowel. This technique of proper bowel distention and compression also facilitates evaluation of the small bowel fold pattern.

Enteroclysis

The intubation/infusion technique of small bowel examination is considered by many to be the most sensitive of the small bowel examinations in detecting even the most subtle of lesions. The advantages of enteroclysis include its ability to fully distend the entire small bowel, simultaneously demonstrating its anatomy both fluoroscopically and by careful compression spot filming (Fig. 3-1).

A standard bowel prep used for barium enema examinations is advisable (without cleansing enemas) to facilitate the passage of barium and to minimize reflux of feces into the terminal ileum.

MATERIALS USED IN ENTEROCLYSIS

Enteroclysis tube. A size 12, SBD-6 Modified Bilboa-Dotter tube, 133 cm in length, with insertable Teflon-coated torque cable (Cook, Incorporated)

Tray
  Either anesthetic mouth spray (Cetacaine) or a topical anesthetic gel (viscous 2 percent Xylocaine)
  Emesis basin
  Tongue depressor
  Lubricant for the duodenal tube

Contrast agents
  Micropaque powder (Picker Corporation) blended 50/50 with water to produce a 300 ml 85% W/V suspension
  HD-85 (Lafayette) 600 ml barium mixed with 900 ml water (1 to 1.5 mixture) producing a 34% W/V suspension
  Carboxymethyl-cellulose (CMC) solution (E-Zm EM)

Infusion System
  Hemodialysis pump (Renal Systems Mini Pump: R.S.-7800) or
  50 ml syringes
  Y-Connector and two enema bags for use with two contrast agents.

Intubation can be performed by an oral or transnasal route in the upright position. A guidewire is intro-

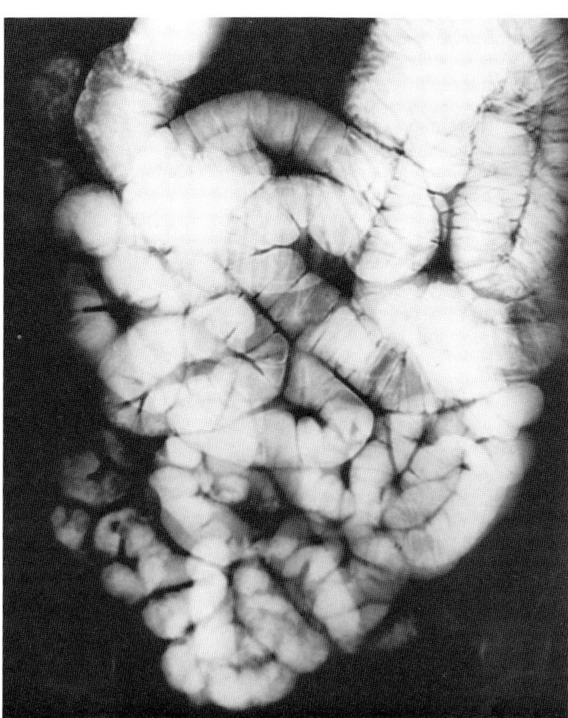

Fig. 3-1 Normal enteroclysis exam. Note optimal distension of the small bowel. Use of two contrast agents makes the bowel appear transparent.

duced after the tube tip has been successfully advanced into the stomach. The patient is then placed in a supine RPO or lateral position, and the tube is advanced to the distal duodenum or proximal jejunum to minimize subsequent reflux of contrast materials. One of the barium mixtures is introduced either by rapid manual injection with 50 ml syringes, or more efficiently with a renal dialysis pump at an infusion rate of 80 to 120 ml/min. (If Micropaque is used, infuse only 200 ml of the solution.) Cooled methylcellulose is used immediately after the instillation of Micropaque for a double-contrast examination of the small bowel. The use of HD-85 requires no additional methylcellulose and produces a single-contrast examination.

As the contrast materials are introduced, compression and fluoroscopy are performed, with filming of well-distended segments of the bowel. Obtain prone and supine overhead 14 × 17 inch films of the abdomen in the middle and at the end of the small bowel filling. The exam lasts 15 to 25 minutes, including intubation.

In addition to the identification of potential mass lesions and ulcerations, the valvulae conniventes are evaluated. Folds are normally 1.5 to 2.0 mm thick. Fold thickening can be readily assessed using this technique. The bowel wall, which normally measures 1 to 1.5 cm in width, can also be assessed.

The Dedicated Small Bowel Meal

The role of the dedicated small bowel meal study appears to be an alternative to the enteroclysis examination, when difficulties with tube placement or poor patient cooperation prevent the latter study from being performed. It is essentially a meticulously performed small bowel follow-through without precedent examination of the more proximal upper gastrointestinal tract. The technique has already been outlined.

Peroral Pneumocolon

The peroral pneumocolon (PPC) is useful in the evaluation of the distal small bowel and the ileocecal area, as well as the ascending colon. The examination is an adjunct to the small bowel follow-through or the dedicated small bowel meal. Patient preparation is identical to that used for colonic examination.

When barium is observed in the right colon, the patient is returned to the fluoroscopic suite, and a small rectal catheter is inserted. Air is inflated until distension of the ileum and cecum are observed fluoroscopically (1.0 mg intravenous glucagon may be administered to achieve further relaxation of the cecum and distal small bowel. In addition, glucagon has been shown to be effective in promoting reflux across the ileocecal valve). When adequate air reflux and barium coating of the bowel have occurred, compression spot films are obtained.

Water-Soluble Contrast Material for Small Bowel Evaluation

The role of water-soluble contrast continues to be controversial, the subject of occasional differences of opinion between radiologists and clinicians. The most common application of the problem occurs when the patient presents with a potential small bowel obstruction, and a water-soluble contrast examination is requested to identify the level of the obstruction. Fear that barium may become impacted in the small bowel has no basis in fact. Considerable evidence in animal studies suggests the opposite. Available water-soluble contrast agents are hypertonic; in some instances they have an osmolality four to five times greater than that of serum plasma. As a result, considerable amounts of fluid are drawn into the bowel, which may exclude any possibility of visualizing a lesion because of the considerable amount of dilution that occurs. The exact level or nature of the obstruction may, therefore, be totally impossible to determine. (In the presence of an intestinal tube that has been placed for decompression, water-soluble contrast may not result in such severe limitations, if the tube is within a short distance of the actual obstructing site.)

The overall experience with this controversial procedure has lead us to conclude that barium is preferred for the evaluation of potential small bowel obstruction. When the colon is known to be normal and a small bowel obstruction is clinically suspected, barium is the contrast agent of choice. The use of water-soluble contrast material is indicated solely in situations of questionable perforation.

MALABSORPTION

The term malabsorption refers to the abnormal absorption of food products (fat, water, protein, carbohydrates) from the small intestine. This creates symptomatology manifested by steatorrhea; frequent, foul smelling stools; weight loss; and abdominal distension.

The small bowel is comprised of mucosal folds, the so-called "valvulae conniventes" on which numerous fingerlike projections, the villi, are located. The villi measure approximately 1 mm in length and are further composed of microvilli that are 1 μ long. This intricate architecture increases the surface absorptive area 600 times that which would be present should the small bowel be a simple, featureless tube. The villi are lined with a single layer of columnar epithelium, below which are located capillaries and lymphatics. Complicated transport mechanisms in the surface epithelium allow nutrients to be taken up by the submucosal vasculature. Carbohydrates are broken down into monosaccharides, proteins into amino acids, and peptides and fats into fatty acids and monoglycerides. All are primarily absorbed in the duodenum and proximal jejunum, as are water and electrolytes.

There are a number of diseases that cause malabsorption clinically. Depending on the pathogenic process involved, the radiographic appearances of these diseases can vary.

The small bowel has a limited number of alterations in its appearance, although it is affected by a wide variety of disease entities. Many diseases have similar radiographic appearances in the small bowel. A logical stepwise approach to the assessment of the small bowel can often lead to a correct diagnosis. Listed below are criteria used when evaluating the small bowel for malabsorption.

1. *Diameter:* The small bowel has a maximal normal diameter of 3 cm. In the absence of intubation or glucagon, diameters greater than 3 cm are considered abnormal.
2. *Fold thickness:* The valvulae conniventes normally measure 1.5 to 2.0 mm. Measurements greater than 3 mm should be considered pathologic.
3. *Wall thickness:* The distance between two loops of bowel comprises the thickness of two bowel walls. Each wall should measure 1 to 1.5 mm in thickness.
4. *Secretions:* There should be no appreciable amount of fluid in the small bowel. Excess secretions can be noted as dilution of the barium column and segmentation.
5. *Transit time:* The normal time period during which barium traverses the small bowel and enters the colon is 3 hours on the average. Variations occur from as little as 30 minutes to as long as 8 hours.

One popular method of evaluating the small bowel for malabsorption is to use the algorithmic approach popularized by Goldberg (1976) (see Fig. 3-2).

When evaluating the small bowel, it is important to simplify one's approach, identify the most striking finding on the small bowel series, and determine the extent and location of the abnormality. Finally, one must integrate the radiographic findings with the clinical and laboratory data available. This simplified version, popularized by Lichtenstein, may be more

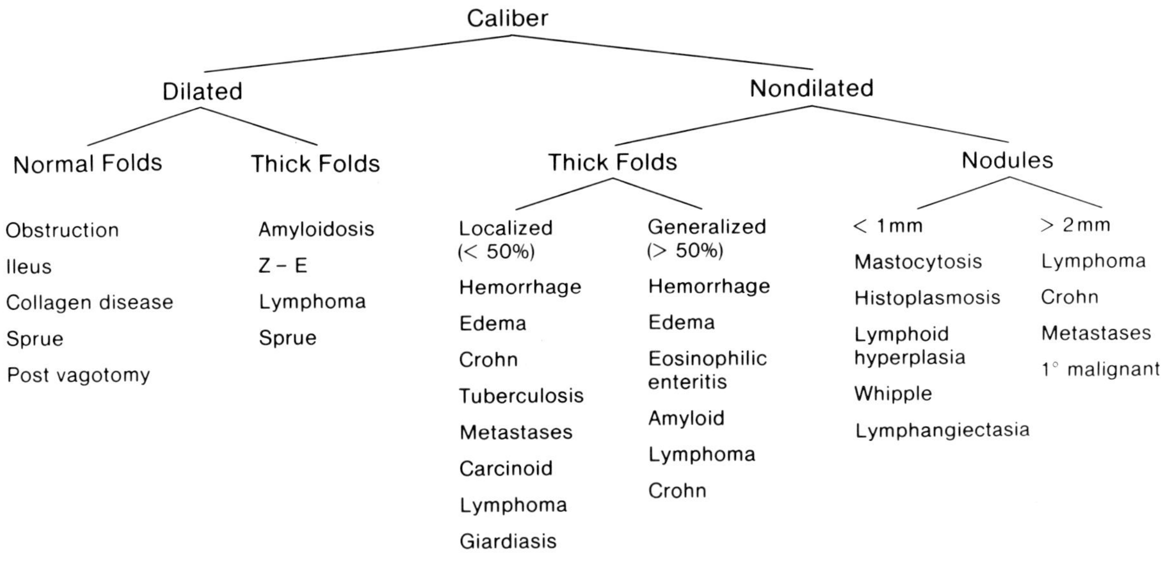

Fig. 3-2 Algorithm for small bowel disease.

practical than the more complicated algorithmic approach.

A SIMPLIFIED APPROACH TO SMALL BOWEL EVALUATION

Dilatation
  Obstruction/ileus
  Scleroderma
  Sprue
  Collagen vascular disease
Fold prominence/nodularity
  Crohn disease
  Lymphoma
  Edema
  Whipple disease
  Lymphangiectasia
  Amyloidosis
  Nodular lymphoid hyperplasia
  Primary and secondary neoplasia
  Hemorrhage/ischemia
  Giardiasis
Hypersecretion
  Sprue
  Whipple disease
  Lymphangiectasia

Sprue

The term sprue is given to three disease entities with similar pathology. These are celiac disease seen in children, nontropical sprue, and tropical sprue in adults. Tropical sprue has no known etiology, but its clinical presentation and histologic presentations are identical to the other forms. Patients respond to folic acid with B_{12} and antibiotic therapy, generally tetracycline. Celiac disease and nontropical sprue are virtually the same disease process identified at different times of life. There appears to be some geographic predilection in that there two entities occur more commonly among people from northern Europe. Although no genetic pattern of transmission is evident, there may be familial tendencies. The disease occurs more commonly in women.

Nontropical sprue is caused by an intolerance of the protein gluten. Gluten is found in wheat, rye, and barley. Some consider that patients with sprue have an enzyme deficiency, although many now feel that there is an abnormal immune response to this protein. When gluten is removed from the diet, the patient's symptoms usually improve dramatically. Clinically, patients have diarrhea and steatorrhea. Malabsorption occurs in addition to weight loss, retarded growth, and various mineral and vitamin deficiencies.

Pathologically, there are marked changes in the villi. The villi may be flattened and broadened, or there may be virtual loss of these structures. The total surface area of the villi is markedly diminished. Pathologic changes are also noted in the epithelial mucosal cells, which become flattened and cuboidal. The cells are not only morphologically abnormal, but their chemical function is altered so that transport across cell membrances is significantly prolonged. These histologic changes have been noted to reverse when appropriate therapy is instituted. Tropical sprue tends to heal more slowly and in some cases incompletely. The altered radiographic patterns are variable, reflecting the disease activity at any given time.

Radiographically, a variety of abnormalities may be evident. These may vary between patients, and sometimes different patterns present in the same patient during different times in the course of the disease. One of the most typical findings in sprue is dilatation of the small bowel. This is more typical in the midbowel. In general, the caliber increases with the severity of the disease. The etiology of the dilatation is unknown, although it has been postulated that is reflects a combination of the slight hypokalemia caused by decreased electrolyte absorption and a decrease in tonicity of the small bowel wall (Fig. 3-3).

The transit time of the barium column can be quite variable in sprue, although there is a tendency for slight prolongation related to the flaccidity and diminished contractility of the bowel. Rarely will it be more rapid than normal.

One of the most difficult areas in evaluating sprue is the variability in the fold pattern. In some instances, the folds are more prominent, caused by the increased secretions as well as the associated hypoalbuminemia from protein malabsorption. This abnormality is most commonly appreciated in the duodenum. The fold pattern of the ileum may be prominent, creating the so-called jejunalization appearance of the ileum. Occasionally, the fold pattern is diminished. In rare circumstances, the fold pattern is completely lost, creating the "moulage" sign. This term is derived from the French term *moulage,* meaning casting, describing the effacement of folds in such a way that it resembles a tube into which wax has been poured and allowed to harden. The moulage sign develops when increased secretions obsure the mucosal folds (Fig. 3-4).

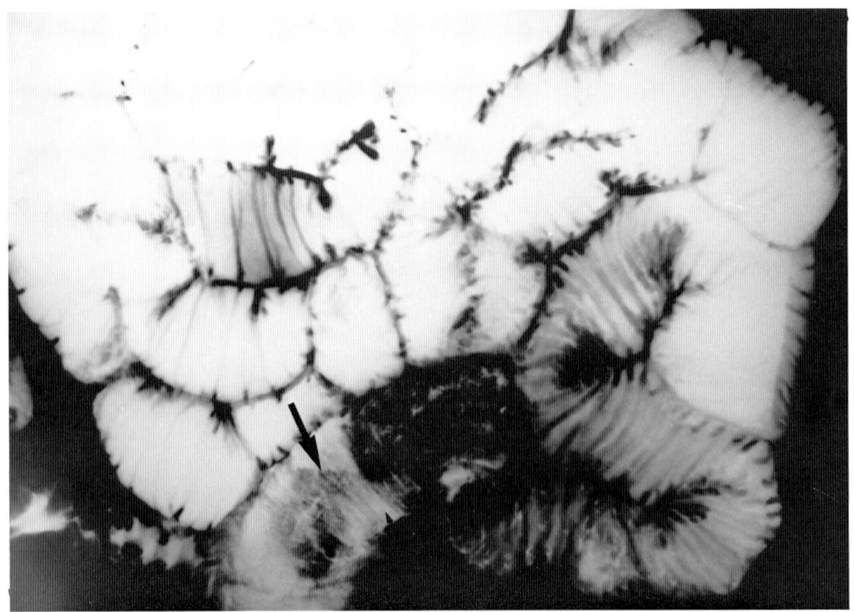

Fig. 3-3 Sprue. The bowel is dilated. Intussusception is present in the midjejunum *(arrow).*

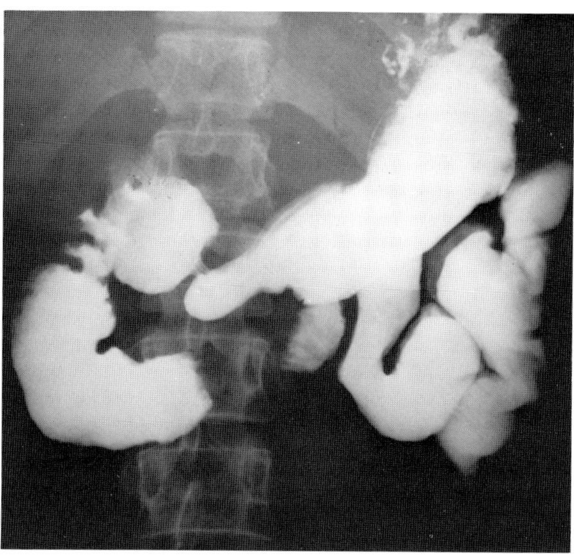

Fig. 3-4 Moulage sign in a patient with sprue. The duodenum and jejunum are completely featureless, a characteristic appearance of advanced disease.

Increased secretions are typical of the patient with sprue. These excess secretions play a part in the radiographic feature of segmentation. Segmentation refers to a separation of the barium column into several large clumps. Flocculation of barium associated with increased secretions is no longer appreciated with the new barium suspensions.

Patients with sprue also exhibit transient intussusception, the typical "coiled-spring" appearance of which can occasionally be demonstrated radiographically. Ulceration is rarely evident in sprue, although it has been reported.

There is an association between sprue and the development of intestinal malignancy. It would appear that patients with a long history of sprue are more likely to develop carcinomas of the small bowel. Lymphomas have also been reported. Whether adherence to a gluten-free diet will decrease the likelihood of malignant degeneration has been debated.

Scleroderma

Scleroderma is a systemic connective tissue disease with characteristic skin changes, arthropathy, and Raynaud's phenomenon developing usually early in its course. In the latter stages of the disease, abnormalities of the gastrointestinal tract occur. These changes are secondary to replacement of the muscular layers of bowel with collagen and fibrous tissue, resulting in muscular atrophy. Mesenteric vascular arteritis has been noted. Virtually the entire intestinal tract can be affected. Although the small bowel can be involved at any time in the course of the disease, its development is generally preceded by the extraintestinal manifestations listed above.

The most dramatic change is a marked alteration in bowel motility. Normal peristaltic activity is diminished with secondary dilatation of bowel. The hypomotility seen in scleroderma develops as the muscular layers are replaced with fibrous tissue. The diminished motility causes stasis of bowel contents.

Clinically, these patients experience malabsorption, presumably from resultant bacterial overgrowth with changes in the bile acids. Occasionally, patients will respond to antibiotic therapy.

A commonly noted abnormality of the small bowel is dilatation, particularly in the duodenum, which can be quite massive. In the jejunum and ileum, the most striking feature is hypomotility, with varying degrees of dilatation (Fig. 3-5). The mucosal folds are generally normal, or thinned and straightened, appearing closer together, the so-called "hide-bound" appearance caused by the submucosal fibrosis. Increased secretions are generally not present.

Pseudosacculation of the small bowel may occur when intermittent areas of fibrosis create outpouchings of the more normal intervening segments. Rarely, intramural pneumatosis can occur for reasons that are not clearly understood (Fig. 3-6).

Whipple Disease (Intestinal Lipodystrophy)

This entity was first described at the turn of the century by Whipple, who identified patients as those with malabsorptive complaints, diarrhea, steatorrhea, abdominal pain, weight loss, fever, adenopathy, and altered skin pigmentation. An important feature of this disease is a nondeforming arthritis.

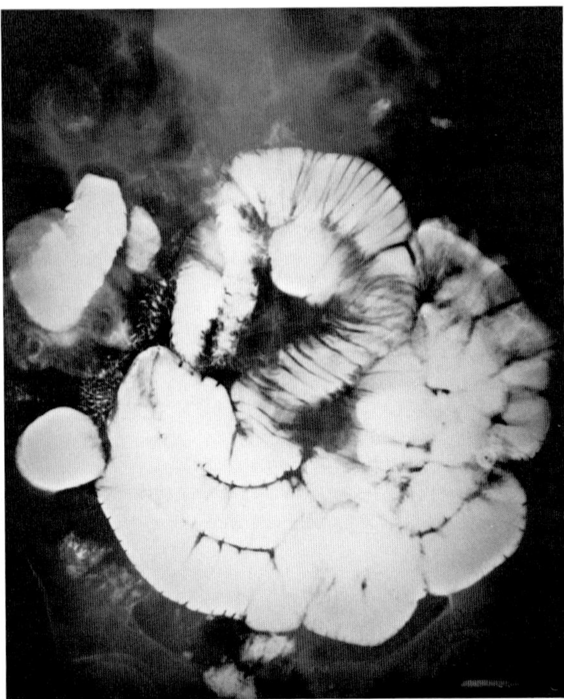

Fig. 3-5 Scleroderma. In addition to dilatation, the folds are thinned and more closely approximated than normal (compare this with sprue in Fig. 3-3).

The hallmark of Whipple disease is the presence of foamy PAS-positive staining macrophages in the lamina propria of the small bowel. These glycoprotein-laden macrophages may also be found in mesenteric and peripheral lymph nodes. Electron microscopic examination usually reveals remnants of rod-shaped bacilli in macrophages, supporting the concept that Whipple disease is infectious in origin. These patients also have a good response to broad-spectrum antibiotics. The bacteria, however, have not been isolated and may be secondary invaders rather than primary pathogens.

Radiographic examination of the small bowel reveals a diffuse thickening of the folds of the small bowel, predominantly in the jejunum (Fig. 3-7). On close inspection, the mucosal surface has a sandlike nodularity caused both by infiltration of the villi by macrophages and concurrent intestinal edema. The lumen of the small bowel may be normal in caliber, or slightly dilated. Because adenopathy may occur, a focal extrinsic mass effect can be noted along the mesentery. Some increased secretions may be present. Whipple disease is often difficult to differentiate from intestinal lymphangiectasia, hypogammaglobulinemia, amyloidosis, and systemic mastocytosis. The diagnosis is ultimately made by small bowel biopsy.

Amyloidosis

Classically, amyloidosis has been divided into primary and secondary types. Recently, this distinction

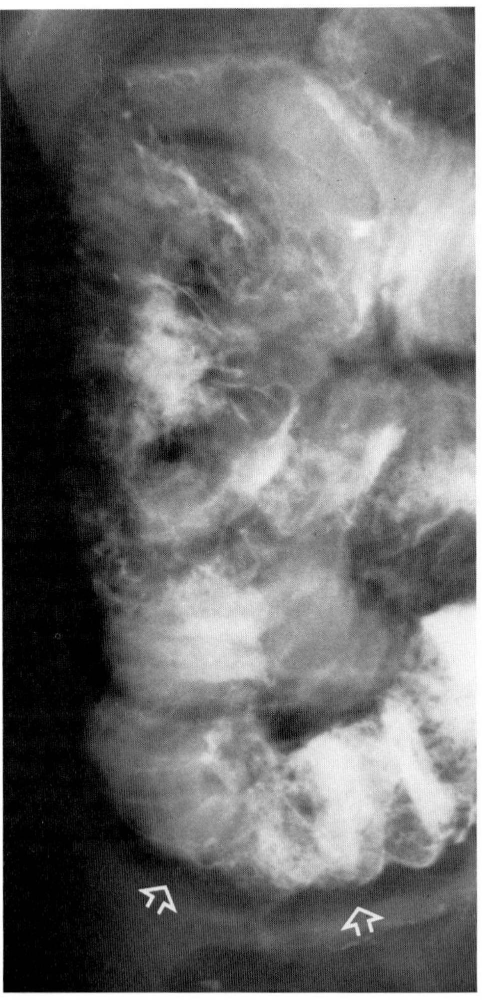

Fig. 3-6 Intramural pneumatosis in a patient with scleroderma *(arrows)*. The etiology may be the connective tissue disorder or steroid therapy. When these air cysts rupture, patients present with benign pneumoperitoneum.

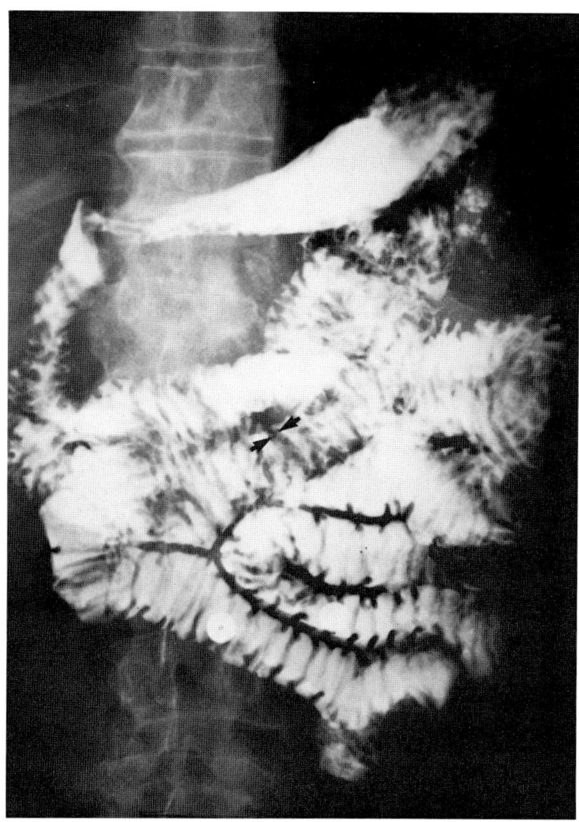

Fig. 3-7 Whipple disease. The folds are uniformly thickened *(arrows)* and are slightly indistinct owing to infiltration of the villi with glycoproteins.

has been less commonly used. It has been suggested that all cases of amyloid are the result of plasma cell dyscrasias, such as multiple myeloma.

All areas of the intestinal tract can be involved by this disease. Clinically, these patients may have diarrhea, malabsorption with steatorrhea, protein loss, intestinal pseudoobstruction and vascular insufficiency.

Histologically, much of the amyloid is diffusely deposited about the submucosal arterioles. The epithelial cells may be flattened or even destroyed in cases of extensive amyloid deposition.

The most typical roentgen finding is diffuse thickening of the folds. This thickening is usually in a symmetric pattern, extending from the jejunum to the ileum (Fig. 3-8). On occasion, the distribution can be

patchy and uneven. The caliber of the small bowel is generally normal, but as the disease progresses, mild dilatation may occur. Findings of ischemic disease associated with arteriolar compression may become apparent. The motility of the bowel is often diminished, owing to impaired motor activity.

Intestinal Lymphangiectasia

Lymphangiectasia is a disease manifested by malabsorptive symptomatology, hypoalbuminemia, and hypogammaglobulinemia.

Histologically, the bowel wall is filled with dilated lymphatics. Abundant PAS-negative macrophages are present in the mucosa. The disease can be congenital, manifesting itself in infancy or acquired, presenting late in life. Steatorrhea is the result of damaged and thickened mucosal cells, possibly the result of chronic leakage of chyle into the bowel lumen. Protein loss is

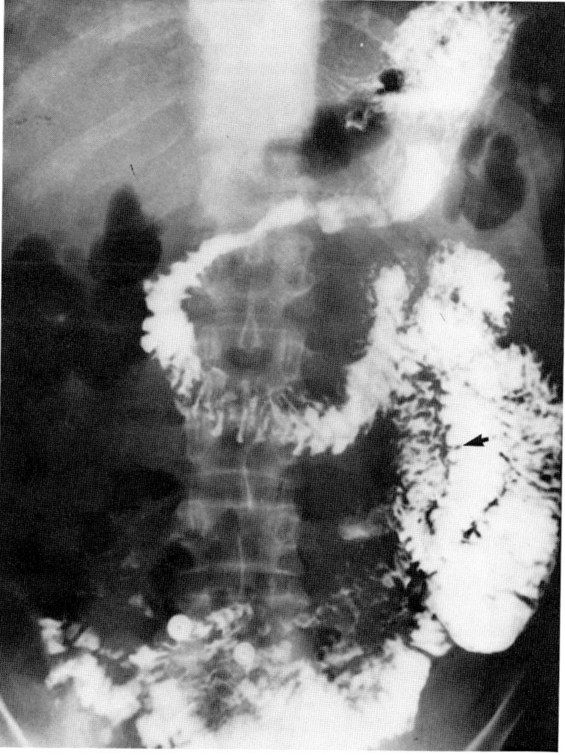

Fig. 3-8 Amyloidosis. The folds are thickened. In profile they appear peripherally "clubbed" *(arrow).*

probably secondary to rupture of the dilated lymphatics. Therapy is a low-fat diet, which theoretically decreases lymph production.

Radiographically, the mucosal folds are diffusely thickened, as a result of the hypoproteinemia. A fine nodularity, reflecting the dilated mucosal and submucosal lymphatics, is also present. Increased secretions dilute the barium column (Fig. 3-9).

Eosinophilic Gastroenteritis

Eosinophilic gastroenteritis is a disease characterized by a peripheral eosinophilia accompanied by mucosal, submucosal, and serosal eosinophilic infiltration of the intestines with concurrent edema. There is a history of food allergy in approximately two-thirds of patients. This disease entity must be clinically distinguished from parasitic infections, which can also present with a peripheral eosinophilia. The disease is more common in younger patients who develop recurrent attacks of abdominal pain, vomiting, and diarrhea.

The stomach and small bowel are most commonly affected, with the colon rarely involved. The folds are markedly thickened and appear almost polypoid. Spasm and irritability are present in advanced cases.

Immunoglobulin Disorders

Immunologic defenses to diseases can be divided into two distinct categories: humoral and cellular immunity.

Humoral immunity is dependent on the serum components known as immunoglobulins or antibodies. These gammaglobulins are subdivided, according to antigenic specificity, into IgA, IgD, IgE, IgG, and IgM. Immunoglobulin G comprises the majority of serum globulin; IgA is formed in the intestinal mucosa and, therefore, plays an important role in local

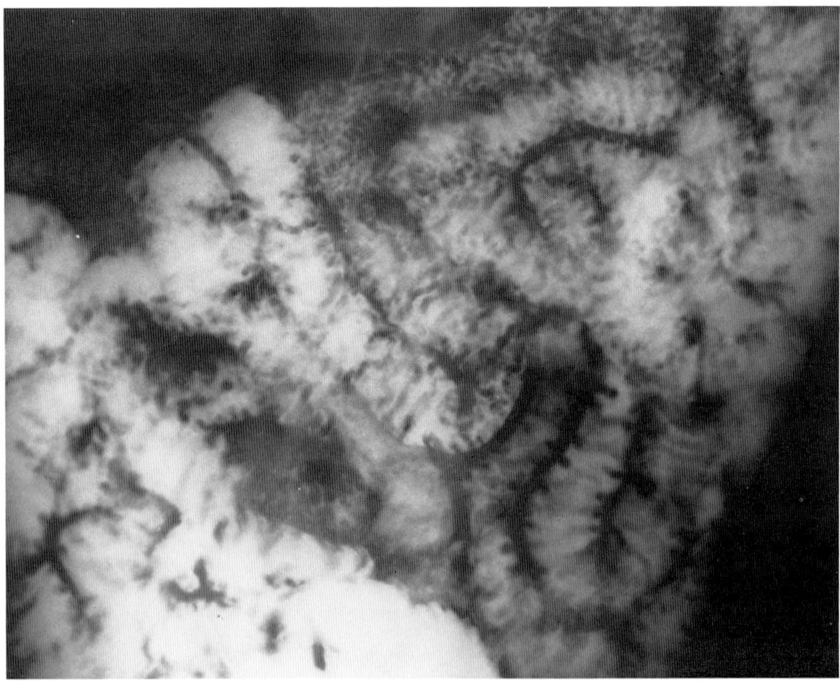

Fig. 3-9 Lymphangiectasia. The folds are thickened secondary to the hypoproteinemia that occurs in these patients. The barium column is diluted by the chyle present in the bowel lumen.

defense mechanisms. Primary IgA deficiency can result in IgA-deficient sprue (associated with gluten enteropathy) or diffuse nodular lymphoid hyperplasia. Immunoglobulin deficiency states are associated with an increased tendency to infections.

Neoplastic processes such as multiple myeloma and Waldenström macroglobulinemia involve the plasma cells and may have prolific effects on specific immunoglobulin levels.

The second form of the body's immunologic defense is cellular immunity, which resides in the lymphocytes. This type of immunity does not affect the gastrointestinal tract.

The radiographic features of immunoglobulin disorders vary. Patients afflicted with gammaglobulin deficiency states exhibit nodular lymphoid hyperplasia manifested as tiny 1.0 to 2.0 mm nodular filling defects in the small bowel. This appearance can also be seen in patients with giardiasis, who commonly have a variable immunoglobulin deficiency state.

Patients with IgA deficiency sprue manifest identically to those with other forms of sprue.

Waldenström macroglobulinemia results in a finely granular pattern along the small bowel folds. Diffuse thickening of the small bowel folds themselves, secondary to infiltration of the mucosa with plasma cells and lymphocytes, is commonly appreciated.

Mastocytosis (Urticaria Pigmentosa)

Mastocytosis is an uncommon disease characterized by mast cell proliferation of the dermis, reticuloendothelial system, and the bowel wall. The mast cells contain histamine, the secretion of which elicits fibrosis. The intestinal tract may be variably infiltrated with mast cells. Villous atrophy has been described in advanced cases.

Clinically, patients have abdominal pain, diarrhea, and nausea. They present with a pruritic macular rash. Half of the patients have hepatosplenomegaly.

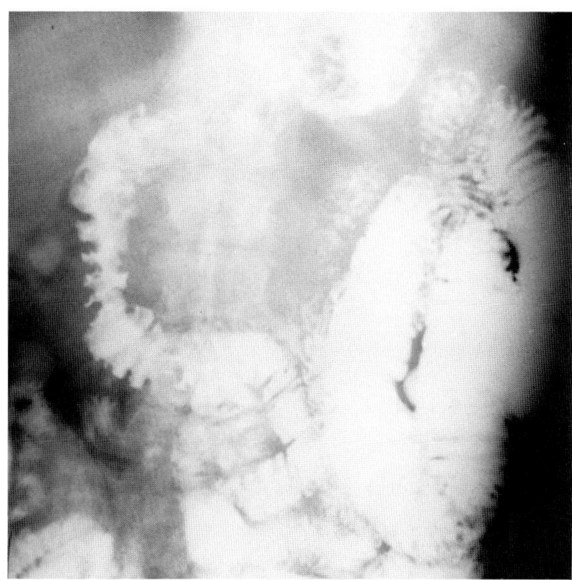

Fig. 3-10 Mastocytosis. This adolescent presented with a history of allergies and a peripheral eosinophilia. The nodular thickening in the proximal small bowel is caused by an urticarial reaction in the mucosa.

The radiographic examination shows a coarse nodular thickening of the small bowel folds caused by the cellular infiltrate, and resultant urticarial mucosal reaction (Fig. 3-10).

Patients with mastocytosis are at an increased risk for developing peptic ulcer disease related to histamine release by the mast cells. H_2 blockers are used to treat these patients.

Incidentally, the bones of many patients are diffusely sclerotic.

Graft Versus Host Disease

In patients who receive allogeneic bone marrow transplants, it is not uncommon to identify changes in the small bowel, colon, and esophagus after several days, weeks, or months. The transplanted histocompatible bone marrow may elicit a reaction of donor T lymphocytes against surface antigens in the host, producing crypt-cell necrosis, ulcerations, vascular dilatation, and edema. Commonly involved tissues are skin, liver, and bowel.

On barium studies, abnormalities occur throughout the entire gastrointestinal tract, particularly in the ileum where severe edema, ulceration, mucosal nodularity, and fold effacement produce an appearance identical to inflammatory bowel disease (Crohn disease). Therapy includes putting the bowel to rest and administering steroids, as well as Imuran and Cyclosporin. It is important to rule out infectious enteritis *(Yersinia, Camphylobacter, Candida)* prior to therapy.

Miscellaneous Causes of Malabsorption

CYSTIC FIBROSIS

In patients with cystic fibrosis, abnormalities can be identified within the small bowel and colon. Often, there is a coarse nodular thickening of the mucosa, particularly in the duodenum and proximal jejunum, reflecting glandular enlargement with inspissated mucoid material (Fig. 3-11).

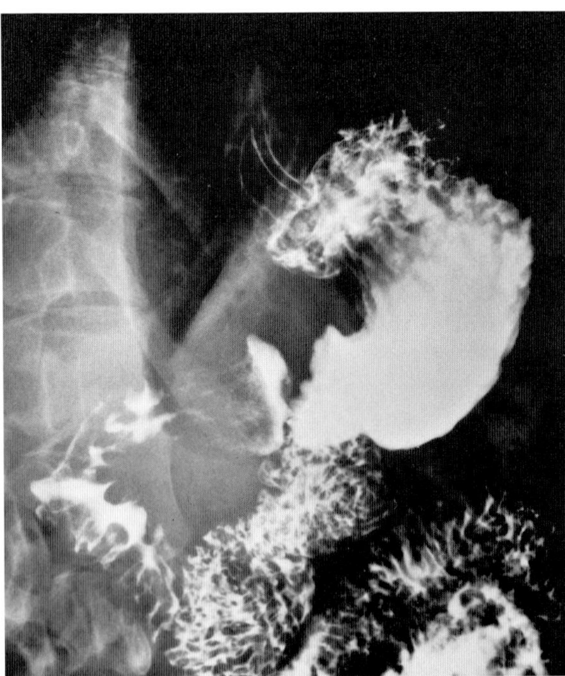

Fig. 3-11 Cystic fibrosis. This young adult with a history of chronic lung disease presented with diarrhea. The nodular fold thickening in the duodenum is secondary to enlargement of the mucosal glands filled with inspissated mucus.

PANCREATIC INSUFFICIENCY

Patients with chronic pancreatic disease may develop malabsorption caused by a deficiency of pancreatic enzymes. A certain number of these patients will have increased small bowel secretions. The small bowel folds are generally normal, and the caliber is unaffected by the increased intraluminal contents.

DIABETES

Patients with diabetes can have clinical symptoms of malabsorption, although the exact etiology of this manifestation is uncertain. On small bowel examination, the bowel may appear slightly dilated. In some instances, there are spruelike changes with increased secretions, segmentation, and fold abnormalities.

LACTASE DEFICIENCY

Absence of the enzyme lactase produces symptoms of malabsorption after ingestion of milk products. The routine small bowel examination is normal. However, after lactose is added to the barium mixture, the small bowel becomes edematous and fluid filled, diluting the barium column dramatically.

VASCULAR DISORDERS

Ischemia

Abnormalities in the arterial and venous supply to the small bowel result in a variety of clinical and radiographic presentations. Etiologies include atherosclerosis, thrombus formation secondary to birth control pills or venous stasis, emboli, and several vasculitides (thromboangitis obliterans, collagen vascular diseases, polyarteritis nodosa, and rheumatoid arthritis). Impairment of the blood supply affects the entire bowel wall. Initially, the mucosa, which is extremely sensitive to alterations in its blood supply, begins to ulcerate. Hemorrhage and edema cause nodular thickening of the submucosa. Peristalsis is absent within the involved segment. Subsequently, healing may be complete or may produce areas of fibrosis and stricture formation.

Clinically, patients present with symptoms that reflect the severity of the vascular compromise. When

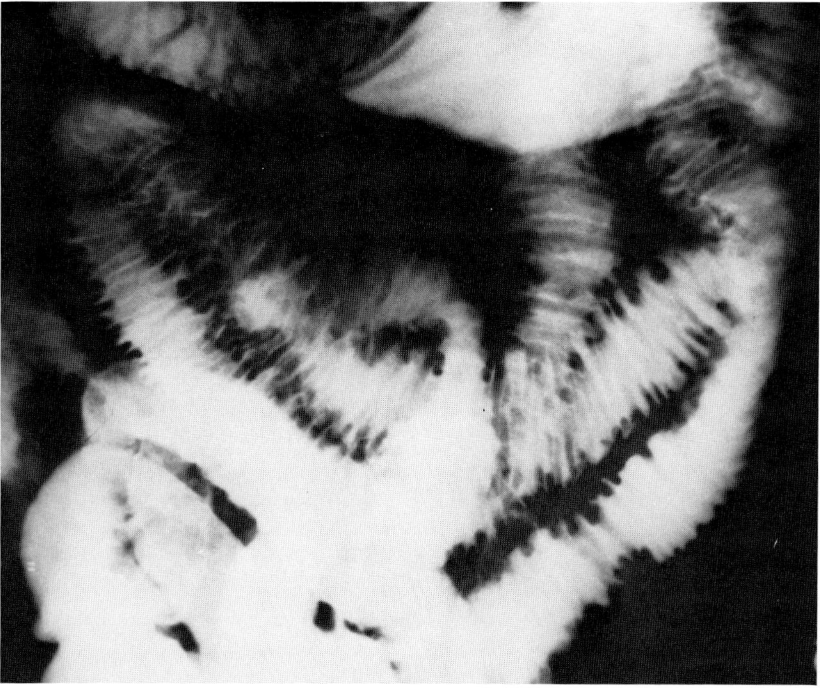

Fig. 3-12 Stacked-coin appearance of submucosal hemorrhage. This pattern is indistinguishable from ischemia, edema, and various infiltrative disorders.

blood flow impairment solely affects absorption, patients present with "intestinal angina" or postprandial abdominal pain. However, when there is occlusion of the mesenteric vessels, patients suffer severe abdominal pain, tenderness, and distension. Passage of blood in the stools is frequently present as well.

Radiographic changes may also help to quantitate the severity of vascular compromise. The plain film of the abdomen may well be abnormal, revealing rigid, narrowed, and thickened loops of small bowel. The thickening caused by submucosal edema and hemorrhage may be minimal, creating the "stacked-coin" appearance of symmetrically thickened valvulae conniventes (Fig. 3-12). As the edema progresses, the valvulae appear to have been replaced with a scalloped wall, compromising the intestinal lumen. This appearance is termed "thumbprinting" (Fig. 3-13). Localized areas of perforation appear as linear or punctate collections of intramural gas or "pneumatosis intestinalis" (Fig. 3-14). Fistulas and sinus tracts can also occur.

With incomplete healing, normal submucosal layers may be replaced with fibrotic tissue and result in subsequent stricture formation (Fig. 3-15). Fibrosis can occur within several weeks of the acute event. Asymmetric stricture formation can cause outpouching of intermediate segments of bowel, thus forming sacculations or "pseudodiverticula."

Angiography during the acute event can be useful when the occlusion originates in a major mesenteric branch.

Intramural Hemorrhage

Bleeding into the bowel wall can be associated with a variety of causes. Trauma, coagulopathies (hemophilia, vitamin K deficiency), Henoch-Schönlein purpura, thrombocytopenia (idiopathic thrombocytopenic purpura), hypofibrinogenemia, anticoagulant therapy, disseminated intravascular coagulopathy, and a variety of malignancies (leukemia, lymphoma,

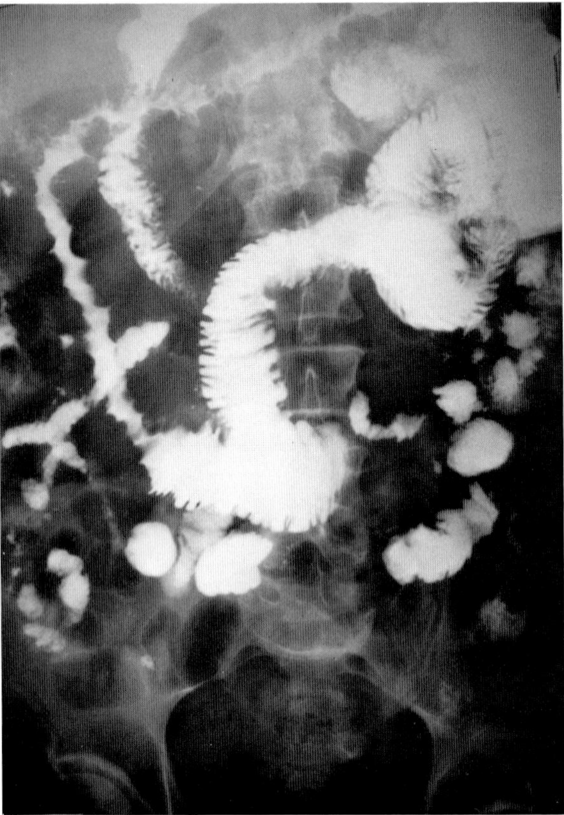

Fig. 3-13 Thumbprinting in an elderly man who presented with ischemia of the jejunum and ileum secondary to embolic disease.

metastatic disease of the bone marrow) have all been implicated.

Blunt abdominal trauma, including seat belt injuries, particularly affect the duodenum because of its fixed retroperitoneal location. Hemorrhage into the bowel wall can be extensive and, with sufficient trauma, perforation can occur, extruding duodenal contents into the right anterior pararenal space (Fig. 3-16).

Henoch-Schönlein purpura is an acute arteritis that develops within weeks of a streptococcus infection in younger patients. Multiple organ systems are affected (i.e., a purpuric skin rash and nephritis are common). Intestinal disease presents with abdominal pain associated with focal or diffuse areas of hemorrhage and edema.

Hemophilia is an inherited bleeding disorder caused by deficiency in the precoagulant activity of antihemophilic globulin (factor VIII). The gene is sex-linked recessive. Female carriers transmit the disorder to half of their sons and the gene to half of their daughters. Exsanguinating hemorrhage may follow injury or surgery. Spontaneous bleeding episodes are characteristic in severe cases. The basis of therapy is the transfusion of materials containing factor VIII precoagulant activity, which temporarily corrects the specific defect.

Idiopathic thrombocytopenic purpura is a disorder of children and young adults who develop acute onset thrombocytopenia with purpura over the limbs and upper torso. When intermittent, gradual bleeding persists for 6 months or more, the disease is considered to represent a chronic form. Treatment includes splenectomy and, occasionally, immunosuppressive therapy.

Anticoagulant drugs include coumarin derivatives and heparin. The coumarins antagonize the action of vitamin K and lead to the same clotting abnormality as that induced by vitamin K deficiency. They prolong prothrombin as well as partial thromboplastin times, and reduce the level of prothrombin and factors VII, IX, and X. Heparin inactivates thrombin, preventing its action on fibrinogen. Coumarin-induced hemorrhage is treated by administering vitamin K and plasma. The action of heparin is reversed with protamine sulfate infusions.

A variety of malignancies that affect the bone marrow lead to a depletion of platelets and, thus, produce spontaneous hemorrhage. The most common of these are the leukemias and multiple myeloma. Lymphomas and metastatic disease to the marrow can also produce thrombocytopenic states.

Differentiation of the radiographic changes of mesenteric vascular occlusion from intramural hemorrhage is difficult. In general, the stacked-coin appearance and the lack of spasm favor hemorrhage, whereas thumbprinting generally indicates ischemia. Neoplastic diseases can be distinguished by the localized presence of tumor nodules, focal areas of dilatation, and ulcerations. (Neoplastic diseases will be discussed later.)

Radiation Enteritis

It is appropriate to discuss radiation changes of the small bowel after a discussion of vascular disorders since the major underlying changes are vascular in nature. The small bowel can be affected by radiation, especially following surgery, with resultant adhesions fixing the small bowel within the radiation port. The amount of radiation necessary to produce damage varies among individuals and is somewhat dependent on the patient's underlying vascular status. Doses of 5,000 to 6,000 rads will often produce radiographic changes of radiation enteritis, but doses as low as 1,500 rads have been known to produce clinical symptoms. Both acute and chronic pathologic changes occur with radiation. In the acute phase, there is mucosal damage; the mucosa becomes edematous and ulcerates. Vascular injury occurs in the initial phase, creating submucosal edema and hemorrhage. Later, fibrosis develops within the submucosal and muscular layers of the bowel. Obliterative endarter-

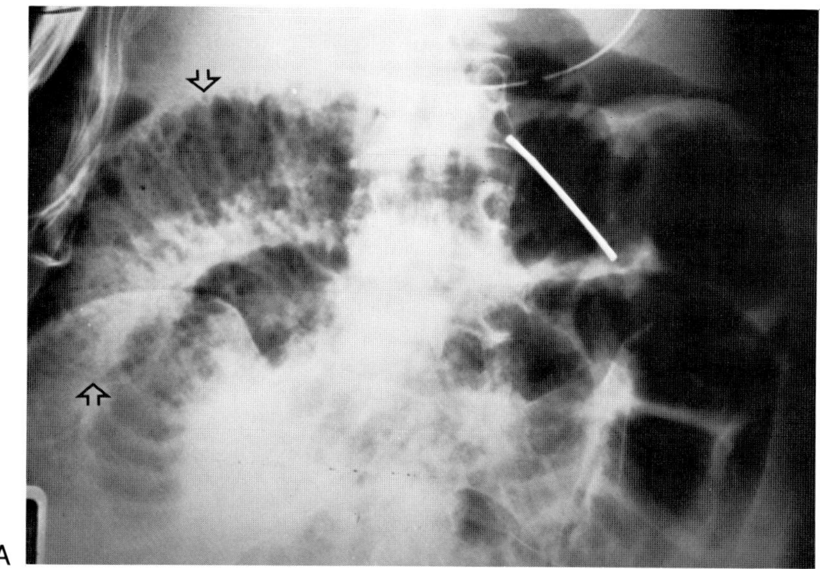

A

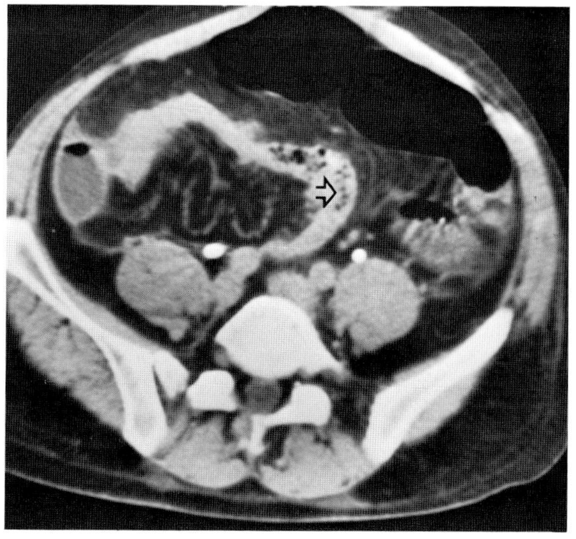

B

Fig. 3-14 (A) Intramural pneumatosis of the small bowel appears as fine, punctate, and linear gas collections *(arrows)* following the contour of the bowel. This patient had infarction of his entire small bowel. **(B)** CT scan of the same patient reveals the intramural gas collections *(arrows)*.

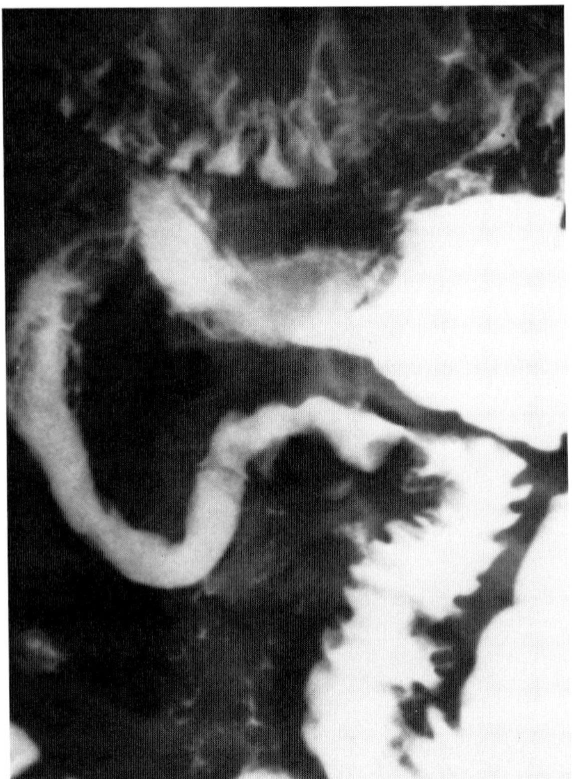

Fig. 3-15 Fibrosis and stricture formation occur as late sequela of ischemic enteritis.

itis, caused by endothelial proliferation, compounds the ischemic changes.

Clinically, patients in the acute phase experience bloody diarrhea and abdominal pain.

Radiographically, the folds are uniformly thickened initially. In severe cases, thumbprinting may become evident. The bowel becomes irritable and spastic. Ulcerations are superficial and usually are not radiographically apparent. Gradually, effacement of the folds, narrowing of the bowel lumen, and rigidity and fixation of the affected segments occur. The more normal proximal gastrointestinal tract dilates (Fig. 3-17).

CROHN DISEASE

Crohn disease was first described as an inflammatory condition involving the terminal ileum, in 1892.

In the early 1960s, the features of colonic involvement were appreciated. Now we realize that virtually any part of the gastrointestinal tract can be affected.

The small bowel is involved with a frequency equal to that of the colon (70 percent). Duodenal involvement occurs in 20 percent of cases.

There are two peaks of incidence; the first occurs in the 15- to 30-year-old age group and the second, which is less common, occurs in the elderly. Familial trends have been identified in the Ashkenazi Jewish population.

The etiology is unknown. One theory suggests an immunologic basis, whereas the other, a viral or bacteriologic agent.

The initial process involves the submucosa. Lymphoid tissue becomes hyperplastic and obstructs the lymphatics with resultant lymphedema (Fig. 3-18). The overlying epithelium of the hyperplastic nodules degenerates and discrete or aphthoid ulcerations form. These ulcers can be as large as 3 mm in diameter and have an average depth of 1.0 to 2.0 mm. The ulcers are irregularly scattered throughout the gastrointestinal tract with intervening areas of normal mucosa creating "skip areas." The ulcerations enlarge and fuse with one another, growing in length and depth, to give the intervening edematous mucosa a "cobblestone" appearance (Fig. 3-19). As the ulcers deepen, they involve the entire thickness of the bowel wall, occasionally forming sinus tracts or even fistulous communications with other epithelialized surfaces, most commonly other segments of bowel. Fistulas can also form to the bladder, vagina, and abdominal wall. Adjacent lymph nodes enlarge. Abscess formation, especially in the ileocecal region, is common as the sinus tracts enlarge and essentially wall off. The terminal ileum is the most commonly affected segment of the small bowel in Crohn disease. The incidence decreases as one examines the alimentary tract proximally.

Fibrosis develops in eccentric areas of the bowel wall, creating pseudodiverticula. Strictures can also occur, resulting in variable degrees of obstruction (Fig. 3-20).

Two phases of small bowel disease are identified on the small bowel examination — the nonstenotic and stenotic. These do not necessarily correspond to the duration and severity of the disease process.

The nonstenotic phase consists of thickening and irregularity of the mucosal folds caused by the inflammatory process. Ulcerations are identified that form longitudinal and transverse fissures creating a cobblestone effect. Advanced disease may leave behind scattered islands of mucosa or "pseudopolyps" (Fig. 3-21). Scarring or fibrosis produces a rigid and featureless bowel, with a patchy, eccentric distribution being a constant feature throughout the acute and chronic phases.

The stenotic phase is characterized by strictures that cause areas of obstruction. (The string sign of high-grade ileal narrowing represents spasm, and not fibrosis as is commonly thought.)

Comparative studies of the enteroclysis technique and routine small bowel follow-through have shown the superiority of the former, particularly in demonstrating the earlier signs of disease. The earliest sign of edema, and the subsequent superficial ulcerations, are well demonstrated using the enteroclysis technique.

Preoperative regression of disease is rare. Crohn disease generally progresses locally with time. Following surgical resection, recurrence is common, frequently occurring within 2 years postsurgery (Fig. 3-22).

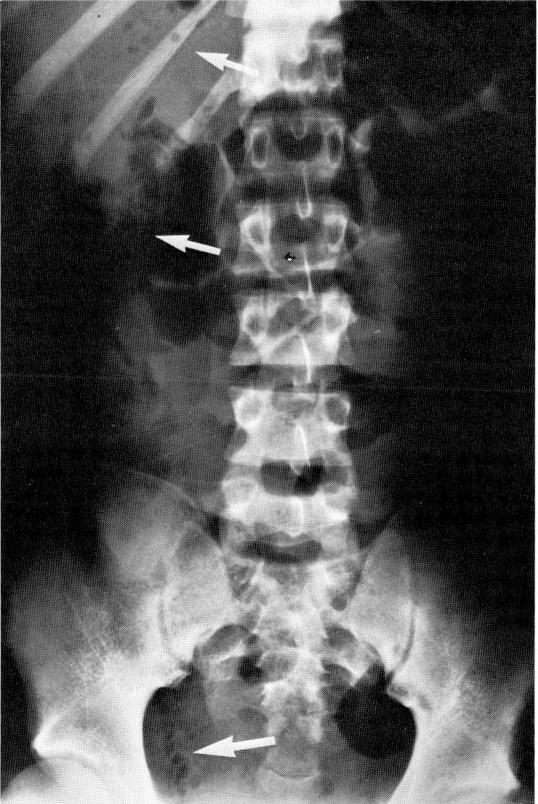
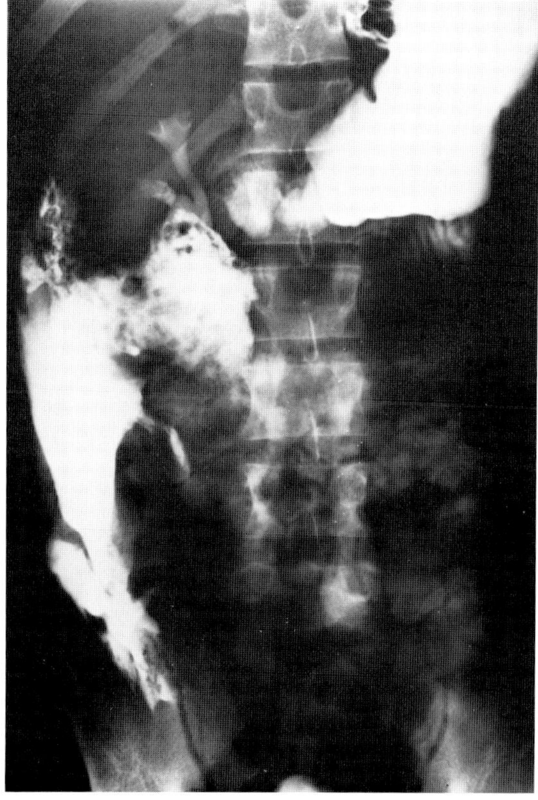

Fig. 3-16 **(A)** This 18-year-old, black male presented after blunt abdominal trauma with low-grade fever and abdominal pain. This KUB revealed extraluminal gas *(arrows)* in the right abdomen and pelvis, which, on a subsequent IVP, proved to be in the retroperitoneum. **(B)** A Gastrograffin upper gastrointestinal exam identified a duodenal tear, with extrusion of contrast into the right anterior pararenal space (note dye in the right renal collecting system from the recent IVP).

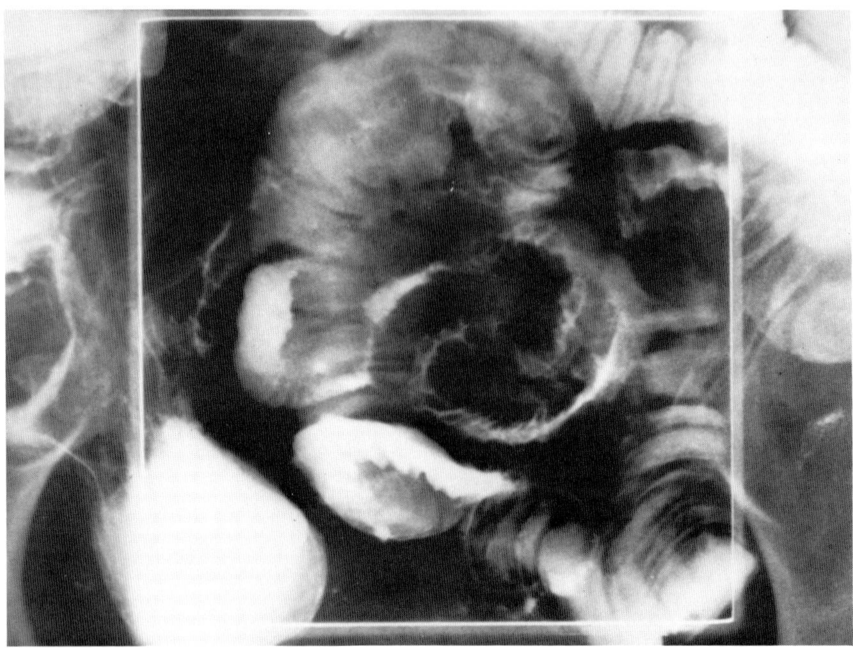

Fig. 3-17 Radiation enteritis. The ileum is narrowed, thickened, and fixed in an area that corresponds to the radiation port. Note the symmetry of the thickening, which helps to differentiate this entity from metastatic involvement, which is generally asymmetric in distribution.

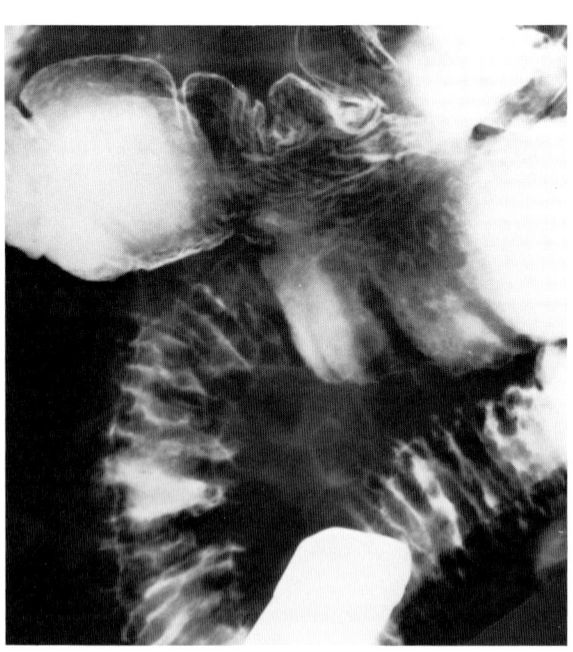

Fig. 3-18 Early Crohn disease. There is focal edema of the jejunum as the earliest sign of small bowel involvement. Ulcers develop subsequently.

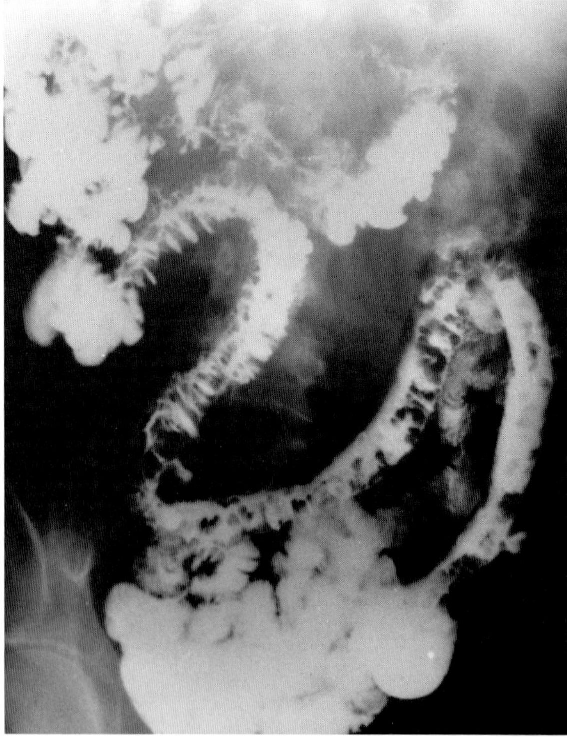

Fig. 3-19 Advanced Crohn disease. The ulcers are identified as deep longitudinal and transverse fissures throughout the ileum. The mucosa has a cobblestone appearance.

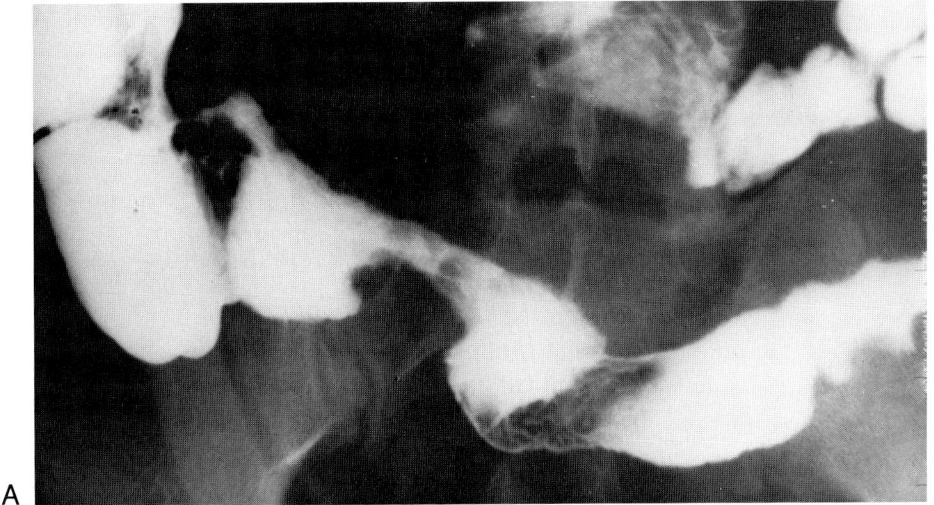

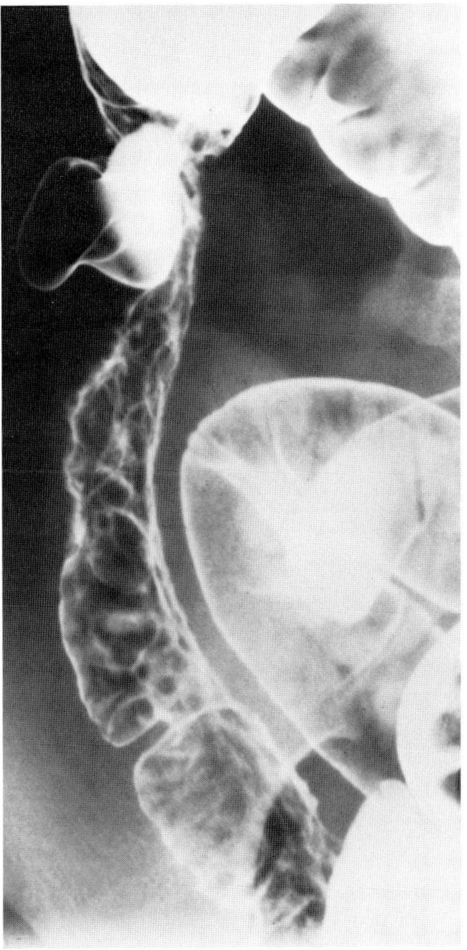

Fig. 3-20 **(A)** Pseudosacculation of the terminal ileum is secondary to asymmetric scarring. **(B)** The terminal ileum, on this peroral pneumocolon exam, reveals the changes of chronic Crohn disease. There is asymmetric scarring and complete loss of the normal fold pattern.

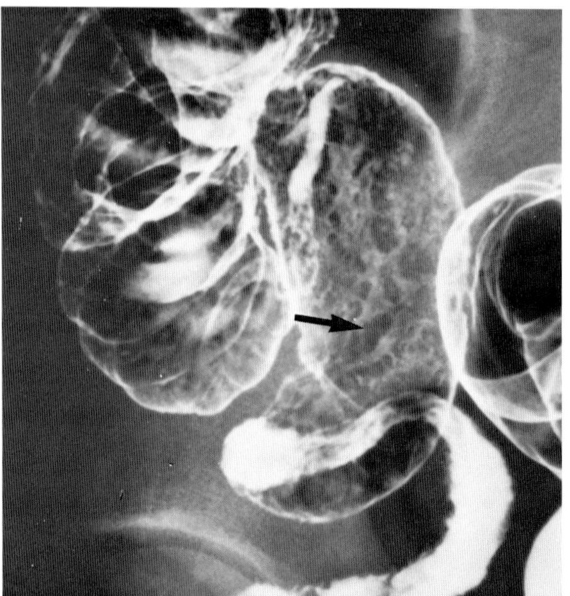

Fig. 3-21 Pseudopolyps *(arrow)* represent islands of normal mucosal tissue scattered between areas of denuded mucosa.

PARASITIC DISEASES OF THE SMALL BOWEL

Giardiasis

Giardia lamblia is a flagellated protozoan whose trophozoites attach to the mucosa of the small bowel, primarily the duodenum and proximal jejunum. It is a common commensal organism of the small bowel; however, on occasion, it can be associated with diarrheal malabsorptive illness. The disease can be acute in onset, or run a chronic course, depending on host-related factors such as nutritional status, age, and the presence of intestinal bacteria. Patients who develop clinical symptoms associated with the disease often have an underlying immunoglobulin deficiency. Giardiasis is also encountered in children and postgastrectomy patients.

Histologically, the mucosa becomes inflamed, with distortion of the villi and damage to the epithelium. The mechanism of the malabsorption that occurs is unknown and is not dependent on the severity of mucosal damage.

Radiographically, the duodenal and jejunal infestation reflects the changes of mucosal edema with distortion and thickening of the folds. There is invariably a marked degree of spasm and irritability present. Secretions may be increased but rarely sufficiently to dilute the barium column.

In patients with hypogammaglobulinemia, nodular lymphoid hyperplasia results in a fine nodular appearance of the fold pattern. At times, this may be the only abnormality detectable on the small bowel series (Fig. 3-23).

Patients respond to quinacrine (atropine) therapy.

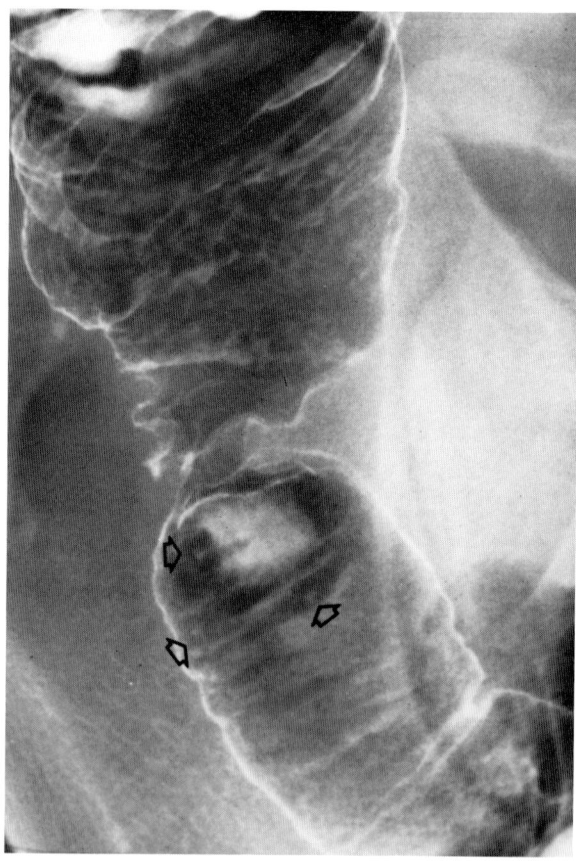

Fig. 3-22 Distal ileum recurrence of Crohn disease *(arrows)* just proximal to the ileocolic anastomois. These aphthous ulcers represent early superficial disease.

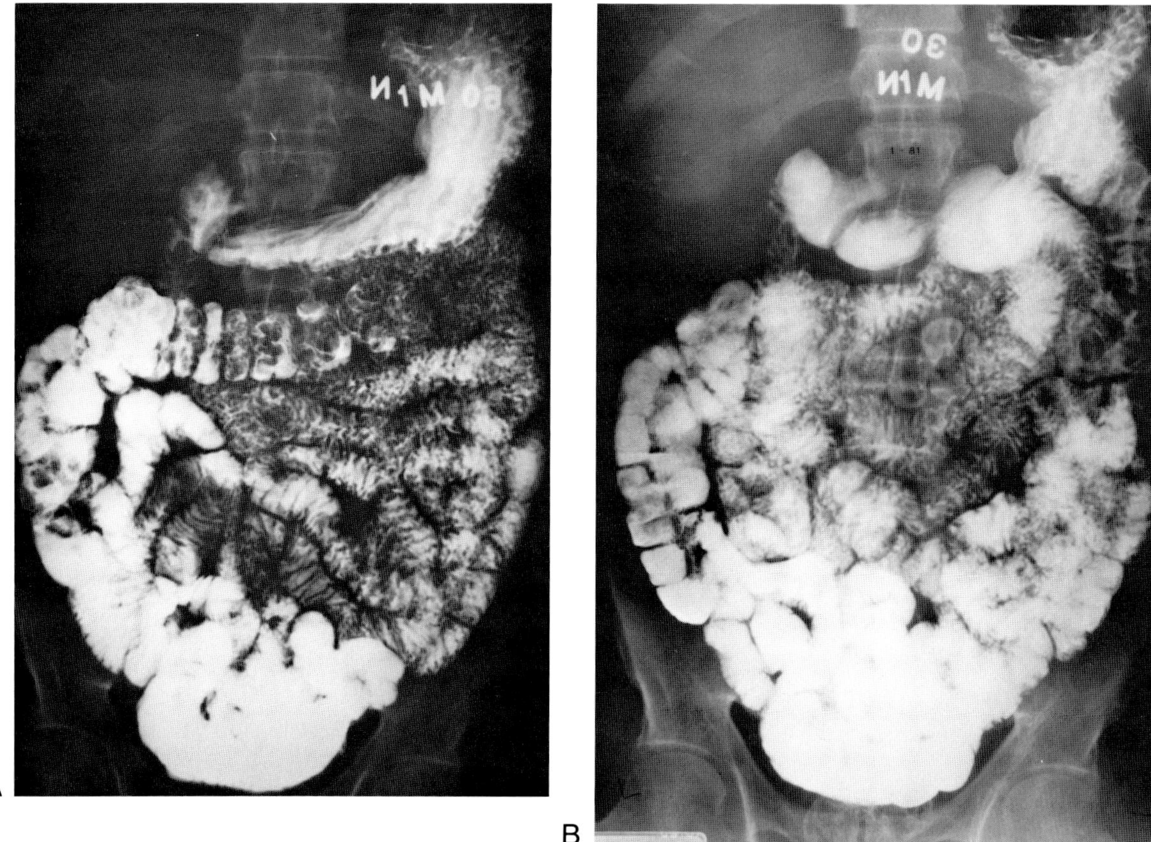

Fig. 3-23 (A) Giardiasis. A small bowel exam is 1977 revealed a diffuse nodularity throughout the distal duodenum and jejunum secondary to lymphoid hyperplasia in response to the infestation. The patient had an immunoglobulin deficiency. **(B)** Follow-up small bowel exam, in 1980, after quinacrine therapy reveals no evidence of disease.

Hookworms

Common hookworms that may infest the small bowel include *Necator americanus, Acylostoma brazilenzi,* and *A. duodenale.* They produce a chronic infestation with clinical symptoms of pain, abdominal tenderness, and diarrhea. Hookworms have a life span of several years and reside within the proximal small bowel. Fertilization occurs within the bowel. Ova are passed into the feces, hatching in the soil. Larvi are then absorbed by the skin, entering the bloodstream and reaching the lungs, where they are coughed up and swallowed, once again entering the intestinal tract. The worms attach to the mucosa, and their buccal capsules elicit severe mucosal edema.

Radiographic changes are similar to those seen in giardiasis, with thickening and irregularity of the fold pattern, along with irritability, producing fragmentation of the barium column. The administration of tetrachlorethylene is the treatment of choice.

Tapeworms

Taenia species are known to infest the distal small bowel. Symptoms are rather nonspecific and chronic in nature. On occasion, the adult tapeworm may be visualized as a long filling defect in the barium column. It does not have an intestinal tract, and ingested barium is not visualized, as it is within the roundworm.

Ascariasis

Ascaris lumbricoides is a large, intestinal roundworm. Because of its propensity to amass in large numbers, symptoms of intestinal obstruction are not uncommon. The parasite can be detected radiographically as a coiled filling defect in the barium, and its fine, linear intestinal tract can be visualized as it ingests the contrast agent (Fig. 3-24).

INFECTIOUS ENTERITIS

Yersinia Enterocolitica

This gram-negative bacterium is found throughout the Western Hemisphere and induces intestinal and nodal infections in children and young adults. The terminal ileum appears to be the most commonly involved site, although the entire small bowel and colon can be involved in severe cases. Clinical symptoms may mimic acute appendicitis, although the appendix itself is rarely involved pathologically. Early in its course, there is irregular thickening of the mucosal folds, aphthous ulceration, and eventual cobblestone appearance of the small bowel mucosa. At this stage,

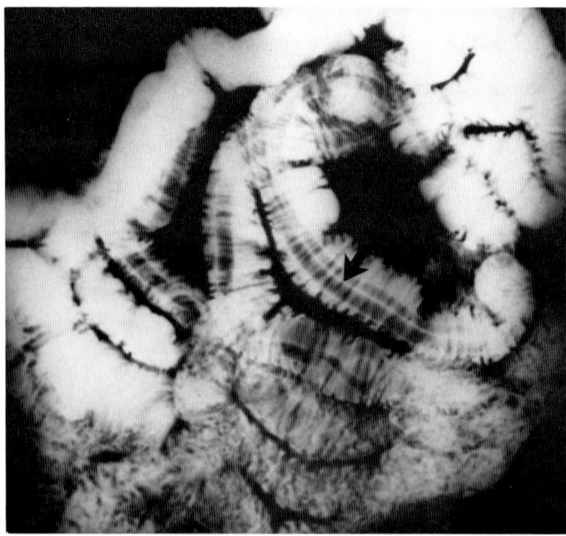

Fig. 3-24 Ascariasis. The roundworm is readily identified in the jejunum. Its linear intestinal tract is filled with barium *(arrow)*.

the radiographic changes are identical to those of Crohn disease. The bowel can also focally dilate during the acute edematous stage. Within weeks, the infection usually subsides on antibiotic therapy, with gradual resolution of the inflammatory changes.

Tuberculosis

Tuberculosis is still the most common cause of inflammatory bowel disease in underdeveloped, nonindustrialized countries. The ileum and proximal colon are the most common intestinal sites of infection and may be the only areas of involvement in some patients. Less than 50 percent of patients with intestinal involvement have lung disease. Infection occurs after infected milk or sputum is swallowed or by hematogenous and lymphatic spread from the lungs.

Patients present with abdominal pain, weight loss, and diarrhea. In advanced cases, symptoms of obstruction or perforation may occur.

The intestinal lesions are initially obstructive, with eventual stricture formation. It is difficult, if not impossible, to distinguish tuberculosis from Crohn disease radiographically in any phase of the disease process, although some authors have noted that the ulcers in tuberculous ileocolitis are annular, as opposed to longitudinal as in Crohn disease (Fig. 3-25). Therapy is the same as that for the pulmonary disease.

Histoplasmosis

The fungus *Histoplasma capsulatum* can be a systemic agent that can affect the small bowel as well as the lungs. Symptoms include diarrhea, vomiting, and abdominal pain. Malabsorption may also be present to some degree.

Radiographically, there is a diffuse, fine, nodular thickening of the small bowel folds.

Typhoid Fever

The bacterium *Salmonella typhosa* can produce severe and acute gastrointestinal symptoms of bloody diarrhea and abdominal pain. The agent is transmitted by eating contaminated food or drink.

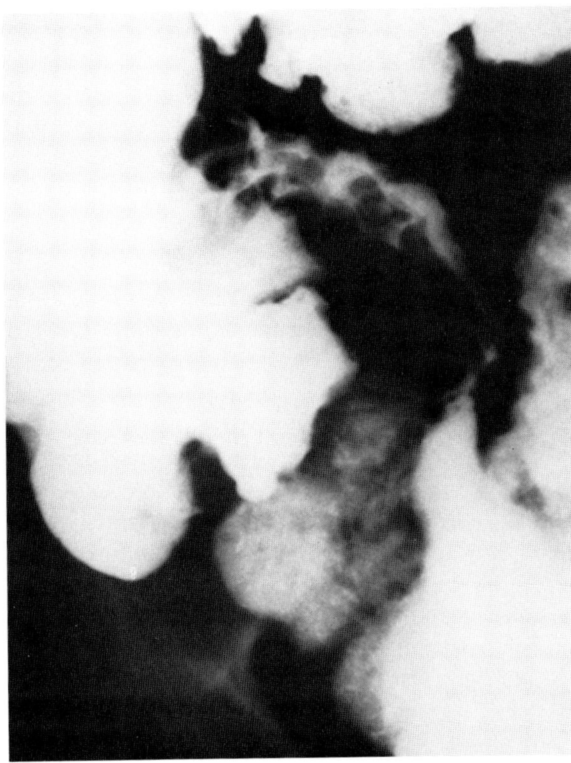

Fig. 3-25 Tuberculous ileitis. The inflammatory changes in the terminal ileum are nonspecific but identical to those seen in other infectious processes and Crohn disease.

Radiographically, there is mucosal edema with narrowing of the distal small bowel. The folds of this region are markedly thickened and ulcerations are commonly present. *Salmonella typhosa* infection is indistinguishable from Crohn disease, *Yersina,* and tuberculous enteritis.

Cytomegalovirus

This virus can be seen infecting several areas of the gastrointestinal tract. Its involvement is identified almost solely in patients with acquired immunodeficiency syndrome (AIDS). As AIDS is encountered more frequently, the incidence of this unusual infection increases.

Early in its course, it produces thickening of the folds with irritability and increased secretions. As it progresses, it can lead to ulceration and perforation.

Cryptosporidiosis

This unusual parasitic infection of the bowel is seen only in patients with AIDS. Nonspecific focal or diffuse inflammatory changes can be seen throughout the entire small bowel with thickening of the folds and intermittent irritability (Fig. 3-26). Patients present with choleralike diarrhea.

Herpes and *Candida albicans*

Patients who are immunosuppressed, most commonly those with lymphoma and leukemia, may be diffusely infected with Herpes or Candida. Case reports of ileocolitis resembling early Crohn disease describe aphthous ulcerations and mild edematous changes.

NEOPLASMS OF THE SMALL BOWEL

Primary neoplasms of the small bowel are uncommon. Malignant tumors are even rarer, comprising less than 1 percent of all malignant intestinal neoplasms. The reason for this low neoplastic rate is un-

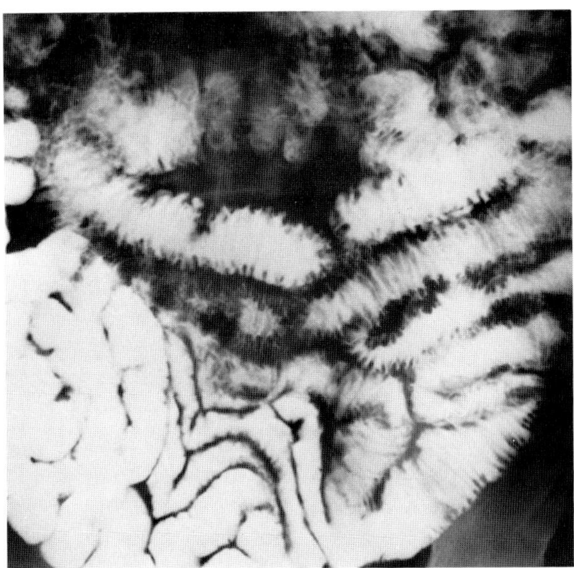

Fig. 3-26 Cryptosporidiosis. This AIDS patient presented with severe watery diarrhea. The jejunum revealed edematous changes.

certain, but several explanations have been postulated. These include the rapid transit of contents through the small bowel, the sterility and neutral composition of small bowel contents, as well as the extensive immune system present in the small bowel.

The diagnosis of these tumors is often difficult as symptoms can be rather vague. Symptoms include abdominal pain, often poorly localized; gastrointestinal blood loss, nausea; vomiting; and diarrhea. With the advent of enteroclysis techniques, the potential for the early diagnosis of these lesions exists.

Benign Tumors of the Small Bowel

Benign tumors of the small bowel are much more common than their malignant counterparts. They are often asymptomatic and are generally discovered incidentally at autopsy, or at surgery. Obstruction and hemorrhage are the more common symptoms observed. Obstruction results from intussusception of the neoplasm, which serves as a leading point in the bowel lumen. Bleeding from these tumors is often associated with superficial ulceration. Ulcerations result from mechanical injury, intussusception, or focal ischemia. Blood loss from benign tumors can occasionally be massive.

In some series, adenomas are the most common tumors, whereas in others, leiomyomas predominate. Other benign tumors, in decreasing order, are the lipoma, fibroma, neurogenic tumor, and hemangioma. These neoplasms have many features in common. They can be singular or multiple, sessile or pedunculated, and can ulcerate. Distinguishing characteristics do, however, exist. Consequently, these neoplasms are described separately.

ADENOMA

Adenomas are one of the most common small bowel tumors. They occur in the duodenum and proximal jejunum (Fig. 3-27). Since they are mucosal tumors, they grow into the lumen of the bowel and, when pedunculated, are likely to intussuscept and produce symptoms of obstruction. Being extremely vascular, they bleed readily. Ulcerations are superficial, however. It is uncertain whether adenomas of the small bowel degenerate into carcinomas. Although the po-

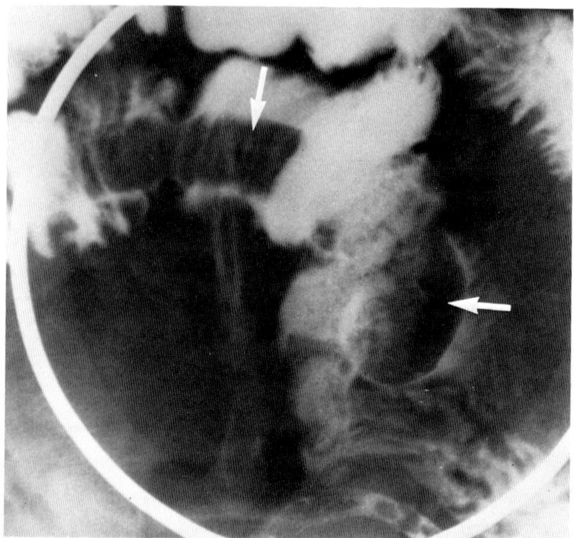

Fig. 3-27 A pedunculated adenoma is identified as a smooth filling defect in the jejunum *(arrows)*.

tential does exist, this occurrence is felt to be rare. Villous adenomas of the small bowel are described as well. They are characteristically lobulated, irregular, and larger than simple adenomas. They are more fre-

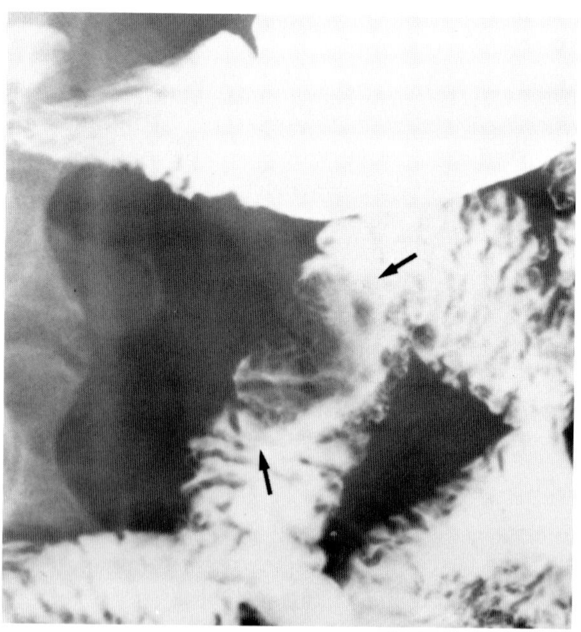

Fig. 3-28 This jejunal villous adenoma *(arrows)* has all the features of its colonic counterpart.

quently found in the duodenum, and the possibility of malignant degeneration of these lesions also exists. In many ways, their radiographic and clinical features are similar to colonic villous adenomas (Fig. 3-28).

LEIOMYOMAS

These smooth muscle tumors of the small bowel originate in the submucosa and appear as smooth, oval, filling defects. They may even have a dumbbell type of growth pattern, with both intra- and extraluminal components. When intraluminal, they mimic adenomas and lipomas and can frequently intussuscept. As they enlarge, they can compress the bowel contour.

The distribution of these lesions is even throughout the small bowel, although the jejunum is slightly favored. These tumors are quite vascular and will often undergo central necrosis, resulting in marked gastrointestinal hemorrhage. They can often be diagnosed, at angiography, by a swirl-like pattern of blood vessels. It is difficult to distinguish leiomyomas from leiomyosarcomas, both radiographically and histologically. Size is often a determining feature, although this is inprecise. Both tumors will have similar clinical and radiographic features.

LIPOMAS

Although fatty tumors of the small bowel arise from the submucosa, they are often found as intraluminal lesions. They are soft tumors, and their growth is in the direction of least resistance; i.e., toward the lumen of the bowel. Radiographically, they appear as smooth, intraluminal filling defects. They are often compressible. Lipomas are occasionally pedunculated and frequently intussuscept. They ulcerate noticeably on radiographic examination. Lipomas are found anywhere within the small bowel, but are most frequently identified within the ileum.

HEMANGIOMAS

Vascular tumors of the small bowel are rare. There are several types of hemangiomas: (1) capillary (composed of capillary plexuses), (2) cavernous (blood-filled endothelial-lined spaces), or (3) a mixture of the two. The small bowel is the most common location for intestinal hemangiomas, being more frequent than in other regions of the gastrointestinal tract. Typically, they are found in the jejunum. Hemangiomas can be multiple. There is an associated increased incidence of these tumors in patients with Turner syndrome (amenorrhea, coarctation of the aorta, and neck webbing), Osler-Weber-Rendu (hereditary hemorrhagic telangectasia), tuberous sclerosis, and blue rubber bleb–nevus syndrome.

Radiographically, they are often not distinguishable from other benign tumors, although phleboliths have been identified within them. These lesions are best identified at angiography.

NEUROGENIC TUMORS

Neurogenic tumors (neurofibromas, ganglioneuromas) of the small bowel are uncommon. They arise from neurogenic tissue in the bowel wall and are, thus, submucosal in origin. When multiple, they are often associated with generalized neurofibromatosis (von Recklinghausen disease). The majority of isolated neurofibromas are found in the ileum. Clinically, they present with bleeding and intussusception.

Radiographically, they are indistinguishable from other benign mesenchymal tumors.

MISCELLANEOUS BENIGN TUMORS

Lymphangiomas

These rare lesions are frequently multiple and present as intraluminal or intramural filling defects. They are identical in appearance to other benign submucosal tumors.

Hyperplasia (Brunner's Gland Adenoma)

Hyperplasia of a Brunner's gland occurs in the duodenum, presenting as a single, smooth, frequently large, intraluminal filling defect. It can be sessile or it can elongate, protruding into the lumen of the duodenal sweep.

Heterotopic Pancreatic Tissue

Ectopic pancreatic tissue, although most commonly found in the antrum of the stomach, can be found along the duodenal sweep. The appearance is identical to a gastric lesion with a smooth outline and central dimple (representing a pancreatic duct remnant).

Polyposis Syndromes Involving the Small Bowel

PEUTZ-JEGHERS SYNDROME

This inherited autosomal dominant syndrome is associated with pigmented lesions of the skin and buccal membranes. The polyps are histologically hamartomatous, containing all of the cellular features of the small intestinal mucosa. The polyps are predominantly found in the small bowel, being most common in the jejunum (Fig. 3-29). A small percentage of patients will also have polyps in the stomach and colon as well. The size of the polyps can vary considerably, with many being small and beyond the scope of routine radiographic detection. As with many of the polyposis syndromes, the appearance of these le-

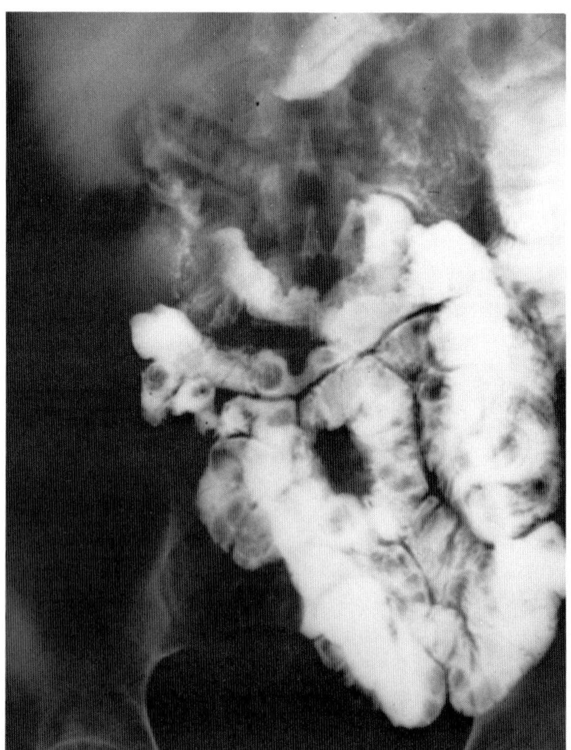

Fig. 3-29 Peutz-Jeghers. The small bowel is filled with numerous hamartomatous polyps.

sions begins in early adulthood. For the most part, the patients may remain asymptomatic. Symptoms of obstruction do occur and are secondary to intussusception. Intermittent bleeding has also been reported.

There is convincing evidence that a small percentage (3 to 5 percent) of these patients will develop malignancies within the duodenum. Additional evidence exists regarding malignant degeneration of the more distal small bowel and colonic polyps. There are also associated polyps of the ovary, and the nasal and bronchial passages.

CANADA-CRONKHITE SYNDROME

This syndrome is associated with polyps of the gastrointestinal tract, malabsorption with loss of protein and ectodermal changes of alopecia, skin discoloration, and dystrophic nail changes. Histologically, the polyps are inflammatory and usually develop in the fifth and sixth decades. The colon and stomach are predominantly involved, but a large number will also have small bowel polyps. There is no apparent genetic transmission. Symptoms include abdominal pain and diarrhea. The clinical course is poor, owing to the malabsorption.

OTHER POLYPOSIS SYNDROMES

Many of the other hereditary polyposis syndromes have been associated with polyps of the small bowel. Both familial polyposis coli and Gardner syndrome, transmitted in an autosomal dominant fashion, can present with adenomatous polyps of the small bowel.

Juvenile polyposis can also infrequently involve the small bowel with hamartomatous polyps.

Carcinoid Tumors

Carcinoid tumors arise from enterochromaffin (argentaffin) cells and are descendants of the APUD cell system. They can be found in any area of the gastrointestinal tract as well as the bronchial tree. A large percentage of these tumors (20 to 35 percent) do occur in the small bowel and as such constitute the largest group of tumors of the small bowel, occurring primarily in the ileum. It should be noted that the appendix is the most common location for carcinoid

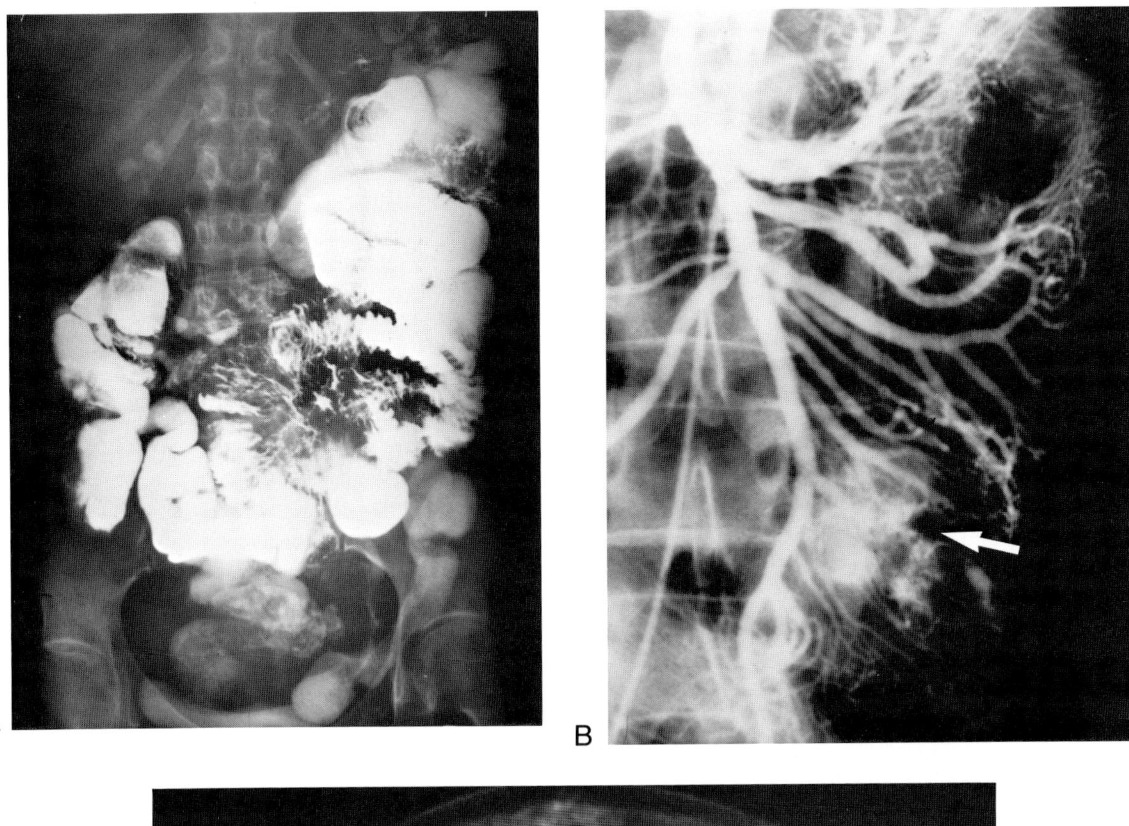

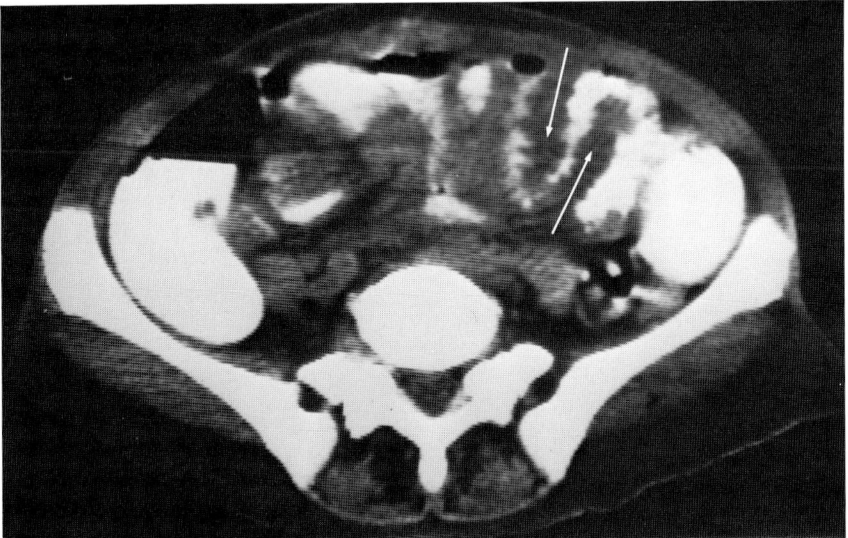

Fig. 3-30 **(A)** Carcinoid. There is an intense desmoplastic response in the proximal ileum, with acute angulation of the thickened small bowel radiating toward the tumor. The carcinoid itself was not apparent on this examination. **(B)** An intense blush of the tumor is present at angiography *(arrow)*. **(C)** CT scan revealed localized thickening of the ileal loops *(arrows)*.

tumors. They are virtually unknown in the esophagus. The carcinoid tumor can be found in almost any age group, although it is usually diagnosed in the adult population. Carcinoid tumors are capable of secreting a wide variety of peptides and hormones, including serotonin, kallikrein, and histamine. These hormones are responsible for producing the well-known clinical "carcinoid syndrome."

The classic carcinoid syndrome is characterized by intermittent stress- or pressure-induced flushing of the face and neck, occasionally with associated cyanosis and wheezing. The exact cause of the flushing is uncertain. It was once thought to be caused by the release of serotonin, but recent evidence suggests that kallikrein converted to bradykinin in the bloodstream is the more likely etiology. Wheezing and bronchospasm are also related to serotonin release. The syndrome also includes attacks of watery diarrhea and abdominal cramps, results of the effect of serotonin on the intestinal smooth muscle. Liver metastases are invariably present in patients with carcinoid syndrome, when the tumor originates in the small bowel. In the normal liver, serotonin is inactivated by monoaminoxidase, and thus, is not released into the general circulation. In the presence of liver metastasis, inactivation may not occur.

Since serotonin and bradykinin are in high concentrations in the circulation, they can effect endocardial inflammation and subendocardial fibrosis, leading to tricuspid insufficiency and pulmonary valvular stenosis. The left side of the heart is spared, presumably by the deactivation of serotonin by monoaminoxidase in the lungs.

The classic laboratory finding is excess 5-hydroxy-indoacetic acid (5-HIAA) in the urine. Serotonin is converted, by monoaminoxidase, to 5-HIAA which, in turn, is excreted in the urine. Elevated urine levels of 5-HIAA reflect the amount of serotonin produced in the body.

As with other small bowel tumors, carcinoid may also present clinically with occult gastrointestinal blood loss or intussusception.

As a general rule, the degree of malignant degeneration varies with the site of the tumor. Those in the appendix or stomach rarely metastasize, whereas those arising in the small bowel have the highest incidence of metastasis. By the time of initial diagnosis, 33 to 50 percent of patients will have metastatic involvement.

This primary mucosal tumor grows into the wall of the small bowel, and is, therefore, indistinguishable radiographically from other submucosal lesions. It can occur singly or in multiples and can be widely scattered throughout the small bowel.

The strong desmoplastic reaction produced by serotonin release causes kinking and angulation of the adjacent small bowel loops, often in a spoke-wheel pattern (Fig. 3-30). The tumor itself may not be identifiable. Fibrosis can occur either focally or throughout, creating intermittent areas of obstruction. Mucosal ulceration is uncommon.

The tumor spreads slowly, by infiltration, through the bowel wall to the mesentery and adjacent lymph nodes. Distant spread occurs by lymphatic and vascular channels.

Carcinoids are intensely vascular at angiography. Small bowel ischemia has been reported secondary to vascular compromise by the intense desmoplasia and resultant fibrosis.

Recommended therapy is wide resection of the involved small bowel segment. The prognosis is generally favorable.

PRIMARY MALIGNANT NEOPLASMS OF THE SMALL BOWEL

Malignant neoplasms, primarily involving the small bowel, are quite rare and account for less than 1 percent of all malignant tumors of the gastrointestinal tract. There are two important primary neoplasms to consider — adenocarcinoma and lymphoma. Each has a slightly different distribution, and the radiographic characteristics also serve as differentiating points.

Adenocarcinoma

Adenocarcinomas of the small bowel are rare. They generally occur in the duodenum and proximal jejunum. There is a diminishing incidence of this neo-

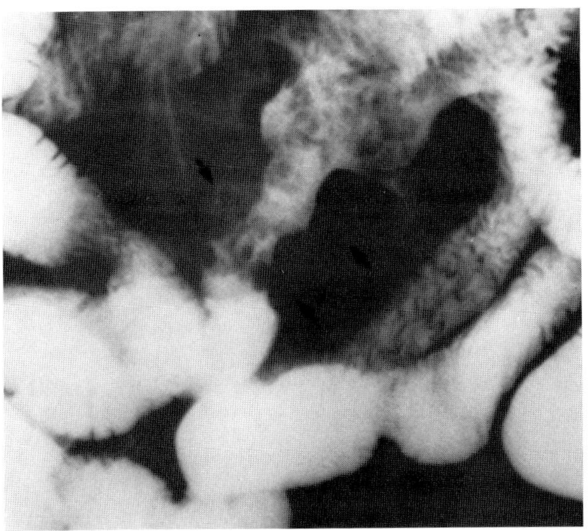

Fig. 3-31 Primary adenocarcinoma of the jejunum. The arrows point to an annular, ulcerating mass.

plasm beyond the ligament of Treitz. This is in contrast to lymphoma and carcinoid tumors, which are more common in the ileum. Adenocarcinomas are usually found in patients over the age of 50 and are more common in males. There is a known increased incidence of these tumors with sprue, as well as with regional enteritis.

Most lesions are symptomatic at the time of discovery, usually the result of localized pain secondary to obstruction, or to hemorrhage. Carcinomas present in the duodenum can obstruct the common bile duct or cause gastric outlet obstruction.

Radiographically, adenocarcinomas are indistinguishable from metastases. In fact, the pathologist can often not distinguish a primary adenocarcinoma from metastatic adenocarcinoma from a distant site. Most often, these lesions are annular, producing a short, segmental stricture often with ulceration (Fig. 3-31). They may, at times, have a scirrhous appearance with infiltration of a longer segment of bowel. Occasionally, they can be polypoid.

Lymphoma

Malignant lymphoma is one of the most common malignant neoplasms encountered in the small bowel, the other being metastatic disease. Lymphoma may be primary, or it may represent a manifestation of diffuse systemic involvement. Intestinal lymphoma is invariably of a non-Hodgkin type, often histiocytic. Hodgkin disease, involving the small bowel, is very rare. Involvement can be seen in any age group although, typically, it is seen in adults. A primary neoplasm of the small bowel in the younger patient is statistically more likely to be lymphoma than carcinoma. As with carcinoma, lymphoma is also reported to occur with increased frequency in patients with sprue.

Lymphoma can mimic a wide variety of small bowel pathology, particularly in its diffuse or nodular forms. Inflammatory processes such as Crohn disease commonly mimic lymphoma. Ischemia or hemorrhage can produce similar patterns as well. Metastases can also be indistinguishable from lymphoma. Radiographically, several manifestations of lymphoma have been catagorized.

MULTIPLE NODULES

Multiple intramural nodules of varying size involve large segments of the small bowel. These nodules are generally found in the ileum and frequently ulcerate. They can be distinguished from lymphoid hyperplasia by their larger size and asymmetric distribution (Fig. 3-32).

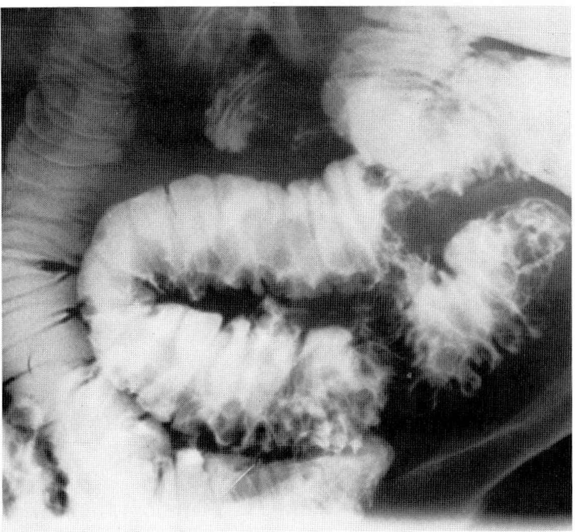

Fig. 3-32 Nodular form of lymphoma. Multiple polypoid filling defects are scattered throughout the small bowel.

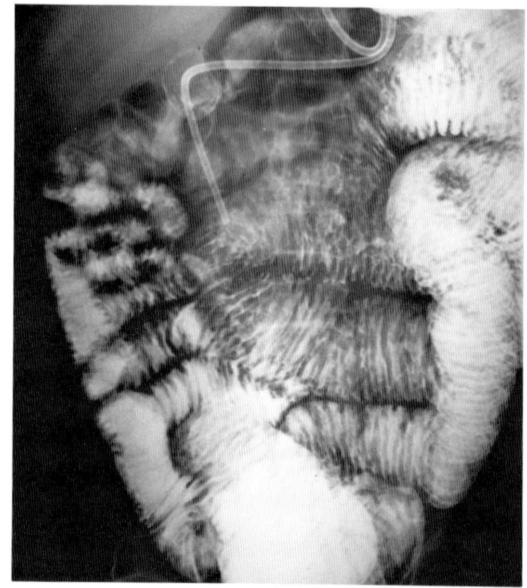

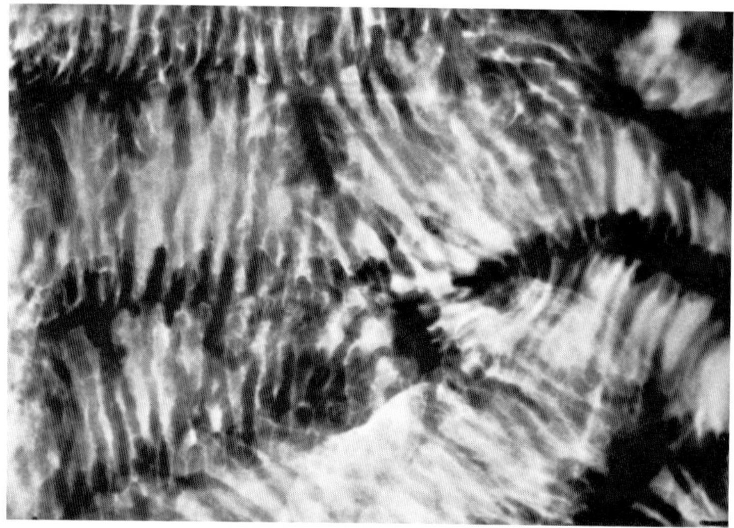

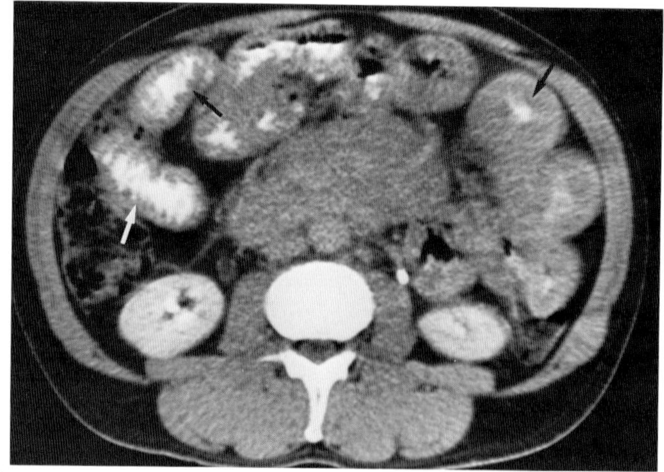

Fig. 3-33 (A) Infiltrating form of lymphoma. Enteroclysis exam reveals diffuse nodular thickening throughout the entire small bowel. **(B)** Coned-down view. **(C)** CT scan confirmed the thickened small bowel wall *(arrows)*.

INFILTRATING FORM

The small bowel becomes diffusely thickened with effacement of the normal fold pattern and separation of the bowel loops (Fig. 3-33). In advanced cases, the bowel lumen can be narrowed by submucosal tumor, or it may become dilated and "aneurysmal." This latter appearance occurs when the entire wall is replaced by tumor, with pooling of barium within the atonic segment. This radiographic appearance is virtually pathognomonic of small bowel lymphoma.

POLYPOID FORM

Occasionally, lymphoma can appear as a large intraluminal filling defect, sometimes expanding the lumen of the bowel. This form often presents clinically with intussusception.

ENDO-EXOENTERIC FORM

Massive lymphomatous infiltration of the bowel can produce complete destruction of the bowel wall with a resultant large mass. Fistulas to other portions of the

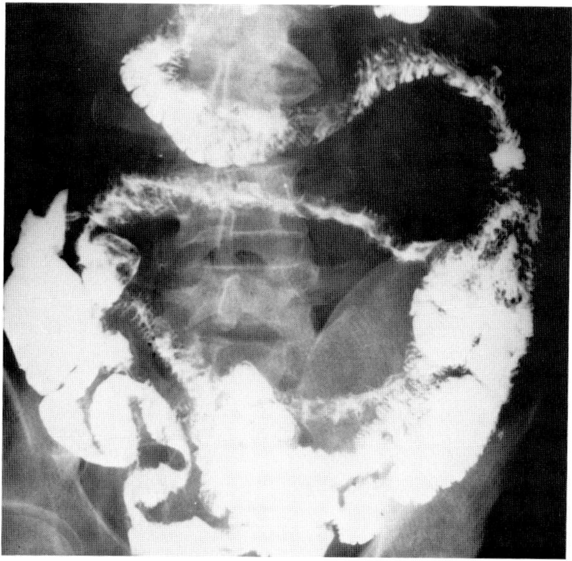

Fig. 3-35 Invasive mesenteric form of lymphoma. The small bowel is displaced by huge mesenteric lymphomatous masses.

bowel may also be present. The appearance of a large, ulcerating mass of the small bowel is commonly seen not only in lymphoma but also in metastatic disease (particularly melanoma) (Fig. 3-34).

INVASIVE MESENTERIC FORM

The tumor becomes massive and grows in an extraluminal fashion, displacing bowel loops and other abdominal structures. The bowel is displaced but not fixed, as it would be in metastatic disease. Obstruction does not commonly occur (Fig. 3-35).

Sarcoma

Other primary small bowel malignancies are the sarcomatous counterparts of the previously mentioned mesenchymal tumors. The most common form is the leiomyosarcoma. Fibrosarcomas and neurofibrosarcomas have also been reported. They are often indistinguishable from their benign counterparts. Leiomyosarcomas have large extraluminal components with minimal intraluminal extension. These tumors are usually vascular and can be diagnosed at angiography. It should be noted that, as a group, sarcomas are extremely rare.

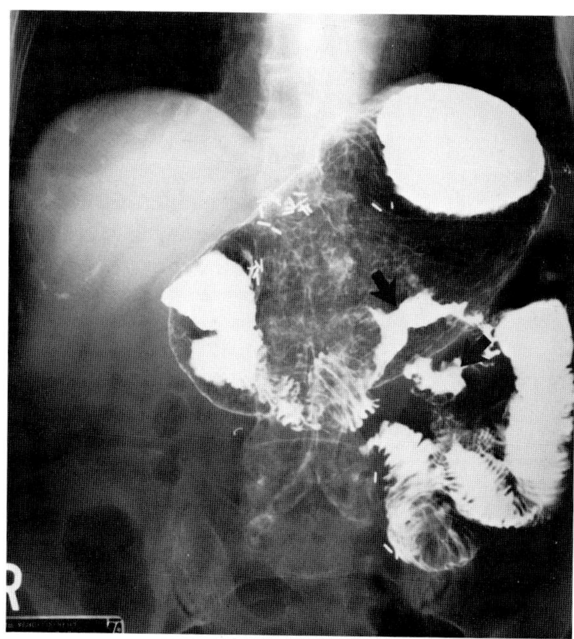

Fig. 3-34 Endo-exoenteric form of lymphoma. Two adjacent ulcerating masses are present on either side of the ligament of Treitz *(arrows)*.

Metastatic Disease to the Small Bowel

Secondary tumors to the small bowel are common and, along with lymphoma, represent the most common neoplasms encountered in the small bowel. Commonly, metastatic lesions are multiple, although radiography may only detect a small number of the lesions present.

There are several radiographic patterns of metastatic disease to the small bowel. Metastases can present as intramural nodules. These may ulcerate and produce a "bull's-eye" or "target" lesion (Fig. 3-36). This is commonly seen in melanoma as well as metastases from the breast and kidney, spindle-cell tumors, and Kaposi sarcoma. They may also appear as masses primarily involving the mesentery with mural involvement of the adjacent small bowel. Another presentation is a combination of both intramural and

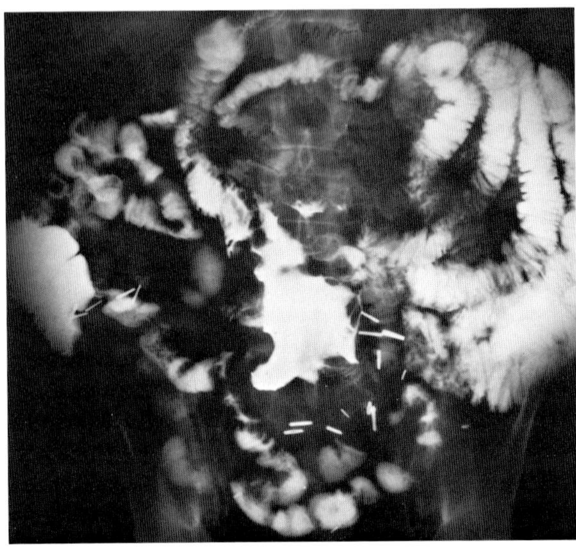

Fig. 3-37 Metastatic melanoma. A large ulcerating mass is displacing adjacent loops of small bowel. This lesion is identical to lymphoma, primary adenocarcinoma, and other metastases.

intraperitoneal masses. Metastases can mimic certain other processes, such as lymphoma of inflammatory bowel diseases. Usually in the clinical context, the diagnosis can be made. A number of primary tumors are known to metastasize to the small bowel via a *hematogenous route.* These are invariably extraabdominal tumors. The most common primary tumor to do this is melanoma followed by lung in males and breast in females (Fig. 3-37). With the increasing incidence of AIDS, it is likely that more cases of metastatic Kaposi sarcoma will also be encountered.

When metastases occurs via a hematogenous route, they often arise from the antimesenteric side of the bowel.

Metastatic melanoma has a propensity to invade the lumen, often producing massive ulceration of the tumor mass.

Primary tumors that arise in the abdomen can secondarily involve the small bowel by either intraperitoneal seeding, direct invasion, or lymphatic extension. Of these, *intraperitoneal seeding* is the most common.

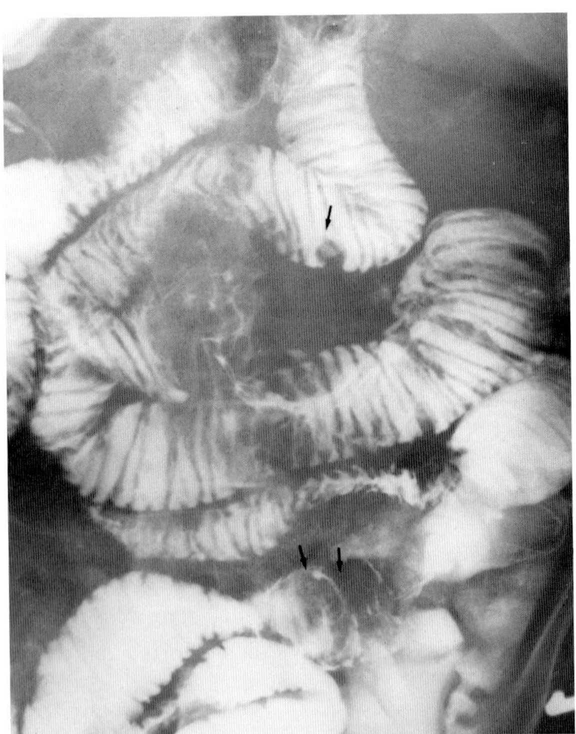

Fig. 3-36 Metastatic breast carcinoma to the small bowel *(arrows)* presents as bull's-eye lesions (seen best in the proximal jejunum).

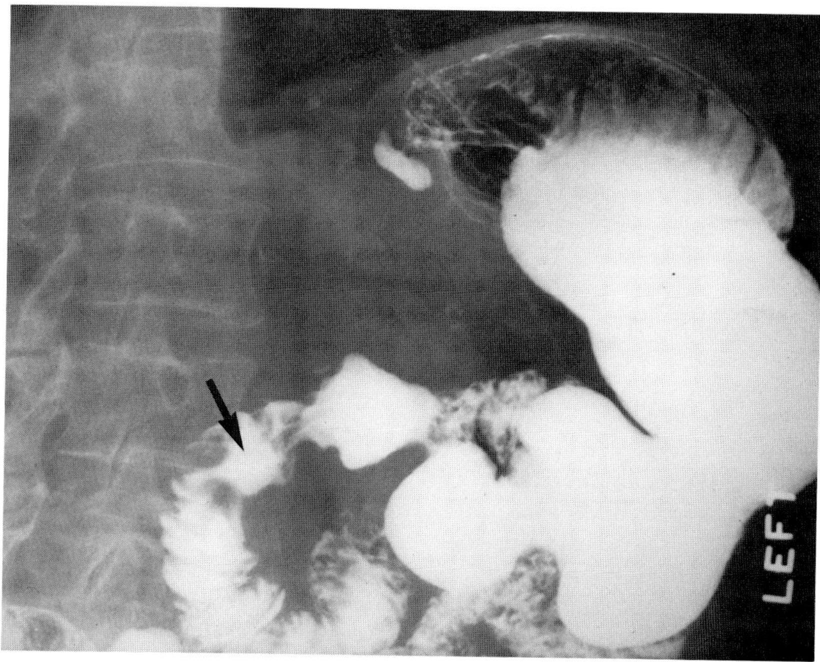

Fig. 3-38 Carcinoma of the pancreas with direct extension into the adjacent duodenum. The arrow reveals an ulcer, representing transmural invasion of the carcinoma.

Certain patterns of this form of metastatic spread do occur and are dependent, to some degree, on the type of primary tumor. Malignant cells will be transported in the ascitic fluid, which circulates throughout the abdomen. The cells will collect in certain areas of stasis and result in the growth of metastatic nodules. The most common site is within the pelvic cavity, particularly the pouch of Douglas. Small bowel metastases also develop along the recesses of the small bowel mesentery. The mesentery extends from the duodenojejunal junction obliquely to the ileocecal region. Tumor cells "cascade" toward the ileocecal region and produce metastatic deposits in the right lower quadrant. The most common tumors to produce intraperitoneal seeding are tumors of the genital tract in the female (usually ovarian) and gastrointestinal tumors in both sexes (particularly from the stomach, pancreas, and colon).

Tumors arising from the kidneys may involve the small bowel by *direct extension,* as can tumors arising from the pancreas (Fig. 3-38). Tumors of the stomach, liver, or colon are much less likely to do this.

DIVERTICULA OF THE SMALL BOWEL

One of the most commonly encountered structural abnormalities in the small bowel is the diverticulum. These rarely cause symptoms. A number of clinical problems are occasionally encountered with diverticula, and these will be briefly discussed.

Duodenal Diverticulum

These are true pulsion diverticula that usually arise from the medial wall of the duodenal sweep, most commonly in the second portion. They increase in frequency with age and have been reported in up to 20 percent of upper gastrointestinal examinations. These diverticula rarely give rise to symptoms, although bleeding and perforation have been reported. The ampulla of Vater can occasionally be obstructed by large diverticula, causing biliary and pancreatic symptomatology.

Intraluminal Duodenal Pseudodiverticulum

This entity is extremely rare and represents a congenital web or diaphragm. Bowel contents produce distension and ballooning of this web, resulting in a "windsock" appearance.

Jejunal Diverticulum

These pulsion diverticula usually occur along the mesenteric border of the small bowel. They are typically encountered in older patients. Jejunal diverticula are most common near the ligament of Treitz, and their incidence decreases distally. They do not usually produce symptoms but have been known to bleed, perforate, obstruct, and produce malabsorption. The malabsorption produced by characteristically large, small bowel diverticula is caused by stasis of small bowel contents, with resultant bacterial overgrowth. Bacteria in the upper small bowel are few and usually aerobic. However, in situations of stasis, as in small bowel diverticulosis, anaerobes proliferate. This bacterial overgrowth produces two problems: (1) resultant steatorrhea secondary to bacterial deconjugation of bile salts, as well as hydroxylation of fatty acids; and (2) the development of a megaloblastic anemia caused by bacterial competition for and absorption of vitamin B_{12}. Antibiotic therapy can often ameliorate the symptoms.

Ileal Diverticulum

Diverticula involving the terminal ileal region are occasionally encountered. Again, these are pulsion-type diverticula. Rarely, they have been known to perforate.

Meckel Diverticulum

The Meckel diverticulum is a remnant of the vitelline duct. It is a congenital lesion and not acquired, as are other small bowel diverticula. It is the most frequent congenital anomaly of small bowel, occurring in 1 to 3 percent of patients at autopsy. Meckel diverticula are located along the antimesenteric border of the ileum, usually within 50 to 100 cm of the terminal ileum. Most patients with Meckel diverticula are asymptomatic. The most frequently encountered symptom is bleeding, often seen in the pediatric age group. Approximately 20 percent of these diverticula will contain ectopic gastric mucosa, which produces ulceration. Technetium pertechnetate scans are extremely sensitive in detecting Meckel diverticula containing ectopic gastric mucosa. Meckel diverticula can also contain ectopic pancreatic or colonic tissue. Another common symptom of Meckel diverticula is inflammation. Clinically, this may be indistinguishable from appendicitis. Occasionally, these diverticula have been known to invaginate into the lumen and produce obstruction by intussusception.

Radiographically, Meckel diverticula are notoriously difficult to detect. However, with the use of small bowel enteroclysis, they can be identified with a greater accuracy rate.

POSITIONAL ABNORMALITIES OF THE SMALL BOWEL

Rotational Abnormalities

It is important to know the embryologic development of the digestive tract in order to appreciate the abnormalities that may be encountered in the positioning of the bowel. The intestines develop outside the fetal abdominal cavity, and as growth continues, they return within the abdomen. This is accomplished by a counterclockwise rotation of the intestines, with the superior mesenteric artery acting as a central axis point. There is a 270-degree turn of the bowel before it reaches its final position, with the jejunum located in the left upper quadrant and the cecum and terminal ileum in the right lower quadrant. There are a variety of abnormalities that can occur owing to failure of proper rotation.

Nonrotation

If the intestines fail to rotate as they return to the abdomen, the entire colon, including the cecum, is positioned on the left, whereas the jejunum and ileum are on the right (Fig. 3-39). Often, the ligament of Treitz is not present, and there may be some positional abnormality of the duodenum as well. The term "common mesentery" in this instance refers to the presence of a single large mesentery. Many times,

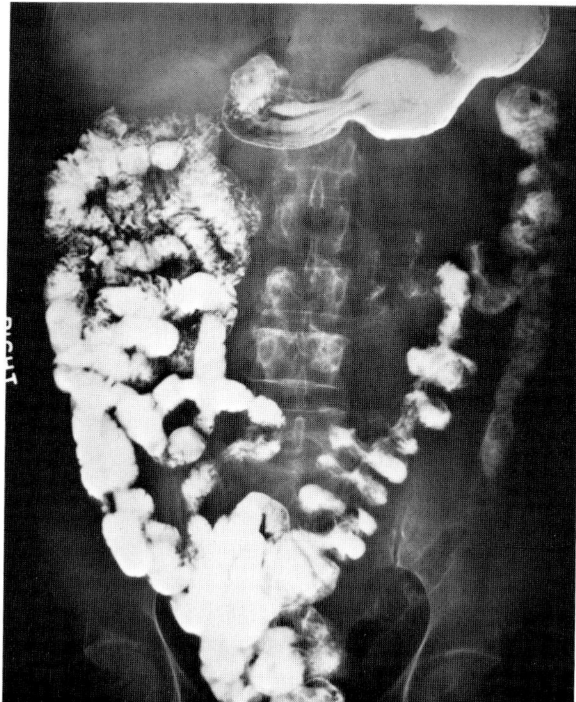

Fig. 3-39 Nonrotation of the bowel. Failure of intrauterine rotation of the intestines causes abnormal positioning of the small bowel in the right side of the abdomen and the left side of the colon.

this condition is asymptomatic and is incidentally discovered. The bowel is at increased risk of developing a midgut volvulus, which commonly occurs in infants. Also, there can be a variety of adhesive bands producing partial obstruction.

Malrotation

Virtually any arrest of rotation of the intestines can result in some degree of malrotation. Depending on the type and severity, they produce symptoms associated with subsequent obstruction volvulus. A common anomaly is a high-positioned cecum, with bands arising from it, crossing toward the liver (Ladd's bands) to produce obstruction of the duodenum.

Internal Hernias

Intraabdominal herniation occurs as the result of defects in the mesentery and peritoneal reflections.

These congenital anomalies incarcerate the small bowel and may, on rare occasion, compromise the vascular supply or cause obstruction. Internal hernias, which more commonly occur, include the following.

1. Paraduodenal hernias (left and right)
2. Small bowel mesentery
3. Sigmoid mesentery
4. Transverse colon mesentery
5. Foramen of Winslow
6. Paracecal hernia

Paraduodenal hernias are far and away the most common of the congenital internal hernias. These are the result of a defect in the parietal peritoneum at the ligament of Treitz. The defect can occur to the left or to the right of the duodenum as it emerges from the retroperitoneum. Left paraduodenal hernias are more common.

Radiographically, internal hernias are recognized as displaced loops of bowel that are tightly bunched together in a localized area of the abdomen. Proximal dilatation can be identified if obstruction is present. Right paraduodenal hernias displace the stomach and ascending colon leftward, the latter being due to an associated malrotation or common mesentery. Left paraduodenal hernias displace the stomach to the right, and the transverse colon inferiorly.

Herniation of the small bowel can also occur through surgical defects in the anterior abdominal wall (ventral hernias). Radiographically, these are best identified on lateral views of the abdomen.

Herniation of the bowel or mesentery through the diaphragm can occur either through the Bochdalek (posterolateral) or Morgagni (anterior) foramina, or as the result of a traumatic diaphragmatic tear. The Bochdalek foramen is the result of incomplete closure of the pleuroperitoneal membrane. In addition to bowel, portions of the spleen or left kidney may enter the chest. The foramen of Morgagni is an anterior muscular defect behind the sternum. Small bowel, omentum, colon, and portions of the left lobe of the liver may herniate into the chest.

Inguinal hernias are divided into direct and indirect types. Indirect hernias are more common. The indirect hernia represents a failure of fusion of the processus vaginalis peritonei after the testis has descended into the scrotum, thereby allowing abdominal contents to enter this peritoneal diverticulum. The direct inguinal hernia protrudes lateral to the border of the rectus muscle and inferomedial to the inferior epigastric vessels as the result of a weakness in the transversalis fascia in the floor of the inguinal canal. Uncommonly, direct hernias may dissect through fascial planes into the scrotum.

Femoral hernias descend through the femoral canal beneath the inguinal ligament. Because of their narrow necks, they are prone to incarceration and strangulation. These hernias occur more commonly in women and are less common than inguinal hernias in general.

The Spigelian hernia is a spontaneous ventral hernia through the linea semilunaris, a confluence of the sheaths of the lateral abdominal muscles and the lateral rectus muscle. Small bowel or sigmoid colon is identified, projecting laterally and anteriorly at the lower level of the iliac crest. Although, barium studies frequently identify the various hernias, CT can be particularly useful in the diagnosis of hernias.

PNEUMATOSIS INTESTINALIS

Air may occur in the wall of the bowel in association with a variety of pathologic entities. It may accumulate as multiple submucosal cysts (found more commonly in the colon, e.g., pneumatosis cystoides intestinalis) or as linear collections of gas.

In most patients with pneumatosis cystoides, there are few symptoms. Some patients have associated chronic obstructive pulmonary disease (COPD). In these patients, air from the ruptured alveoli dissects into the mediastinum, down into the retroperitoneum, and along the mesentery to the small bowel wall. Other patients may have associated ischemia or ulcerative bowel conditions. A significant number of patients have no identifiable underlying abnormality. The diagnosis is made on plain films, barium studies, or on CT.

Linear gas collections in the bowel wall generally indicate the presence of bowel infarction, especially when associated with acute abdominal symptomatology (Fig. 3-14). In infants, pneumatosis intestinalis is associated with necrotizing enterocolitis. Linear pneumatosis can also be seen in patients who have undergone jejunoileal bypass surgery for obesity. Patients with collagen vascular disease, especially scleroderma, can develop intramural gas for unknown reasons (Fig. 3-6). Steroids and various chemotherapeutic agents, nonobstructive ileus, and patients who have undergone endoscopy can also develop pneumatosis.

Radiographically, the intramural linear gas collections are generally slightly blacker than the intraluminal gas presumably because the intramural air is isolated from the intraluminal fluid contents. Portal venous gas is commonly associated with bowel infarction and can help in differentiating the causes of intestinal pneumatosis.

When the submucosal gas collections rupture through the serosa, releasing gas into the peritoneal cavity, free air can be identified on upright films of the abdomen. Because the intraluminal fluid contents are not extruded, peritonitis does not occur. This condition is, therefore, termed "benign pneumoperitoneum."

SMALL BOWEL IN THE PEDIATRIC PATIENT

There are a variety of conditions of the small bowel that are predominantly encountered in the pediatric patient, particularly in the neonate. Although this section will not attempt to cover all aspects of small bowel disease in the pediatric patient, several of the most commonly encountered conditions will be briefly discussed.

Atresia and Stenosis

The digestive tube in utero is not always a hollow structure. Early in its development, the tube is a solid core of cells, and a lumen gradually develops late in the first trimester of pregnancy. Modern theory favors that atresias and stenoses develop from focal, vascular compromise of the developing gut, probably due to some form of intrauterine stress. The most common location for atresia is the distal ileum, occurring in 60 percent of cases, whereas 40 percent occur in the distal duodenum or proximal jejunum.

There are three forms of atresia: imperforate diaphragm, fibrous strand, and multiple blind ends of bowel separated by complete gaps. Bowel loops proximal to or between atretic segments are generally dilated and become gangrenous. Atresias are commonly associated with Down syndrome.

Radiographically, the diagnosis is made on plain films with identification of gas to the stenotic or atretic point (Fig. 3-40). Differentiation from midgut volvulus (associated with malrotation) is made on barium enema examination.

Meconium Ileus

Meconium ileus occurs in one-tenth of all patients with cystic fibrosis. Inspissated meconium caused by a deficiency of pancreatic and enteric enzymes can obstruct the bowel. The meconium can also calcify.

When bowel perforation occurs in utero, the calcium can be identified throughout the peritoneal cavity.

On barium enema examination, a microcolon is identified, associated with failure of passage of bowel contents in utero. Atresias and bowel duplications occur in half of these patients.

Meconium Peritonitis

Meconium peritonitis describes a condition in which meconium escapes into the peritoneal cavity in utero. This condition is seen in a variety of congenital obstructions, including atresias, meconium ileus, volvulus, and peritoneal bands. Clinically, these newborns present with vomiting and abdominal distension. Occasionally, a pneumoperitoneum may be present.

Duplication

Duplications are often referred to as enteric cysts. They occur during recannulation of the gut in utero,

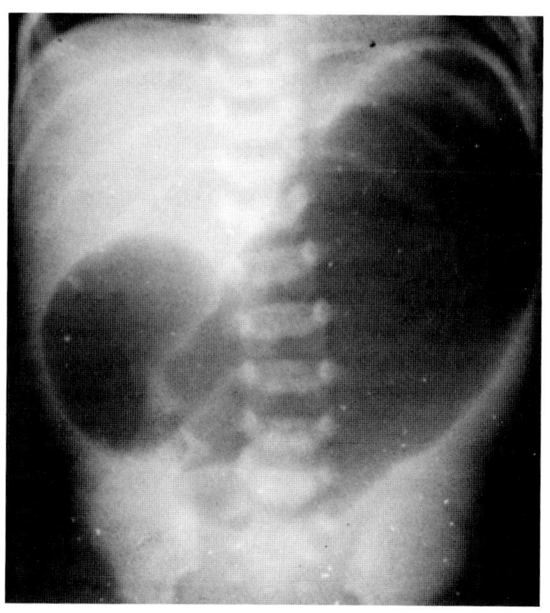

A

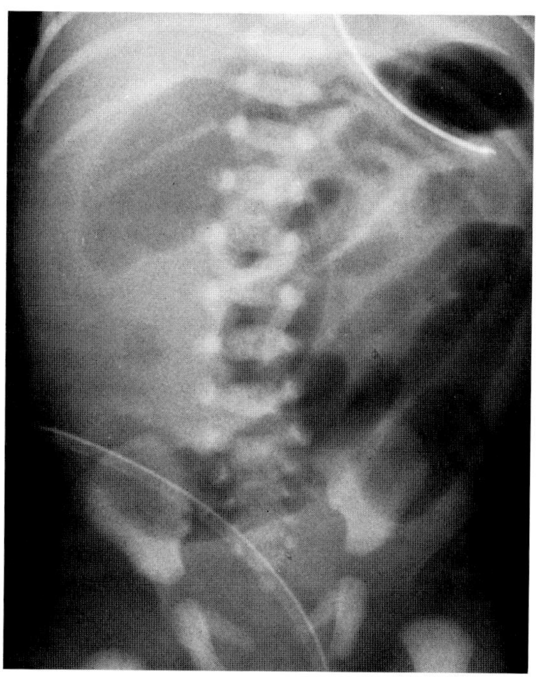

B

Fig. 3-40 **(A)** Duodenal atresia creating the double-bubble sign of a dilated air-filled stomach and duodenal bulb. No gas is present distal to the atresia. **(B)** Ileal atresia. Dilated loops of small bowel are noted throughout the abdomen. No colon gas is present.

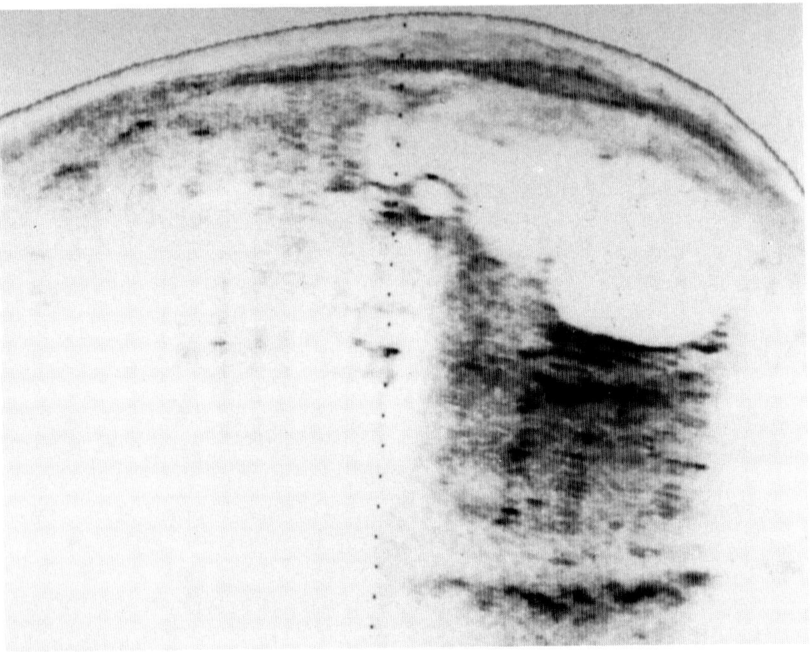

Fig. 3-41 Small bowel duplication cyst. An anechoic, fluid-filled cyst is identified on ultrasound examination. On the barium study, the duplication cyst did not communicate with the true bowel lumen and appeared as an extrinsic mass.

at which time, there is an abnormal development of a dual tubular structure. Sites for intestinal duplication are the ileum and the duodenum, the former being more common. Clinically, duplications are generally asymptomatic. They may produce obstructive cysts or present as a palpable abdominal mass. Most duplications do not communicate with the true lumen and are radiographically evident as extrinsic small bowel masses. Ultrasound and CT may demonstrate a fluid-filled cystic structure (Fig. 3-41).

SUGGESTED READING

Eisenberg RL: Gastrointestinal Radiology. A Pattern Approach. JB Lippincott, New York, 1983

Goldberg HI, Sheft DJ: Abnormalities in small intestine contour and calibre. A working classification. Radiol Clin North Am 14:461, 1976

Herlinger H: Small bowel. p. 423. In Laufer I: Double Contrast Gastrointestinal Radiology with Endoscopic Correlation. WB Saunders, Philadelphia, 1979

Maglinte DDT, Burney BT, Miller RE: Lesions missed on small bowel follow-through. Analysis and recommendations. Radiology 144:737, 1982

Margulis AR, Burhenne HJ (eds.): Alimentary Tract Radiology. CV Mosby, St Louis, 1983

Marshak RH, Lindner AE: Radiology of the Small Intestine. WB Saunders, Philadelphia, 1976

Meyers MA: Dynamic Radiology of the Abdomen: Normal and Pathologic Anatomy. Springer-Verlag, New York, 1982

Osborn AG, Friedland GW: A radiologic approach to the diagnosis of small bowel disease. Clin Radiol 24:281, 1981

Sellink JL, Miller RE: Radiology of the Small Bowel. Modern Enteroclysis Technique and Atlas. Martinus Nijhoff Publishers, Boston, 1982

4

Radiology of the Colon

Dina F. Caroline
Dean D. T. Maglinte

The colon is the most common site of gastrointestinal neoplasms and is also frequently involved in many inflammatory or infectious diseases. Most of the advances in the diagnosis and treatment of colonic diseases, particularly colorectal neoplasm, have been brought about by refinements in fiberoptic endoscopy. In spite of this, the radiologic examination of the colon has remained one of the most valuable examination methods. Shortcomings of the single-contrast barium enema, once the primary radiologic procedure, have been revealed by colonoscopy. These shortcomings brought about refinements in the double-contrast method, which increased the sensitivity and specificity of contrast examinations of the colon. Clinical management relies greatly on radiologic findings and, in certain situations, the diagnosis is based entirely on the radiographic examination.

PHYSIOLOGY AND ANATOMY

Colon Physiology

The proximal half of the colon functions primarily as a water and electrolyte transport system, whereas the distal half is generally involved in evacuation and storage. The transverse colon acts simply as a connection between the right and left sides. In general, sodium and chloride are absorbed, whereas potassium and bicarbonate are secreted.

Anatomy of the Colon

An understanding of normal colorectal anatomy and its common variants is important to the determination of whether a pathologic process is present and also influences the manner in which it is examined.

The colon or large intestine begins at the ileocecal junction and continues to the anus. It is 1.5 m long and is subdivided into several segments. The most proximal is the cecum, a blind pouch — proximal to the ileocecal valve — with the vermiform appendix hanging from its base. Beyond the ileocecal valve, the colon is divided into the ascending, transverse, and descending colons; sigmoid, rectum, and anal canal. The typical morphology of the colon is produced by three bands of longitudinal muscle: the taeniae coli, which originate at the base of the appendix and continue as three separate bands to the rectum, where they fuse and completely encircle the rectum. Between the taeniae and the haustra, sacculations are formed.

The segments of the colon are defined as they course around the periphery of the abdomen between intraperitoneal and retroperitoneal locations. The cecum is at the base of the small bowel mesentery, usually in the right iliac fossa along the ilopsoas muscle. Retention of a mesentery, for a variable distance along the ascending colon, occurs frequently and may create considerable mobility of the ascending colon and cecum, permitting its rotation into the right upper quadrant. The presence of a mesentery in this location predisposes to cecal ileus and cecal volvulus, or twists on its mesentery, leading to obstruction.

At the level of the inferior pole of the right kidney and visceral surface of the liver, the hepatic flexure of the colon turns anteriorly and becomes intraperitoneal at the transverse colon. The transverse colon is suspended by a mesocolon that extends from the pancreas to the transverse colon. It attaches to the transverse colon from the region of the right kidney and duodenum to the tip of the spleen, where it ends as the phrenicocolic ligament. Volvulus of the transverse colon occurs less often than in the sigmoid or cecum.

The phrenicocolic ligament marks the true junction between the intraperitoneal transverse colon and retroperitoneal descending colon. The descending colon lies retroperitoneally in the left paracolic gutter. Retained mesentery to the descending is much less common than to the ascending colon; thus, volvulus of the descending colon is rare.

The sigmoid colon is an intraperitoneal segment lying between the extraperitoneal descending colon and the rectum. Its mesentery attaches it to the posterior pelvic wall. A redundant sigmoid with a long mesentery is the colonic segment most prone to volvulus.

The rectum lies directly anterior to the sacrum. Unlike the remainder of the colon, it is completely surrounded by longitudinal muscle. Most of the rectum lies below the peritoneal reflection; however, the most proximal portion of the rectum has peritoneum on its anterior and lateral surfaces. The reflection of the anterior peritoneum forms the pelvic cul-de-sac, the demarcation between the rectum and sigmoid colon. This region is important inasmuch as it is the most dependent portion of the peritoneum and a prime site for drop metastases, infection, and collection of ascites.

The mucosa of the normal colon is quite featureless on radiographs taken during the double-contrast barium enema examination. Occasionally, very fine, closely spaced transverse lines are identified around the circumference of segments of bowel. These lines are known as the innominate grooves and are a normal pattern.

With good double-contrast technique, tiny (1 to 3 mm) uniform nodules are seen either segmentally or throughout the colon. These nodules represent the normal lymphofollicular pattern of the mucosa, which is seen most commonly in children but may also be present in adults. Enlargement or irregularity in the size of lymph follicles may be seen in lymphoid hyperplasia and may be an early finding in inflammatory or infectious colitides. Multiple, tiny polyps or pseudopolyps may sometimes be confused with the lymphofollicular pattern.

TECHNIQUES OF EXAMINATION

Digital rectal examination and sigmoidoscopy remain the initial procedures in the evaluation of the large intestine. Endoscopy and biopsy complement the radiologic study. The cost-effective barium-contrast examination quickly evaluates the entire colon, and can then guide endoscopy for biopsy and treatment. The barium enema examination and colonoscopy are competitive, but frequently complementary, procedures. Radiology almost always visualizes the entire colon; the mucosa can be shown by double-contrast techniques in exquisite detail with essentially no risk. Colonoscopy, however, can obtain samples of or treat any lesion that is discovered.

The literature of the last decade is replete with reports evaluating the relative merits of these modalities. In general, these reports are flawed because they tend to be presented by highly skilled proponents of one procedure and retrospective, nonrandomized methods of analysis are frequently used. Colonoscopy necessitates a time commitment by the endoscopist, despite which the cecum is only reached in 60 to 90 percent of cases. It is a more expensive modality, has a higher complication rate, and requires greater expertise. The barium enema allows the colonoscopist to anticipate such technical difficulties as a redundant sigmoid or transverse colon, an area of severe diverticulosis, or a stenotic lesion. Barium examination should be regarded as complementary to colonoscopy, since each study has different blind spots, subject to technical failures, and depend on the examiner's expertise. The diagnostic accuracy of both procedures combined is higher than either alone.

Most would agree that a complete large bowel evaluation would entail digital rectal examination, tests for occult blood, sigmoidoscopy, barium enema, and, if indicated, colonoscopy. Many patients will require both the barium enema and colonoscopy for the diagnosis and treatment of diseases of the large intestine. The relative merits of the double-contrast versus single-contrast barium enema study, particularly in the detection of polyps and in the evaluation of inflammatory bowel disease, have also been the subject of controversies. The consensus, at the moment, is that double-contrast studies are far superior and should be the radiologic technique of choice under almost all circumstances.

The main radiologic techniques used to examine the large bowel are (1) the contrast enemas, (2) plain radiographs of the abdomen, (3) peroral pneumocolon, (4) computed tomography, (5) angiography, and (6) radionuclide scintigraphy.

THE COLON CONTRAST ENEMA

The Barium Enema: Double Versus Single Contrast and Clinical Indications

It is now accepted that most carcinomas of the large bowel arise from adenomatous polyps and that the removal of such polyps can reduce the incidence of adenocarcinomas. The sensitivity of polyp detection on double-contrast examination was found to be 87 percent, compared to 59 percent for the single-contrast examination. An error rate of 45.2 percent, using the single-contrast examination, compared to 11.7 percent for the double-contrast method, has been reported in polyp detection. A published series of colon examinations reports a polyp incidence of 9.8 to 13.1 percent, using the double-contrast enema and 1 to 7.8 percent, using the single-contrast examination. Because adenomatous polyps are frequently asymptomatic, routine use of the double-contrast examination

should offer a greater potential reduction in mortality from colorectal cancer. Its greater sensitivity in the detection of inflammatory bowel disease, together with a clearer demonstration of normality, is sufficient reason to adopt the double-contrast barium enema as the standard technique for the radiologic examination of the colon in adults. Proponents of the single-contrast technique point to the extra time expended by radiologists in performing the study. Miller and Maglinte (1982) have described a modified version of the double-contrast technique that significantly reduces examination time and radiation dose. This will be described later. This modification may be particularly applicable to busy practices. It has also been realized that it is easier to teach beginners to perform a high quality double-contrast examination of the large bowel than it is to teach a competent fluoroscopic single-contrast technique. The double-contrast technique can be performed, even on elderly individuals who can move.

The single-contrast barium enema is the technique of choice in emergency situations. It should be the preferred method when large bowel obstruction, acute diverticulitis, acute appendicitis, or a fistula is suspected. With this method, careful fluoroscopy of the advancing barium column is more important than obtaining mucosal detail. The single-contrast barium enema can salvage the occasional failed double-contrast barium enema. The single-contrast barium enema can also be used to clarify questionable lesions noted on double-contrast barium enema (i.e., areas of poor distension or inadequate coating).

A biphasic method of examining the colon has been described and was shown to be significantly superior to the single-contrast examination and, in the presence of diverticulosis, proved to be significantly more sensitive than the double-contrast examination alone. Their contrast material, unfortunately, is not readily available in the United States and other countries. A modified method is described in this chapter under the heading Biphasic Sigmoid Enema: Indications and Technique.

Colon Preparation

The most important factor for any contrast examination of the colon is the bowel preparation. Irrespective of the technique of barium enema employed, the presence of feces may seriously compromise the study. Stool may simulate large neoplasms, small polyps, the irregular mucosal surface, such as that caused by post-inflammatory polyps, and may even obstruct the retrograde flow of contrast. Excessive debris may obscure large colonic lesions. The seriousness of such an error suggests that the radiologist shares the responsibility with the attending physician for ensuring a clean colon.

There is no single way to acheive adequate colon cleansing. The exact combination of diet, laxatives, hydration, and cleansing enemas varies with individual practice. Adequate hydration is common to all methods. The length of dietary restriction and the type of cathartic used vary from one institution to another. A combination of two laxatives appears to give the best results. The main types of cathartics available are the stimulant and the saline groups. The former stimulate peristaltic activity in the large bowel or small intestine, and those used most frequently in practice are castor oil and bisacodyl (Dulcolax). Bisacodyl acts predominantly in the colon; its onset of action is approximately 6 hours after intake. Stimulant cathartics may result in abdominal cramping, mucus secretion, and fluid depletion. The saline group of cathartics are hyperosmolar solutions that attract fluid into the lumen and lead to hyperperistalsis. Adequate oral fluids are necessary, as the loss of fluid into the intestines leads to dehydration. Saline cathartics are contraindicated in patients with cardiac failure or decreased renal function because the fluids lost can lead to increased sodium retention. Magnesium citrate is the most commonly used saline cathartic in practice. Patients with severe constipation may require repeated preparation over several days.

If the scout film shows fecal retention, a 2-L, tapwater cleansing enema, aimed toward filling the entire colon, can be given by experienced personnel. The colon should be examined by air contrast approximately 90 minutes after cleansing.

A popular colon preparation that usually obviates the need for cleansing enemas is based on the hydration technique, using magnesium citrate and bisacodyl. A bisacodyl suppository is used in the morning, prior to the examination. The patient should have nothing by mouth after midnight, if the procedure is to be undertaken in the morning, but may have a clear liquid breakfast if the study is to be done in the afternoon. With this method, a cleansing enema is only needed if the scout film shows considerable fecal debris.

Recently, orally administered gut irrigation has been introduced as an alternative preparation. Although it has been shown to reduce fecal residue, it is associated with less optimal mucosal coating and more retained colonic fluid than observed with the hydration technique using bisacodyl and magnesium citrate. The mucosal coating achieved with the double-contrast barium enema and the oral lavage method is suboptimal. However, if the oral lavage method is used, it should be given early in the evening prior to the examination to ensure sufficient time for all the fluid to be passed.

Use of Hypotonic or Sedative Agents

The administration of a hypotonic agent ensures adequate distension and reduces patient discomfort during the procedure. Glucagon has virtually no contraindications and is the agent of choice. A minimum of 0.75 mg, by the intravenous or intramuscular route, is needed for the colon. Glucagon is useful to prevent or relieve spasm, to distinguish spasm from an organic stricture (Fig. 4-1), and as a possible aid to the retention of barium by incontinent patients.

Light sedation (diazepam and meperidine) is beneficial in combative patients and in those with a total inability to retain contrast because of uncontrollable spasm. An intravenous 10-mg dose of diazepam (Valium) and an intramuscular 25-mg dose of meperidine (Demerol) are adequate.

Rectal Intubation and Use of Rectal Balloon

A rectal examination may provide an assessment of anal sphincter tone and on occasion may disclose an unsuspected lesion in patients who have not had a recent rectal examination. The enema tip should be introduced with care and the rectal balloon reserved

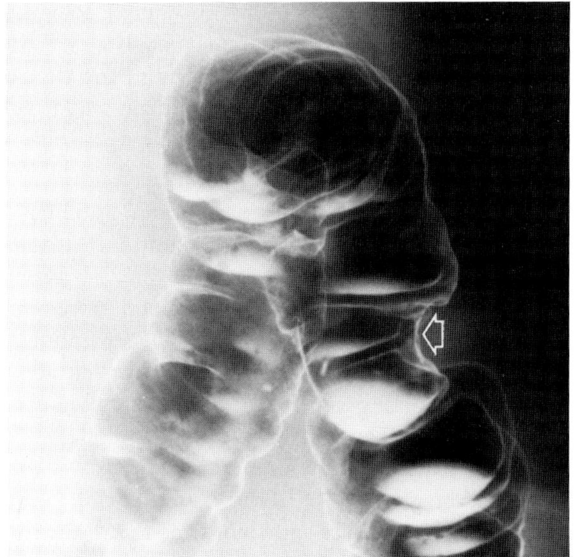

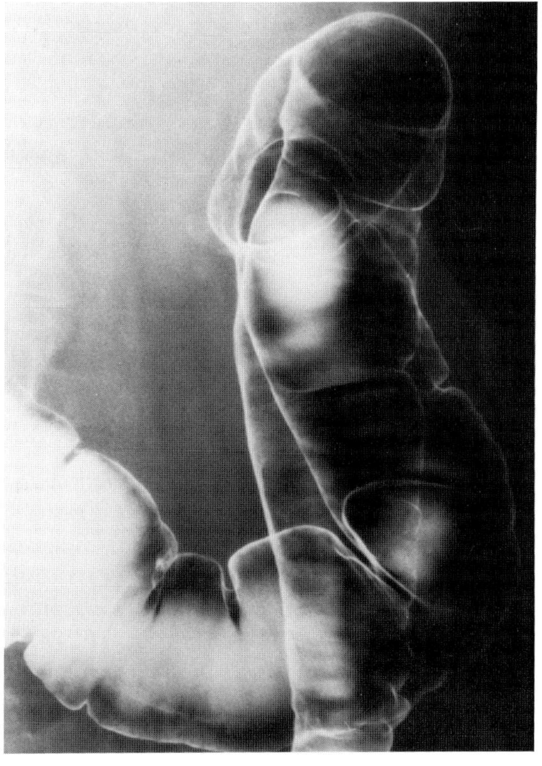

Fig. 4-1 (A) Eccentric polypoid defect in anatomic splenic flexure *(arrow)* simulating a mass. **(B)** Following the administration of 1 mg of glucagon intravenously, no mass is present. The points of transition from intraperitoneal to retroperitoneal segments of the colon can simulate an annular mass (junctional pseudotumor) when the colon is inadequately distended.

for incontinent patients. Inflation of a rectal balloon may obscure a lesion in the lower rectum (Fig. 4-2) and increase the risk of injury. Patients with good anal sphincter tone do not require the use of rectal balloons. The decision as to whether to inflate the rectal balloon is best made on fluoroscopy of the initial flow of barium. Backflow of barium into the anal canal suggests that the balloon should be inflated. This should be done under fluoroscopic control and the inflation stopped when the margin of the distended balloon reaches the side walls of the rectal ampulla. A slight pull on the enema tubing maintains apposition of the balloon against the rectal wall. By taping the buttocks tightly around the enema tube, it may be possible to fill the colon without leakage. In patients with marked rectal pathology (proctitis, stricture, or fissure), a soft rubber catheter or a pediatric enema tip may be used.

Technique of Double-Contrast Examination

There are a variety of ways in which a satisfactory double-contrast barium enema can be achieved. The number of radiographs obtained vary with the experience and preference of the examining radiologist. The essential points are cleansing, coating, sufficient barium to reach the cecum but not enough to obscure, adequate distention with insufflated air, and proper projection so that all surfaces are demonstrated.

Effective colon cleansing is essential. If the barium enema is done after an upper gastrointestinal (UGI) examination, the amount of barium remaining in the colon can be used as a tracer to gauge the efficacy of the colon preparation. A small amount of barium will not degrade the quality of the study; however, moder-

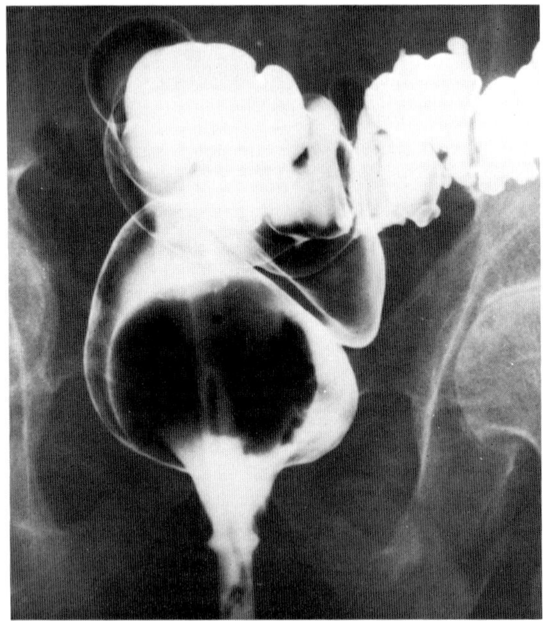

A

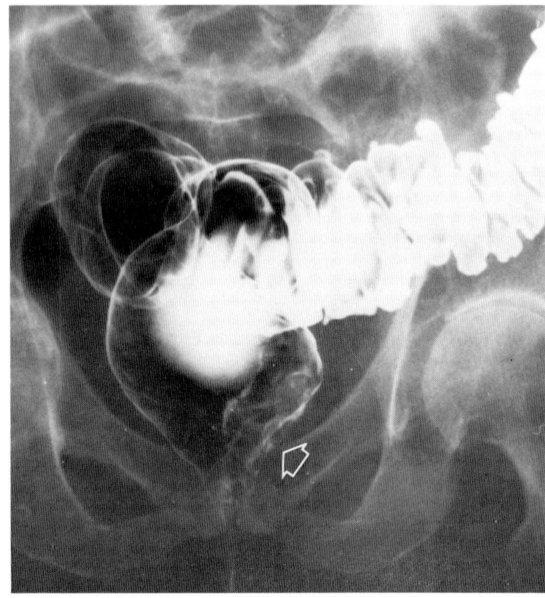

B

Fig. 4-2 (A) Anorectal mass obscured by rectal balloon and barium. **(B)** Following drainage, air insufflation, and removal of the rectal tube, a cloacogenic carcinoma *(arrow)* is apparent.

ate amounts will produce artifacts that may interfere with interpretation.

Viscous barium suspensions of moderately high density (70% to 100% W/V) are used to obtain a uniform opaque mucosal coating. The suspension should have a reasonable rate of flow, maintain its coating properties in the presence of residual water, and be resistant to drying on the colonic mucosa. Commercially prepared liquid barium suspensions, such as HD-85 (85% W/V — Lafayette Pharmacal Inc, Lafayette, IN) and Liquid Polibar or Polibar Plus (100% W/V — E-Z-EM Co, Westbury, NY) give good results. A wide-bore (½ inch) enema tube, measuring 1 to 1.5 feet in length, minimizes the slow rate of flow caused by the high viscosity of the barium suspension. (Faster flowing modifications of the above barium suspensions appear to result in suboptimal coating, particularly of the right side of the colon and especially when a cleansing enema has been given.)

The examination is immediately preceded by the intravenous or intramuscular injection of 0.75 or 1 mg of glucagon. (A retention rectal balloon is inflated only when necessary.) The barium is introduced into

the colon by squeezing the enema bag until the radiologic splenic flexure is reached, with the patient in the prone or left-side down position. This requires 300 to 500 ml of barium. At this point, the enema bag may be lowered and some barium drained from the rectum. Air is then introduced through the attached insufflator. It is important to position the patient in such a way that the barium column stays in front of the air to avoid an airlock that may obstruct the forward flow of barium and compromise the study. The patient is turned slowly onto his right side and then on his back as the fluoroscopist is insufflating with air. The barium should now be at about the level of the hepatic flexure. The patient is turned into a left posterior oblique position and a spot film of the air-filled sigmoid colon is obtained. Additional spot views of the sigmoid, including right posterior and/or lateral views, may be necessary to visualize all loops of the sigmoid with air contrast.

After air-contrast views of the sigmoid are obtained, the patient is turned to his right side and then prone with additional insufflation of air. By now the barium is usually in the ascending colon or cecum. If present, excess barium is drained from the colon and rectum.

Air is reinsufflated and if the patient is able to retain the air, the enema tip may be removed.

The remaining spot films are then taken. These include prone and lateral views of the rectum, erect views of both flexures, and usually two views of the cecum (with and without compression). An erect, lateral view of the rectum and sigmoid may be useful. Additional spot films may be obtained if portions of the colon are obscured by overlapping loops of bowel. (If the patient is not able to retain the air completely, the enema tip may be left in as spot films of the flexures and cecum are obtained, and then removed for spot films of the rectum. Rarely is it necessary to leave the enema tip in place until after the radiographer completes the table films.)

The radiographic technologist takes a series of overhead films after the fluoroscopic examination is completed. This series includes three horizontal-beam films, i.e., right and left lateral decubitus (14″ × 17″) and a prone, shoot-through view of the rectum (8″ × 10″ film). Both supine obliques (right posterior and left posterior) and a prone view are obtained with a vertical beam. A prone angle (Chassard) view of the rectosigmoid is also obtained. Other examiners may include a supine or left posterior oblique, angled view of the sigmoid.

If the colon is redundant or the cecum is not optimally seen on the routine examination, a postevacuation radiograph is often helpful. Any areas of question may be reexamined by reinsufflating air after the patient has evacuated through a soft rubber catheter inserted into the rectum.

The Limited Fluoroscopic Double-Contrast Barium Enema

Recently, Miller and Maglinte (1982) described a method that has reduced examination time, cost, and patient radiation. It can be performed by the skilled radiologist or skilled technologist and is ideal for the resident-in-training who is just starting fluoroscopy. This simplified technique called the Seven Step/Pump Method ensures adequate amounts of barium in the cecum, using less time, barium, and radiation. This technique is based on the usual anatomic positions of the various colon segments, the role of grav-

ity, and the time in each position. Three hundred to 400 ml of barium are first instilled in the rectum. Each step then takes seven full squeezes or pumps on a standard air insufflator in seven different positions. These positions are (1) 7 pumps, prone position; (2) 7 pumps, left lateral position; (3) 7 pumps, left anterior oblique position; (4) 7 pumps, prone position; (5) 7 pumps, right anterior oblique position; (6) 7 pumps, right lateral position; (7) 7 pumps, supine position. After rectal drainage, steps (1) and (7) are repeated before filming. This will ensure adequate distension. Occasionally, additional air and patient positioning under fluoroscopy are necessary to ensure optimal distribution and coating of the barium. All steps may be performed with little fluoroscopy to reduce radiation and shorten examination time. The initial fluoroscopy may be done to ensure that barium is flowing and there is no need to inflate the rectal balloon. Only a final fluoroscopic check is needed to find the 10 percent of patients who need additional maneuvers to place barium in the cecum. The sequence of radiographs, when using conventional fluoroscopic units, are (1) spot radiographs of the sigmoid in various obliquities in the supine and prone positions; and (2) spot radiographs of the cecum and flexures are then taken. The latter are obtained in the upright position. The rectal tube is then removed and overhead radiographs are obtained in the following positions and film sizes.

1. Left lateral rectum 10″ × 12″ view
2. Supine 14″ × 17″ view
3. Right lateral rectum 10″ × 12″ view
4. Prone 14″ × 17″ view
5. Prone 14″ × 17″ view of sigmoid colon with tube angled 30 degrees to the feet
6. Left side decubitus 14″ × 17″ view
7. Right side decubitus 14″ × 17″ view

Imaging each segment of the colon in opposite positions (right and left lateral rectum or prone and supine-angled sigmoid views) allows each segment to be visualized by double contrast, even when a moderate amount of dense barium is present in that segment. This is because the dependent segment in one position is no longer the dependent portion in the opposite position. This also allows the interpreter to utilize, to advantage, the principle of the barium puddle in localizing the site of a lesion. An additional transprone lateral rectal overhead is obtained on patients in whom rectal drainage is inadequate.

Early removal of the rectal tube, prior to overhead radiography, has been shown to improve patient tolerance during the double-contrast barium enema procedure. The use of carbon dioxide instead of room air has decreased abdominal discomfort after the procedure.

The Miller-Maglinte (1982) double-contrast technique is ideally suited for remote-control radiography. An average 2 minutes of fluoroscopic time for the entire procedure is not infrequent. The filming sequence is fairly similar. Angled views of the sigmoid on 10″ × 12″ radiographs in the prone and supine positions and a 14″ × 17″ vertical beam are obtained before the rectal tube is removed. The sequence of filming, film size, and patient position are listed here.

Recumbent

10″ × 12″ left lateral rectum (increase kVp by 10)

10″ × 12″ LPO rectum and sigmoid (angle cephalad)

14″ × 17″ RPO (splenic flexure)

10″ × 12″ right lateral rectum (increase kVp by 10)

10″ × 12″ sigmoid and rectum RAO (angle caudad)

14″ × 17″ prone (include flexures)

10″ × 12″ 2 or 4 on 1 cecum (PA or RAO, AP or LPO) Compress if too much bariun is present.

14″ × 17″ LPO (hepatic flexure)

Erect

14″ × 17″ AP (include sigmoid)

10″ × 12″ LPO (include top of hepatic flexure)

10″ × 12″ RPO (include top of splenic flexure)

10″ × 12″ right lateral or steep oblique (rectum)

The 14″ × 17″ oblique radiographs are substituted by both decubitus views, if the latter adaptation is possible on remote control units. The number of radiographs obtained with remote control radiography ensures at least two views of the anterior, posterior, right, and left lateral walls (dependent walls) of each

segment of the colon. The number of radiographs should be reduced in women of childbearing age. An average of 15 to 20 minutes total procedure time is frequent using remote control fluoroscopy.

The Biphasic Sigmoid Enema: Indications and Technique

The predictive value of the double-contrast study in the detection of sigmoid polyps decreases when extensive diverticula are present. The accompanying muscular wall thickening makes this segment difficult to distend with air. The false-positive and false-negative diagnosis of polyps are most frequent in the sigmoid. Some investigators have shown that a biphasic examination of the colon is more sensitive than the double contrast, done in the presence of diverticulosis. The barium mixture used for this technique is not readily available in North America. A similar result can be obtained by introducing a 1% W/V barium mixture up to the descending colon, after the double-contrast study is completed. The rectal tube should be kept in place once a sigmoid, distorted by diverticula, is noted during the fluoroscopic phase of the double-contrast examination.

There is a significant difference in the biphasic sigmoid films of patients who have diverticula. Frequently there is better distension of this region and less confusion between diverticula and filling defects in the filled phase. The best visualization of polyps in the diverticula are sometimes air contrast and sometimes filled views. The supplementary study, however, is always helpful to confirm a polypoid lesion, or an unfilled diverticulum. The additional filled views (compression supine and prone sigmoid angled views) are a simple cost-effective procedure in this select group of patients and obviates repeat examination or unnecessary endoscopy.

Technique of Single Contrast Examination

The single-contrast or full-column method utilizes high kilovoltage and careful fluoroscopic compression of accessible segments of the barium-filled colon. The rate of barium filling should be slow enough to permit compression and manual palpation to be performed meticulously. A low density (approximately

15% W/V) barium suspension is used. The prime requirement for the barium suspension used is that it should be capable of remaining in suspension for a reasonable period of time. Spot films are obtained of the rectum, sigmoid colon, both flexures, and the cecum. The cecum should be compressed adequately, as a lesion within its wide lumen can be readily overlooked, owing to underpenetration or confusion with residual stool. The addition of a small amount of air may help to penetrate capacious segments, such as the cecum. Following fluoroscopy, 14″ × 17″ film, overhead radiographs are obtained in the prone position; a prone 14″ × 17″ film of the sigmoid, with the tube angled 30 degrees toward the feet, and a 10″ × 12″ lateral radiograph of the rectum are taken. The colon is then drained through the rectal tube (facilitated by a wide-bore enema tubing) by lowering the enema bag to the floor. When drainage has stopped, a supine 14″ × 17″ postevacuation radiograph is obtained. If the colon is still distended with barium, the patient is sent to the toilet and another postemptying radiograph obtained. The postevacuation radiograph is routinely done when the clinical indication is appendicitis or acute diverticulitis, or a sinus tract is suspected, because the increased intraabdominal pressure generated by straining may aid filling of the appendix or a sinus tract.

The Postendoscopy, Postendoscopic Biopsy Barium Enema

A satisfactory double-contrast barium enema can be obtained without difficulty or additional discomfort to the patient following a rigid sigmoidoscopy. Following colonoscopy or flexible sigmoidoscopy, massive gaseous distension of the entire colon hinders filling and is uncomfortable to the patient. The double-contrast barium enema is deferred until the following day. Minimal-to-moderate gaseous filling of the colon, without distension, does not preclude a satisfactory double-contrast barium enema following flexible sigmoidoscopy or colonoscopy.

Barium does not influence the healing of colorectal biopsy sites. Experimental evidence by Maglinte et al (1983) has shown that a superficial mucosal biopsy site is immediately reepithelialized, whereas a deep

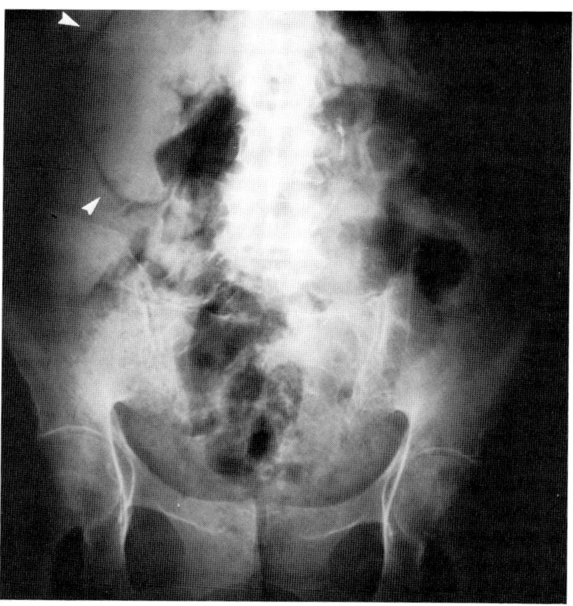

Fig. 4-3 Retropneumoperitoneum following sigmoid biopsy through a rigid scope. Air *(arrowheads)* is seen outlining right kidney. Double-contrast barium enema examination 1 week later shows no evidence of a barium leak or retropneumoperitoneum.

biopsy site takes up to 6 days to completely reepithelialize. The biopsy forceps used during flexible sigmoidoscopy or colonoscopy is generally only capable of obtaining a superficial tissue specimen. Under these circumstances, no waiting period is considered necessary before performing a barium enema. Following biopsy using a rigid sigmoidoscope, it is advisable to wait a week before doing a barium enema examination, unless immediate histologic examination shows a superficial bite. The rectal biopsy forceps commonly used during rigid sigmoidoscopy occasionally enables a deep biopsy bite to be obtained. The subsequent performance of a barium enema may lead to perforation at the biopsy site. The ensuing leakage into the extraperitoneal tissues or peritoneal cavity may prove fatal or give rise to a paracolic abscess. The plain abdominal radiograph should be carefully scrutinized not only for the adequacy of colonic prep or the amount of gaseous distension following endoscopy, but also for subtle evidence of intra- or retropneumoperitoneum following perendoscopic biopsy (Fig. 4-3).

Contraindications to the Barium Enema

Barium examination of the colon is contraindicated in cases of suspected colonic perforation or in patients at risk for intraperitoneal leakage. If a contrast examination is necessary in these patients, iodinated agents such as sodium meglumine diatrizoate (Gastrografin) or sodium diatrizoate (Hypaque) are used as directed. Gastrografin may be substituted with a less expensive water-soluble contrast agent, supplied in 300-ml containers, normally reserved for urographic examinations, such as Urovist (diatrizoate meglumine). Because these compounds are hyperosmolar, they may be used therapeutically in an attempt to relieve fecal impaction in patients with cystic fibrosis, meconium ileus, or meconium plug syndrome. Hyperosmolar water-soluble contrast agents must be used with caution in dehydrated patients, or patients at risk for electrolyte imbalance. These agents should not be passed proximal to an obstructing lesion because intraluminal fluid increases because its hypertonicity increases the risk of perforation. Some of these problems may be reduced as nonionic water-soluble contrast agents become more available.

Complications of the Barium Enema

The barium enema is generally a safe examination. Perforation is a serious complication and occurs in about one in 5,000 examinations. Overinflation of the rectal balloon, traumatic insertion of the enema tip, necrosis or weakening of the colonic wall owing to underlying disease or deep biopsy site, and bursting related to hydrostatic pressure, are the most common causes.

The risk of damage to the rectal wall by an overinflated balloon is greater in the anal canal or rectosigmoid because these segments are less distensible than the rectal ampulla. Incorrect position or eccentric inflation of the rectal balloon predisposes to rectal tear and can be avoided if balloon inflation is performed only under fluoroscopic control. The presence of inflammation, stricture, sinus tract or mucosal lesion in the lower rectum is a contraindication to use of a rectal balloon.

The rectal tube should be inserted by trained personnel. Rigid enema tips should not be used. The risk of impaling the tip on the anterior rectal wall is avoided by directing the enema tip posteriorly, once it has been introduced into the anal canal. The rectal lumen bends acutely backward above the anal canal.

A weakened rectal or colonic wall predisposes to perforation during barium enema. The examination should not be done in patients with toxic megacolon or severe colitis. A necrotic tumor may also predispose to perforation.

Intraluminal pressure measurement during both single- and double-contrast barium enemas has shown that intraluminal pressure is not higher during the double-contrast technique. Air insufflation should be gradual and overdistension avoided by fluoroscopy when patients complain of discomfort. Colon perforation secondary to hydrostatic pressure of the barium is rare. When a single-contrast barium enema is performed, the bag should be kept below 3 feet above the table. The enema bag may be safely raised to 4 or 5 feet, with the viscous barium suspension used for double-contrast barium enema.

Prompt radiographic recognition of perforation is imperative, as the rectum and colon are relatively insensitive to pain and frequently there is no clinical suspicion of perforation. The passage of blood per rectum, subcutaneous emphysema, or the subsequent development of fever, leukocytosis, and shock should arouse clinical suspicion of colorectal perforation. Rectal perforation below the level of the peritoneal reflection after a double-contrast study may extravasate only a small amount of barium, and extraperitoneal air may be difficult to appreciate at fluoroscopy. Hence, immediate diagnosis may be difficult. All radiographs obtained should be examined carefully for extravasation as well as film quality, and searched for pathology before a patient is sent out of the department. Barium extravasation associated with a single-contrast enema is usually massive and is readily diagnosed. The prognosis may be directly related to the amount of barium (and feces) extravasated. As much barium as possible should be drained through the rectal tube. Immediate surgical consultation should be obtained. Immediate laparotomy with thorough saline lavage of the peritoneal cavity and removal of as much barium as possible, repair of the perforation, and diverting colostomy are necessary for intraperitoneal spillage. This is associated with an approximately 50 percent mortality. When retroperitoneal air and no barium is present, conservative management can be tried and surgery reserved for cases that fail to respond. Adhesive complications requiring repeated surgery develop in approximately 30 percent of patients with missed barium and fecal peritonitis.

Barium intravasation is the most lethal, but highly unusual complication. This usually causes death from pulmonary embolism.

The appearance of gas within the portal venous system, after a barium enema, has been seen in patients with inflammatory bowel disease. This is not associated with significant ill-effects.

Inadvertent vaginal intubation can lead to rupture, if it is not recognized.

Transient bacteremia has been shown following a barium enema, but is not accompanied by significant clinical problems.

Barium enema should only be performed with caution in patients with recent myocardial infarction or cerebrovascular accident. Severe coronary artery disease, such as cardiac arrhythmias and evidence of left ventricular ischemia, has been demonstrated following the procedure.

The Colostomy Enema

A technique that prevents leakage of barium around the stoma is needed. A commercial device (E-Z-EM Co., Westbury, NY) is available. It consists of a catheter that is threaded through a flexible plastic cone. A soft rubber catheter (Bardex catheter) may suffice. Inflation of a balloon catheter within the colostomy is avoided to prevent perforation of the wall. The catheter is lubricated and introduced through the stoma for a distance of several inches, or until resistance is met. The cone is then advanced into the stoma until it provides a snug fit, and the patient applies firm manual pressure to the cone to prevent leakage of barium

around it. Double- or single-contrast barium enema can be carried out.

The Water-Soluble Contrast Enema

The use of barium is contraindicated when perforation is suspected. Some radiologists prefer to use water-soluble contrast for suspected acute diverticulitis. Gastrografin or Hypaque are the most commonly used agents. These are hyperosmolar solutions and small amounts may be absorbed. In the very young, debilitated, or elderly, this can cause severe hypovolemia and shock secondary to the large amounts of fluid drawn into the bowel. This contrast should not be used in cases of obstruction. Hypersensitivity may result from the absorbed iodine-containing contrast agent.

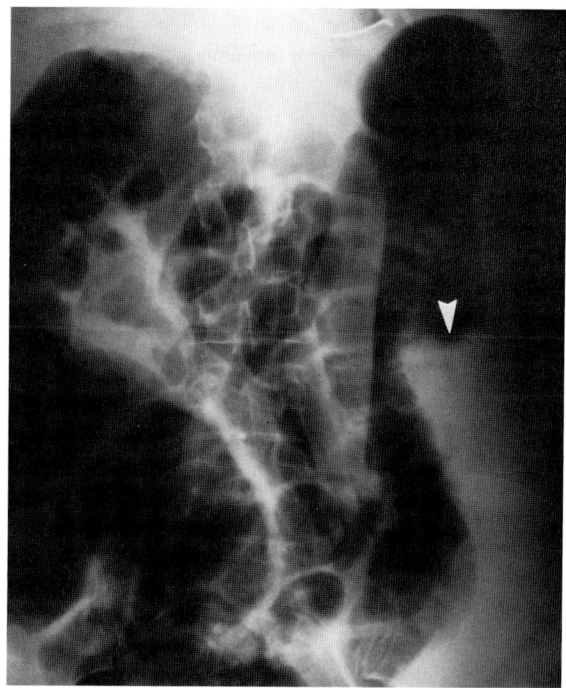

Fig. 4-4 Descending colon carcinoma diagnosed on plain film. Abrupt cutoff of gas column in mid-descending colon by a soft tissue mass *(arrowhead)* permits diagnosis of an obstructing carcinoma. This was confirmed by a single-contrast barium enema examination.

The Peroral Pneumocolon

An assessment of the colon can be achieved by obtaining delayed radiographs 3 hours after the oral ingestion of barium, or later depending on the segment of colon to be evaluated. This technique is valuable when a barium enema fails in the presence of rectal incontinence or severe colitis. It should not be used in suspected colon obstruction. A refinement of this technique is the peroral pneumocolon achieved by the administration of air per rectum when the oral barium has reached the proximal or midcolon. For this technique, a clean colon is desirable and, if possible, the patient should be prepared as for a barium enema. A large volume of low density oral barium (600 to 800 ml 40% W/V) is given. Sorbitol, small amounts of water-soluble contrast, or metroclopramide (Reglan 10 to 20 mg) may be given to speed up transit. If information on the distal small bowel is desired, the use of glucagon (1 mg) decreases pressure in the ileocecal valve and decreases the discomfort of the procedure. The rectal tube should be removed once the adequate amount of air has been introduced.

Plain Film Radiography

Noncontrast radiographs of the abdomen may be diagnostic, or will suggest the treatment or type of examination to be done next (Fig. 4-4). This is usually requested when an acute disorder is suspected. Gas within the colon is an excellent contrast agent. In most patients the course of the colon can be outlined by intraluminal gas. In the supine position gas rises to fill the transverse colon, cecum, and quite often the sigmoid and rectum. With the patient in a left-lateral decubitus position (left-side down, horizontal beam),

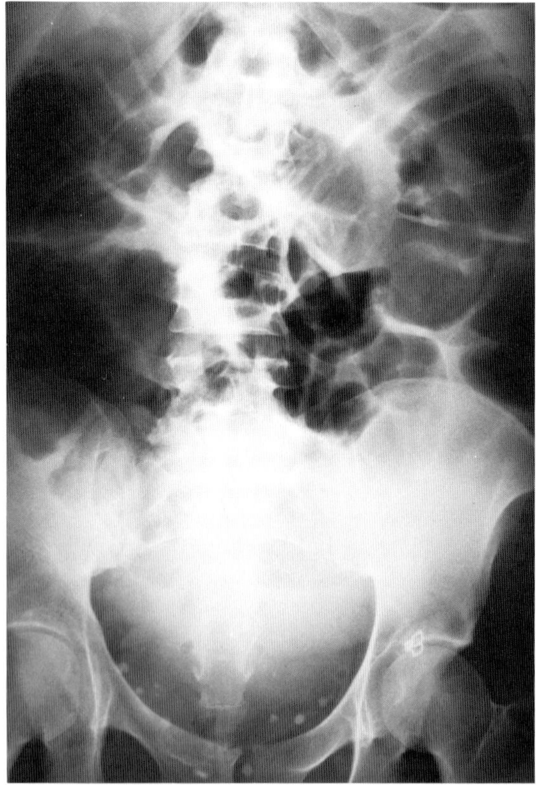
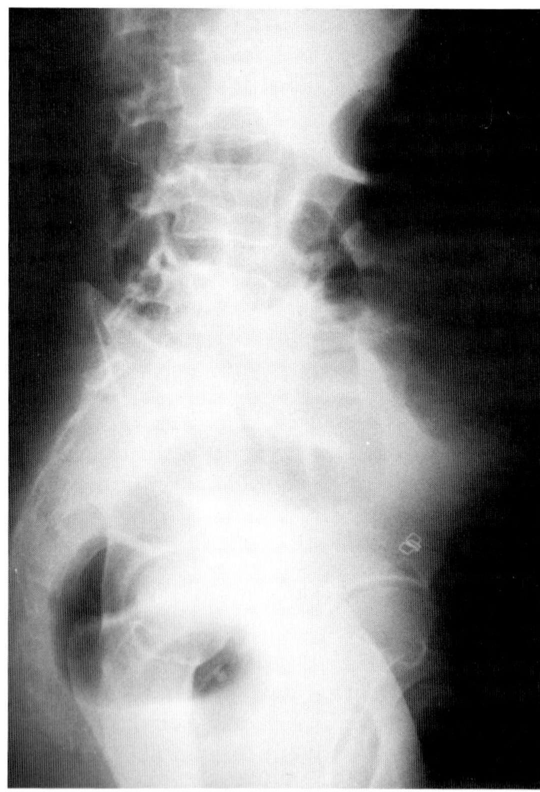

Fig. 4-5 (A) Supine abdominal radiograph of a patient following pelvic surgery. There is no gas in the rectum and distal sigmoid. **(B)** Left-lateral abdominal radiograph. Gas in the rectum and sigmoid confirm the diagnosis of a nonobstructive colonic ileus.

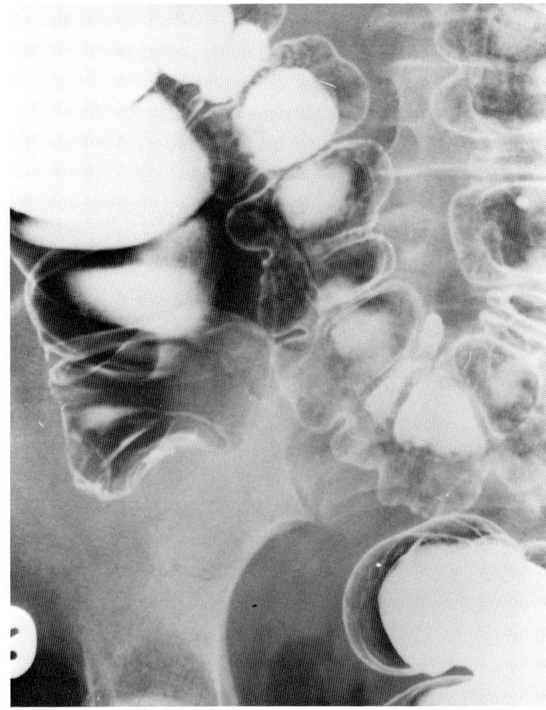

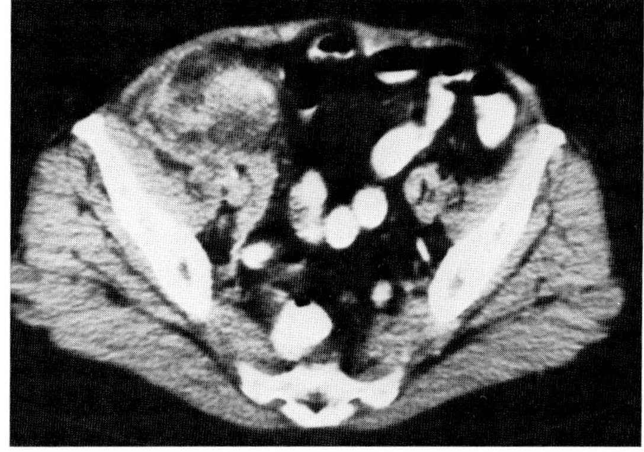

Fig. 4-6 (A) Extramucosal defect in the cecum secondary to an appendiceal abscess. **(B)** CT shows a larger abscess in the right lower quadrant than is apparent on the barium study.

gas fills the ascending colon and cecum. In the left lateral position (left-side down, vertical beam) or right-lateral decubitus view, gas frequently fills the sigmoid colon and rectum. The latter views are valuable projections in differentiating colonic ileus (nonobstructive or adynamic) from left-sided or distal mechanical colon obstruction without resorting to a barium enema (Fig. 4-5). With the patient prone, gas rises into the ascending and descending colon and rectum.

Supine and erect 14″ × 17″ radiographs of the abdomen at low kV are frequently obtained. A left-side down decubitus is substituted for the erect radiograph, if the patient is unable to stand. The inferior rami of the pubic bone should be included in the radiographs so that the presence of gas in the rectum, or external hernias in the groin, can be assessed. Additionally, an erect chest radiograph is obtained; this is the most sensitive view for the detection of pneumoperitoneum. The lateral chest radiograph appears to be more sensitive than the frontal projection in minimal pneumoperitoneum.

Angiography

The localization of the site of acute lower gastrointestinal bleeding and stopping the bleeding are the main roles of angiography in colonic disorders.

Radionuclide Scintigraphy

Radionuclide scintigraphy has its value as a screening test for acute lower gastrointestinal bleeding. Red blood cells or sulfur colloid labeled with technetium 99m are sensitive agents for the detection of active lower gastrointestinal bleeding. It is a noninvasive technique and appears to be more sensitive than angiography. When red blood cells are used, it can be repeated until a bleeding site is demonstrated. Indium 111-labeled leukocyte scintigraphy has been used to assess the extent of involvement in patients with severe idiopathic inflammatory bowel disease too severe to permit barium enema or colonoscopy. This method is infrequently used in practice.

Computed Tomography

The barium enema depicts the luminal surface of the colon. Valuable information is obtained regarding intramural masses or its immediate adjacencies when the masses displace or are adherent to the wall. Extraluminal extension of primary GI disease is frequently better assessed by computed tomography (CT) than by barium study (Fig. 4-6). CT is presently the most informative modality in evaluating extrinsic spread of colorectal disease. Extensive mucosal abnormalities may also be shown by computed tomography. Computed tomography has been shown to be valuable for the recognition of pericolonic or perirectal abscesses in patients with Crohn disease, diverticulitis, or appendicitis. It can be used to determine the extent of tumor spread preoperatively, and the presence and extent of recurrent colorectal carcinoma, particularly after abdominoperineal resection. More recently, double-contrast computed tomography of the colon has been shown to improve detection of mucosal disease. Colon preparation is necessary. Gas can be given by mouth or per rectum. This technique may have practical value in a few selected patients.

Sections at 1 to 2 cm intervals are obtained from the level of the diaphragm to the symphysis pubis following opacification of the gastrointestinal tract. Approximately 700 ml of a 1 to 2 percent solution of Gastrografin or a 1 percent solution of barium sulfate is given 2 to 3 hours before the examination. This is followed by a further 250 ml of oral contrast and an enema of the same contrast agent immediately before the examination is started. Intravenous contrast is not required. The incidence of false-positive diagnoses is decreased if the entire gastrointestinal tract is opacified. The examination should be carefully monitored and additional sections obtained of areas in question.

NEOPLASMS OF THE COLON

Benign Lesions of the Colon

Polypoid lesions cover a wide range of conditions causing protrusion within the lumen of a viscus. Neoplasms, benign and malignant, are the most important of these lesions; however, nonneoplastic conditions may lead to polypoid defects in the colon (as elsewhere). The term polyp is probably best used descriptively rather than to make histologic implications.

Multiple disorders other than primary mucosal lesions may cause single or multiple filling defects in the colon. A normal lymphofollicular pattern and reactive lymphoid hyperplasia (Fig. 4-7) often mimic neoplastic polyps. Other conditions, discussed elsewhere, include infectious and idiopathic colitides and ischemic colitis. Vascular lesions such as hemorrhoids or vascular malformations cause localized, often serpiginous submucosal filling defects. Undigested vegetable matter can occasionally be mistaken for polyps, if the adequate number of radiographs or projections are not obtained. Their appearance often allows one to predict their nature.

Various uncommon conditions present with an appearance of single or multiple filling defects. Pneumatosis coli, caused by intramural gas collections and associated with numerous conditions, may appear as multiple, round filling defects or as linear gas collections. The lucency of these collections and their broad bases generally makes them easily distinguishable from mucosal lesions.

Colitis cystica profunda is probably a postinflammatory condition in which mucus-secreting cysts form

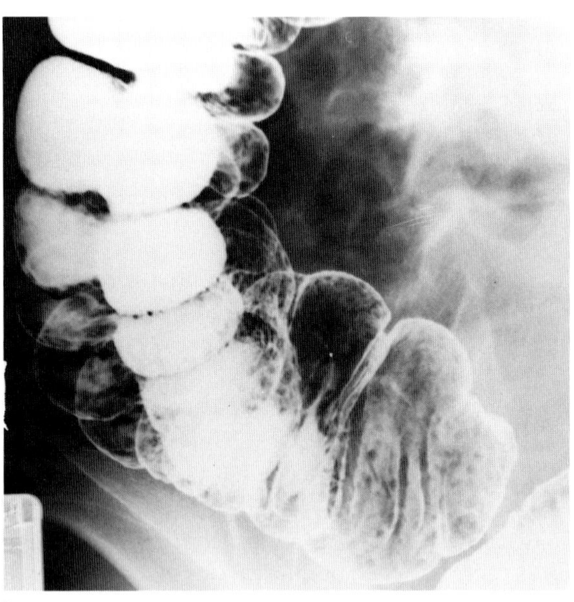

Fig. 4-7 Lymphoid hyperplasia. Multiple, smooth round filling defects were present throughout the colon. These are somewhat larger and less regular in size than those seen with a normal lymphofollicular pattern. This patient had pre-AIDS syndrome.

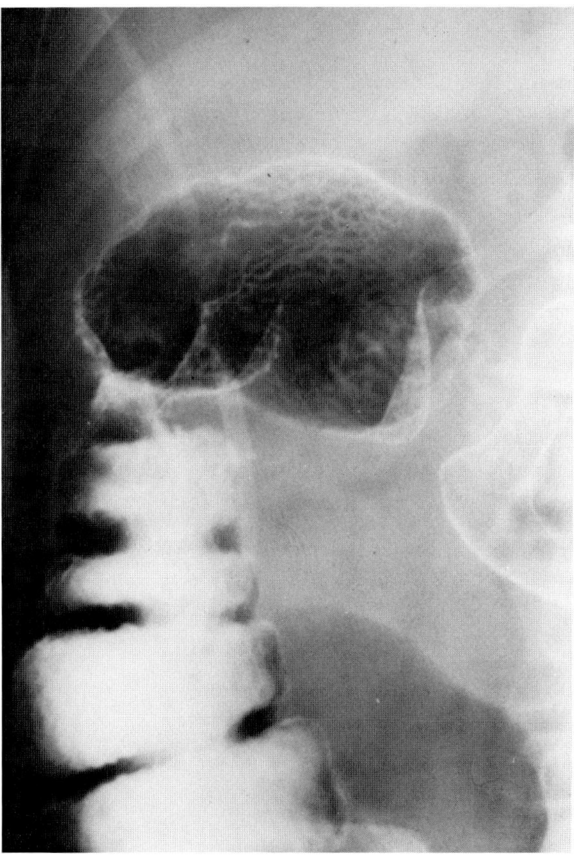

Fig. 4-8 Colonic urticaria pattern. Numerous reticulated raised filling defects are seen proximal to a constricting carcinomas of the transverse colon. (Courtesy of Dr. AC Friedman.)

in the submucosa. The condition usually presents as multiple, submucosal filling defects in the rectum; however, it may occasionally present as a single defect or involve other colonic segments. Diffuse involvement is unusual.

Submucosal edema is another unusual cause of multiple filling defects. The cecum and right side of the colon are affected with multiple, round or angular filling defects. The appearance was first described as colonic urticaria associated with a hypersensitivity reaction. The same pattern has also been seen proximal to a colonic obstruction, with cecal distension and with herpes zoster infection (Fig. 4-8). Amyloidosis may also cause multiple polypoid lesions.

Hyperplastic Polyps

Hyperplastic polyps are the most common polypoid lesions in the colon, accounting for about 90 percent of total lesions. They are not neoplastic but rather are focal proliferations of normal mucosa, sometimes referred to as metaplastic polyps. Because they are not neoplastic, they are frequently omitted from discussions of colonic polyps, and adenomas are listed as the most common polyps.

Hyperplastic polyps are usually small — less than 5 mm — smooth-contoured, and sessile. They may also be single or multiple. On high quality double-contrast examinations, these polyps often have the appearance of a bowler-hat with two intersecting circular shadows, one representing the base of the polyp with a small amount of barium trapped between the base and the colon wall, and the other coating the head of the polyp. Because of their small size, these polyps are detected with much greater accuracy on double- rather than single-contrast studies. The importance of detecting these small lesions is that adenomas, which are true neoplasms with malignant potential, may sometimes have a similar appearance. As endoscopic techniques have improved greatly, the tendency is toward more aggressive removal of even small polyps; thus, their identification on barium studies is useful. Small smooth polyps may be confused with diverticula. Rotation of the patient usually demonstrates extraluminal projection of a diverticulum.

Adenomas

Adenomas are the most common neoplastic colonic polyp. The incidence increases significantly with age. Most polyps occur in the rectosigmoid area; however, several recent studies suggest an increasing number of right-sided polyps.

Polyps are multiple in about 25 percent of patients. Clinically, most patients are asymptomatic. Occult blood in the stool may be present. Histologically, there is proliferation of glandular epithelium into tubules, or villous formation. The polyps are classified, by this appearance, into tubular (glandular), villous, or tubulovillous adenomas. Tubular adenomas are most often pedunculated, whereas villous adenomas tend to be sessile.

Adenomas are considered to be premalignant lesions; thus, their detection is of great clinical significance. Several features have been found to correlate with an increased incidence of malignant degeneration of the polyp. Histologically, the factors include large size, the presence of dysplasia (cellular atypia), and the preponderance of villous, as opposed to tubular architecture. Gross morphologic features appreciated on barium enema are summarized in Table 4-1.

Although the factors predisposing to the development of carcinoma are unknown, the literature supports the concept of an adenoma-carcinoma sequence. They undergo dysplastic changes of increasing severity. Almost all carcinomas are believed to arise in this manner. De novo development of adenocarcinoma (not from an underlying adenoma) is believed to be a rare occurrence, with the possible exception of ulcerative colitis. For this reason, there is an increasing tendency by clinicians to remove all polyps, even those under 1 cm, by colonoscopy. The early diagnosis of colon cancer may be considered an exercise in polyp detection. The radiographic detection of polyps is thus a critical purpose of the double-contrast barium enema.

Polyps may be recognized as fixed filling defects on barium examination. Demonstration of a stalk often defines a polyp (Fig. 4-9). Stalked polyps may have considerable mobility. Therefore, one should define a filling defect carefully before deciding whether a polyp or only fecal debris is present. On double contrast the en face appearance of stalked polyps resembles a target or "Mexican hat"; the barium-coated stalk is seen through the wider head of the polyp. Smooth, sessile polyps may appear as bowler hats, the base forming one semicircular rim and the second formed by the head of the polyp. Some polyps may

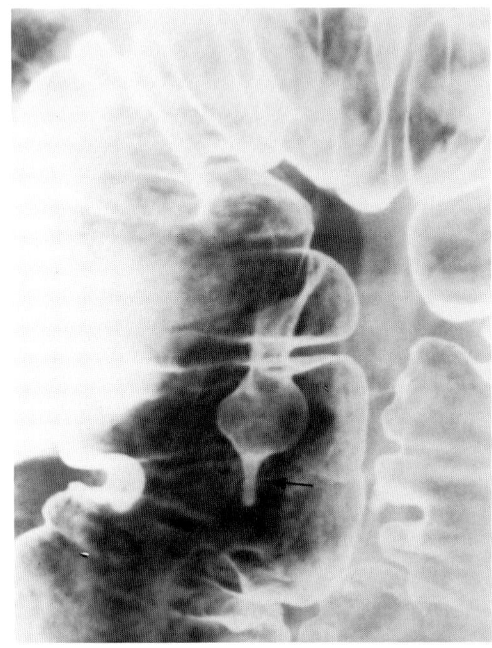

Fig. 4-9 Pedunculated polyp. A droplet of barium *(arrow)* hanging from the head of the stalked polyp—the stalactite phenomenon.

grow to considerable size (Fig. 4-10). Villous adenomas are usually large, flat, broad-based lesions with numerous frondlike projections that trap barium (Fig. 4-11). Small villous tumors are indistinguishable radiographically from tubular adenomas, unless the carpetlike appearance of the frondlike projections are depicted (Fig. 4-12).

Lipomas and Other Mesenchymal Tumors

This group of lesions comprises the nonepithelial, benign neoplasms of the colon, which arise in the

Table 4-1 Evaluation of Polyps for Risk of Malignancy

	Benign	
Size	2.0 cm	2.0 cm (50% malignant)
Contour	Smooth	Multilobulated or irregular
Stalk	Present (pedunculated, long and thin)	Absent (sessile) Short and thick
Underlying colon wall	Smooth	Indented and retracted
Number of polyps	Single	Multiple

submucosal or muscular layers of the colon. Lipomas are the most common tumor of this group and are second to adenomas in the frequency of benign colonic neoplasms. They are most common in the ileocecal region and ascending colon and are often incidental findings at examination. Lipomas are soft lesions that arise in the submucosa and appear as smooth filling defects on barium examination. If a lipoma becomes large enough, it tends to protrude more into the lumen and develops a pseudopedicle to mimic a mucosal lesion. Characteristically, lipomas are distinguishable from other lesions by their softness, pliability, and consequent changeability in shape and size with changes in patient position and compression on barium studies (Fig 4-13). CT, with its

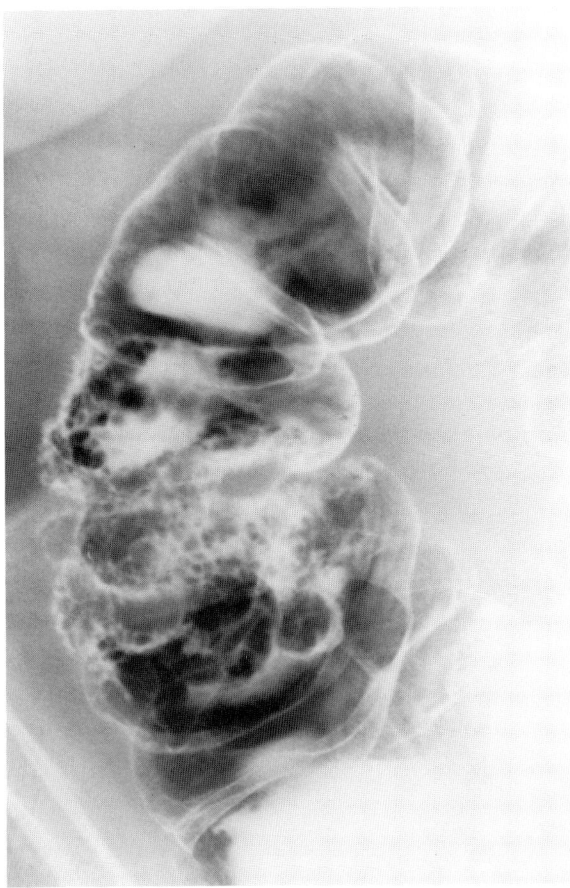

Fig. 4-11 Villous adenoma. Large soft tumor with multiple frondlike projections. Barium trapped between the projections results in the typical appearance of the tumor.

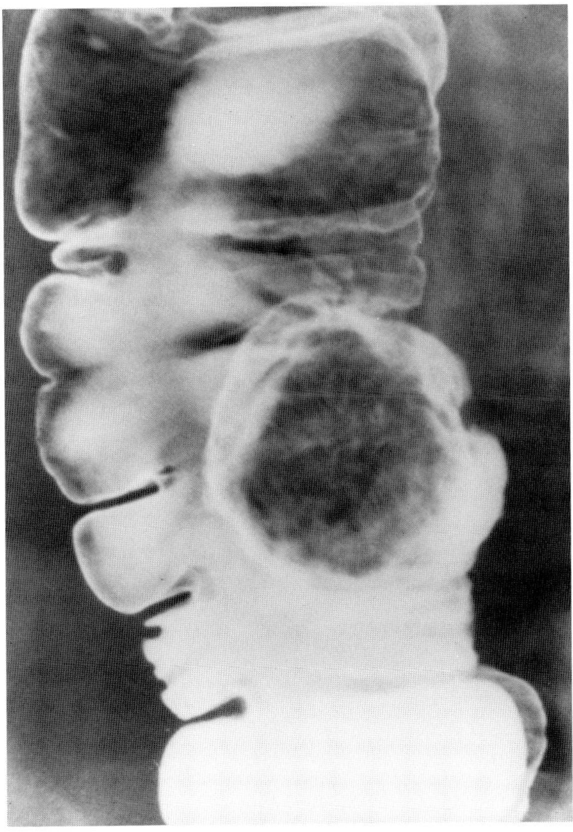

Fig. 4-10 Adenomatous polyp. Sessile polyp, 4-cm in diameter, in ascending colon. This polyp has atypical cells but no invasive carcinoma. Over 50 percent of adenomatous polyps this size are malignant.

ability to measure attenuation, is diagnostic if the lesion is large enough. Lipomas are completely benign; however, symptoms may occur secondary to ulceration, bleeding, or intussusception.

Other mesenchymal tumors, including leiomyomas, neuromas, or neurofibromas are very rare; only 3 percent of leiomyomas of the GI tract occur in the colon. Most of these are in the rectum. They appear as intramural lesions but if they are either under about 5 mm or larger than 2 cm, they may mimic mucosal lesions. Their shape is more fixed than that of lipomas; however, they may also serve as lead points for intussusception and ulcerate. The malignant counterparts of these lesions are exceedingly unusual.

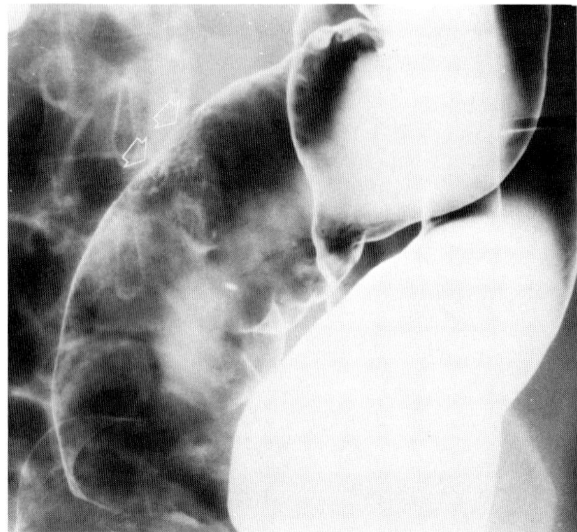

Fig. 4-12 Carpetlike lesion *(arrows)* secondary to a flat villous adenoma in the sigmoid. These lesions are soft. The lesion was missed on initial colonoscopy. Suboptimal radiographs will not show small flat lesions.

Hamartomas and Inflammatory Polyps

Hamartomas are aggregations of normal tissues in an abnormal location. Hamartomatous polyps are unusual in the colon and often associated with Peutz-Jegher Syndrome, which is discussed with intestinal polyposes. Cowden syndrome (multiple hamartoma syndrome), basal cell nevus syndrome, and Turcot syndrome are other rare conditions associated with colonic hamartomas.

Juvenile polyps are also hamartomas, sometimes classified as inflammatory or retention polyps. These are usually solitary lesions in the rectum. Most often seen in children, they occasionally occur in adults. The polyps are usually stalked and lobulated, indistinguishable from adenomas. They may cause intussusception, bleeding or obstruction, or they may prolapse. They may also autoamputate. The rare occurrence of multiple juvenile polyps is discussed with the polyposis syndromes.

Inflammatory polyps formed during the regenerative phase of any inflammatory colitis are mucosal lesions that may vary widely in size and number. They are discussed in more detail elsewhere. Polyps in Canada-

Cronkhite syndrome also are classified as inflammatory.

Carcinoid Tumors

In the colon, excluding the appendix, carcinoids are most often found in the rectum. They are detected as submucosal lesions or may protrude through the mucosa and be indistinguishable from other mucosal polyps. Most of these are found incidentally and behave as completely benign lesions. About 10 percent of rectal carcinoids are aggressive, invading the colonic wall and metastasizing. These represent less than 1 percent of malignant colon lesions. Although found much less frequently than rectal carcinoids, tumors arising elsewhere in the colon tend to be more aggressive and have poorer prognoses.

Endometriosis

Proliferation of endometrial tissue outside its normal location (heterotopia) occurs in about 10 percent of women between 25 and 40 years of age. The pathogenesis is unknown, but it is usually attributed to

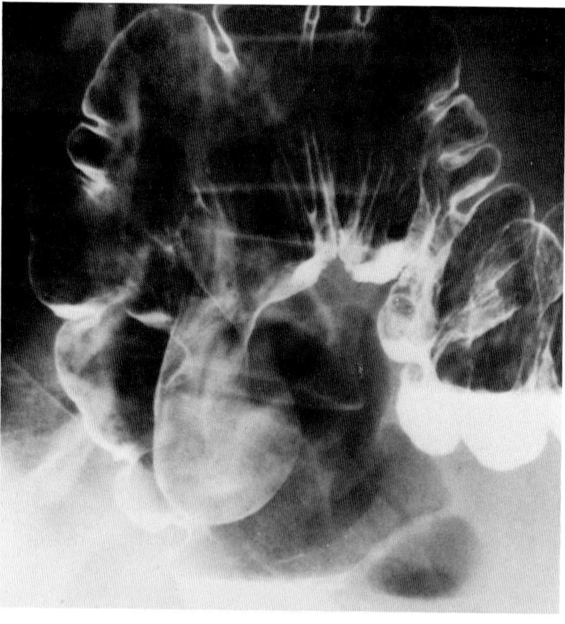

Fig. 4-13 Lipoma. Smooth sharply demarcated soft tissue mass in the hepatic flexure. With the patient erect the lesion appears like a broad-based teardrop. The soft, changeable shape is characteristic of a lipoma.

reflux of endometrial cells through the fallopian tubes and subsequent intraperitoneal spread. Hematogenous or lymphatic dissemination may occur. Others postulate the presence of congenital rests of tissue or differentiation of multipotential mesenchymal cells.

The clinical presentation is variable, most often involving pelvic pain, dyspareunia, and metromenorrhagia. When the colon is involved, there may be constipation, rectal pain, or diarrhea most severe during menses. Cyclical rectal bleeding may be pathognomic but is a rare occurrence and implies mucosal involvement. Involvement of the GI tract occurs most commonly in the pelvis, especially the rectosigmoid and ileocecal regions. Propensity for these areas of involvement is explained either by contiguity with the uterus, ovaries, and their supporting structures, or by intraperitioneal flow as described for metastases.

Endometrial implants originate in the subserosal layer and grow as a result of hormonal stimulations. They may erode through the mucosa. They also are believed to excite a fibrotic response, cause smooth muscle hypertrophy, or both.

A wide variety of radiographic appearances have been described with colonic involvement by endometriosis. Polypoid lesions or endometriomas, often indistinguishable from sessile neoplastic polyps, may occur. Short annular lesions are another appearance that may be difficult to distinguish from carcinoma. Implants in the bowel wall may cause smooth, scalloped lesions. Probably as a result of somewhat deeper invasion, there may be spiculation and puckering of the wall — the surface appearance on the double-contrast examination has been described as crinkled, or crenelated and is identical with the striped mucosal pattern seen with metastatic deposits (Fig. 4-14). Other radiographic appearances in endometriosis include long, tapered strictures. In some cases fibrosis may cause kinking, angulation, and shortening of the bowel. The most common affect of endometriosis on the colon is simply an extrinsic mass effect in the pelvis without any true involvement of the colon.

Polyposis Syndromes

The polyposis syndromes consist of a variety of conditions characterized by the presence of polypoid lesions in the GI tract. Although their histology, dis-

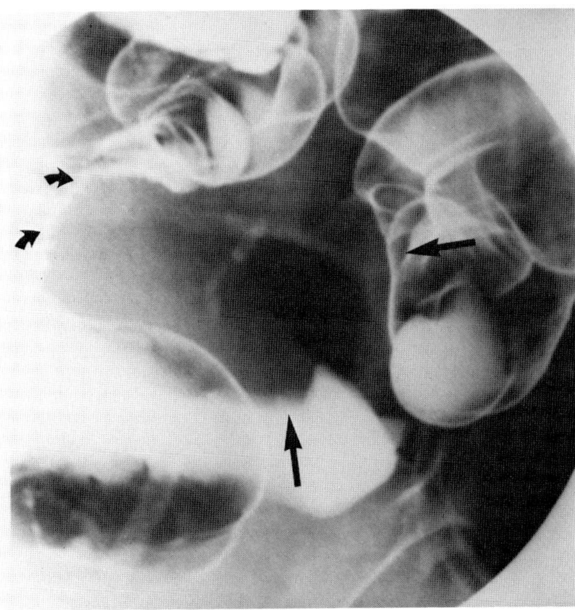

Fig. 4-14 Endometriosis. Pelvic mass causing extrinsic impression on cecum and contrast-filled bladder *(straight arrows)*. Spiculation of the anterior wall of the rectosigmoid *(curved arrows)* indicates mural involvement.

tribution, and inheritance features vary, they are grouped together because of their similarities on radiologic (and endoscopic) examination.

Familial polyposis and Peutz-Jegher syndrome are the most common intestinal polyposes but differ markedly in their characteristics. Gardner syndrome is closely related to familial polyposis and may represent the same disease. The bowel manifestations and consequences are exactly the same. In addition, Gardner syndrome has numerous extraintestinal manifestations. Each of the well-recognized polyposis syndromes is discussed below; their important features are listed in Table 4-2.

Familial polyposis is probably the most important of the polyposis syndromes because the incidence of colon cancer is virtually 100 percent, if the condition is untreated. It is inherited as a non-sex-linked autosomal dominant trait with very high penetrance and occurs in about 1 of 8,000 live births. Symptoms usually begin at about age 30 and include vague abdominal pain, diarrhea, or GI bleeding. Unfortunately, carcinomas are often present at the time of

Table 4-2 Multiple Intestinal Polyposes

Syndrome	Genetic Transmission[a]	Histology	Age Onset	Primary GI Involvement	Extraintestinal Associations	GI Malignancy
Familial polyposis	AD	Adenomas	35	Colon	—	100%
Gardner	AD	Adenomas	—	Colon	Osteomas, soft tissue tumors, sarcomas, ampullary carcinoma	100%
Peutz-Jeghers	AD	Adenomas	Childhood	Small Bowel	Increased skin mucous membrane pigment	Rare
Juvenile polyposis	AD	Hamartomas	Child–20s	Colon	—	?
Canada-Cronkhite	NH	Inflamm. hamartoma	>50	Stomach and colon	Ectodermal change	None
Turcot	?AR	Adenoma	—	Colon	Gliomas	100%
Cowden disease	AD	Hamartomas	Child	Stomach and colon	Circumoral Papillomas Gingival hyperplasia Incidence of breast and thyroid cancer	None

[a] AD = autosomal dominant
AR = autosomal recessive
NH = nonhereditary

diagnosis or develop shortly thereafter. Family members of a patient with familial polyposis, half of whom are also expected to be affected, should be screened for the presence of polyps after puberty.

The polyps are adenomas and a minimum of 100 is found in patients with familial polyposis. The polyps vary in appearance. They may be tiny and carpet the entire colon or they may vary quite widely in size and be scattered, but usually with a preponderance on the left side of the colon. Polyps may be sessile or stalked. When carcinomas develop, they are most likely to be polypoid or annular as with most other colon carcinomas. Adenomatous, hyperplastic, or both types of polyps occur in the stomach or small bowel in about 5 percent of cases.

Treatment, which is usually a total proctocolectomy, is performed when patients are in their twenties. Rectal-sparing procedures, although advocated by some, are controversial because rectal carcinomas may develop despite careful surveillance.

Gardner syndrome is manifested in the GI tract in exactly the same way as familial polyposis. These en-

tities are believed to represent a spectrum of the same disease process or separate mutations at the same allele. The extraintestinal manifestations of Gardner syndrome include osteomas and soft tissue tumors. Osteomas are most common in the head, especially the mandible and sinuses, but occur in the long bones as well. There is often fibrous proliferation manifested by desmoid tumors, peritoneal adhesions, mesenteric and retroperitoneal fibrosis, and keloid formation. Other mesenchymal tumors, including fibromas, leiomyomas, lipomas, neuromas, and occasionally their malignant counterparts also occur. Epidermoid cysts, hyperpigmentation, and a variety of dental abnormalities have been described. There is also reported to be an increased incidence of neoplasms of the ampulla of Vater and the thyroid.

The Peutz-Jegher syndrome is characterized by brownish mucocutaneous lesions, especially on the buccal mucosa, the palms, and the soles, in association with polyps of the GI tract. It is inherited as an autosomal non-sex-linked trait. The incidence is similar to that of familial polyposis. The polyps involve primarily the small intestine and are histologically hamartomas. They vary considerably in size, and large ones may cause obstruction or intussusception. Multiple polyps may be scattered throughout the small intestines. The colon, stomach, or both are involved in about 25 to 50 percent of the cases.

Patients may present with GI bleeding or obstructive symptoms, or they may remain asymptomatic. The hamartomas have practically no evidence of malignant degeneration, but patients with this syndrome may have a slightly increased incidence of stomach, duodenal, and ovarian malignancies. Adenomas as well as hamartomas may be found in the colon. These have the same malignant potential as other adenomas. Therefore, they require careful radiographic evaluation and often need to be biopsied.

Juvenile polyps are usually single and occur sporadically. Occasionally they may be multiple and considered a juvenile polyposis. There have been rare reports of inherited multiple juvenile polyposes. Juvenile polyps present in childhood in the overwhelming majority of cases. Rarely they may present in teenagers or even adults. Histologically, the polyps are hamartomas and are sometimes referred to as retention polyps. They are most common in the rectum and tend to be large, with smooth contours and thin stalks. They may present with bleeding, prolapse, or obstruction. They also tend to undergo autoamputation.

Turcot syndrome is a rare familial association between colonic polyps and gliomas of the brain or spinal cord. The colonic polyps are adenomatous with malignant potential; however, most of the patients succumb to their central nervous system lesions. The inheritance pattern is probably non-sex-linked autosomal recessive, and patients present in their teens.

Cowden disease (multiple hamartoma syndrome) is a rare genetic disorder associated with a wide variety of dysplasias, the most characteristic of which are cicumoral papillomatosis and nodular gingival hyperplasia. Benign and malignant lesions of the thyroid and breast occur. Multiple hamartomatous polyps have been described throughout the GI tract.

The blue rubber bleb–nevus syndrome is a rare angiodysplasia characterized by multiple cutaneous hemangiomas. Polypoid lesions, usually multiple, may be found in the small bowel, colon, and sometimes the stomach. They represent hemangiomas. In addition, other viscera may be involved. The skin lesions are usually apparent at birth. Gastrointestinal bleeding may be a serious complication. Most cases are sporadic, but the syndrome may be inherited as autosomal dominant.

Canada-Cronkhite syndrome is a rare, sporadic polyposis affecting people of middle or older age. The polyps have been described as inflammatory or hamartomas and have no increased evidence of malignancy. The condition may be fatal owing to severe diarrhea, electrolyte imbalance, malabsorption and general debilitation. There are several ectodermal changes in this syndrome, excluding alopecia, dystrophic nail changes, and hyperpigmentation.

Colon and stomach are involved in nearly all cases, whereas the small bowel is involved in 50 percent of cases. The rare presence of polyps in the esophagus has also been described. Myriads of tiny polyps are usually present, but there may also be larger, polypoid lesions.

The important characteristics of the polyposis syndromes are listed in Table 4-2.

Carcinoma

Carcinoma of the colon is the second most frequent cause of cancer-related deaths in the United States. Survival statistics vary considerably with the stage of disease at the time of detection. Adenomatous polyps less than 1 cm in size have less than a 1 percent incidence of malignant degeneration. Polyps between 1 and 2 cm have a 10 percent incidence of malignancy, which increases to 50 percent in polyps over 2 cm in size. Since most symptomatic patients have advanced lesions and most malignancies are believed to develop in preexisting polyps, it is clinically important to diagnose and remove small asymptomatic lesions.

Many groups of patients with a predisposition to colon cancer have been identified. The low-fiber, high-carbohydrate diet of western Europe and the United States appears to be a significant risk factor. Patients with colon cancer have an increased chance of having synchronous or metachronous lesions. The presence of other colonic polyps close to a malignant lesion (sentinel polyps) is also common. Patients with ulcerative colitis and, to a lesser extent, those with Crohn disease have an increased risk for developing colon carcinoma. All of the adenomatous polyposis syndromes carry an exceptionally high risk of colon carcinoma. Patients with other malignancies, a family history of carcioma, and previous ureterosigmoidostomy are also at risk.

It has been emphasized in the past that approximately 50 percent of large bowel carcinomas are diagnosed by digital rectal examination and approximately 67 to 75 percent are diagnosed by rigid sigmoidoscopy. However, recent reports suggest that there has been a change in the distribution of colorectal carcinomas. The site distribution of large bowel carcinomas, as analyzed recently in a large community teaching hospital, is presented in Fig. 4-15. In this study 3.5 percent had synchronous carcinomas. Others have reported as high an incidence as 9 percent. The current literature indicates that from 1937 to 1980 there has been a decrease in left-sided colonic and rectal carci-

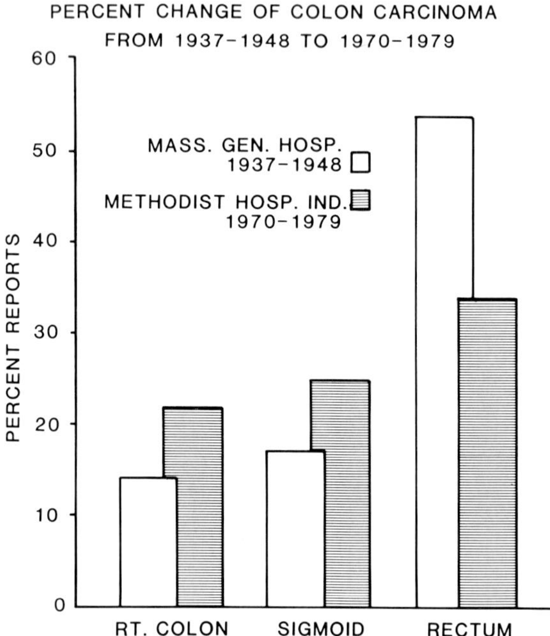

Fig. 4-16 Trends in distribution of rectal and right-sided colon lesions. Comparison of data from two large teaching institutions (Massachusetts General Hospital, Boston—1937 to 1948, and the Methodist Hospital of Indiana, Indianapolis—1970 to 1979). Although 19 percent of lesions are in the ascending colon and cecum, the majority of carcinomas (59 percent) remain in the sigmoid colon and rectum.

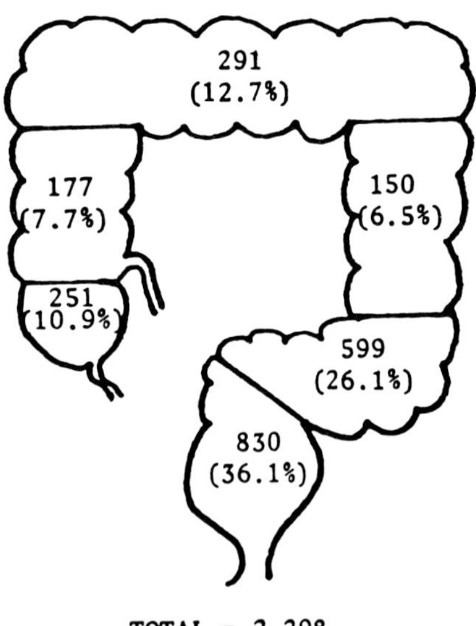

Fig. 4-15 Spatial distribution of colon carcinomas. The result of an analysis of all cases of colorectal carcinoma diagnosed from January 1, 1960 through December 31, 1979 at Methodist Hospital, Indianapolis. (Maglinte DDT, Keller KJ, Miller RE, Chernish SM: Colon and rectal carcinoma: Spatial distribution and detection. Radiology 147:669, 1983.)

noma, and an increase in the number of right-sided colonic malignancies (Fig. 4-16).

Adenocarcinoma accounts for over 95 percent of colonic malignancies. Most of these lesions are polypoid, ulcerative, or annular lesions. Ulceration usually occurs within the tumor mass. Tumor growth can be conceptualized as dysplastic changes in the head of a benign adenoma, which degenerate into frank malignancy and invade the polyp stalk. The polyp and stalk are retracted toward the surface of the lumen and the tumor then invades the colon wall. Disruption of the mucosal pattern is apparent. At this stage, the tumor may appear polypoid. Obstruction and intussusceptions may result from polypoid tumors (Fig. 4-17). As the tumor infiltrates the colon wall and grows around the circumference, it may assume a saddle-like configuration (involving half of the circumference) or an apple-core or annular lesion. Most annular lesions are found in the sigmoid. Intraluminal polypoid tumors,

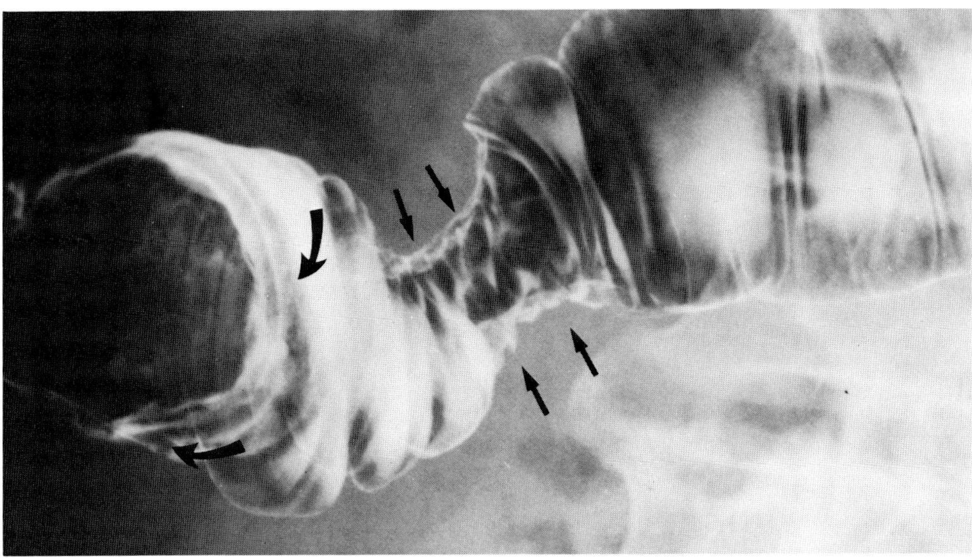

Fig. 4-17 An intussuscepted polypoid adenocarcinoma *(curved arrows)* caused complete obstruction to the flow of barium. A metastatic implant was found distal to the primary lesion *(arrows)*.

which commonly present with bleeding, are more common on the right side of the colon.

These tumors are easily demonstrated by barium examinations. Annular lesions are usually less than 4 cm long. The margins are abrupt, forming a shoulder or shelf with overhanging edges. These most often present with chronic obstructive symptoms. Spasm may mimic annular lesions. In the sigmoid, lesions may be obscured by overlapping loops of bowel. With the double-contrast technique, these lesions may be identified en face through the overlapping loops. Multiple projections with angled views best demonstrate such lesions (Fig. 4-18). Although annular lesions generally represent advanced colonic carcinoma, they usually do not have a significant extramural component. Thus, the barium enema may demonstrate them better than CT (Fig. 4-19).

Plaque-like lesions are another common morphologic presentation of carcinoma. These are relatively flat, irregular lesions, often with ulceration and deformity of the normal contour. These may be difficult to diagnose, if there is no prominent polypoid or ulcerated component. They may be identified by irregularities in surface contour or by barium-etched lines that run in abnormal directions. This corresponds to a slightly raised lesion with an abnormal mucosal surface.

Scirrhous carcinomas (infiltrating or linitis plastica) are rare but virulent tumors that may occur in the rectosigmoid region. Their growth is primarily submucosal, and they may be relatively long (5 to 10 cm). These tumors may mimic ischemic or inflammatory disease. Rarely, metastases from carcinoma of the breast have a similar appearance.

Contained perforation of a carcinoma is a relatively uncommon presentation. A retroperitoneal abscess may be the initial presentation of a colon carcinoma. This should be borne in mind when CT demonstrates an abscess adjacent to the extraperitoneal segments of the colon and appendix. These tumors may have an extraluminal mass effect and focal extravasation. The appearance may be indistinguishable from diverticulitis. If normal mucosal folds can be identified, the diagnosis would favor diverticulitis. Fistulas and obstruction of the small bowel or urinary tract may result.

Mucinous carcinomas have an abundance of mucus-producing cells with multiple hazy or punctate calcifications that may be identified radiographically in the primary or metastatic foci. Although colon carcinoma is uncommon under age 40, when it does occur in young patients it is likely to be of this type and runs a virulent course.

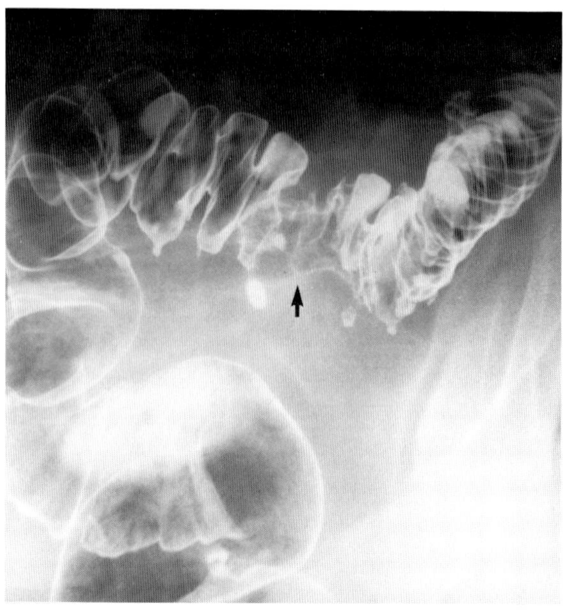

Fig. 4-18 Prone angled sigmoid projection. An area of narrowing with effaced folds *(arrow)* indicates mucosal destruction suggestive of a carcinoma. This should be differentiated from sigmoid diverticulitis (see Fig 4-38).

Cloacogenic carcinoma is another rare, aggressive tumor that arises from transitional cells at the anorectal junction. These are usually plaquelike lesions on the posterior or lateral wall of the rectum (see Fig. 4-2). Squamous cell carcinomas are also very rare.

Recurrence of tumor after resection may be identified by nodularity, eccentricity, and mass effect or narrowing at the anastomosis. Suture line recurrence is more common with colocolic than with ileocolic anastomosis. Pelvic recurrence and recurrence in the tumor bed is often better defined on CT scan than on barium study (Fig. 4-20).

Intraabdominal metastases may spread via the lymphatics with intraperitoneal seeding most often affecting the cul-de-sac, right lower quadrant, and superior aspect of the sigmoid. The radiographic appearance of metastases is the same as other serosal lesions.

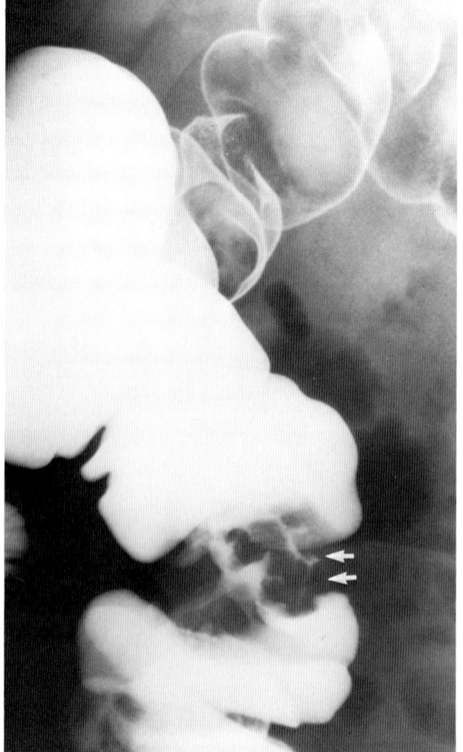

A

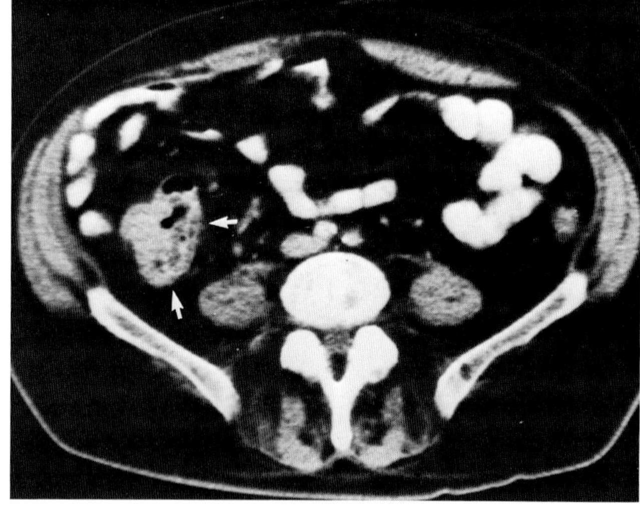

B

Fig. 4-19 Annular carcinoma. **(A)** A short circumferential infiltrating tumor is seen. There is extraluminal tracking of barium through the tumor mass *(arrows)*. **(B)** The lesion is not demonstrated as well on CT *(arrows)*.

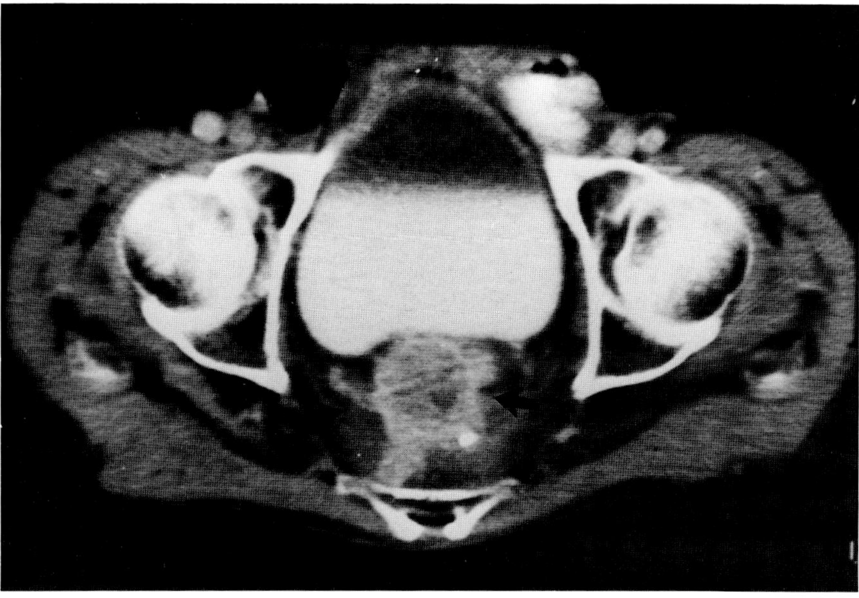

Fig. 4-20 CT demonstrated pelvic recurrence of carcinoma *(arrowhead)* in a patient with a prior abdominoperineal resection and colostomy for carcinoma of the rectum. Pelvic recurrence is common in these tumors and is difficult to detect on barium enema.

Lymphoma

Colonic involvement by lymphoma is unusual. When it does occur, it is most often a result of systemic disease. The stomach and small intestines are more likely to be involved than the esophagus or colon. Primary colonic lymphoma is very rare. Lesions may be large, bulky, fungating, polypoid masses with distortion of the mucosal folds. It usually occurs in the cecum or right colon. Obstruction is uncommon in spite of the tumor's bulk because the lesions are softer than a carcinoma of comparable size. Otherwise, polypoid lymphoma is indistinguishable from carcinoma.

Diffuse colonic involvement can result in multiple submucosal nodules of varying sizes, causing numerous polypoid defects. Folds may be diffusely thickened and have a relatively wide lumen and poor contactility. Unlike lymphoid hyperplasia in which nodules are of uniform size, the nodules in lymphoma vary from very tiny to several centimeters. Radiologically, the appearance is most easily confused with familial adenomatous polyposis (Fig. 4-21). Umbilications in lymphomatous nodules may simulate the

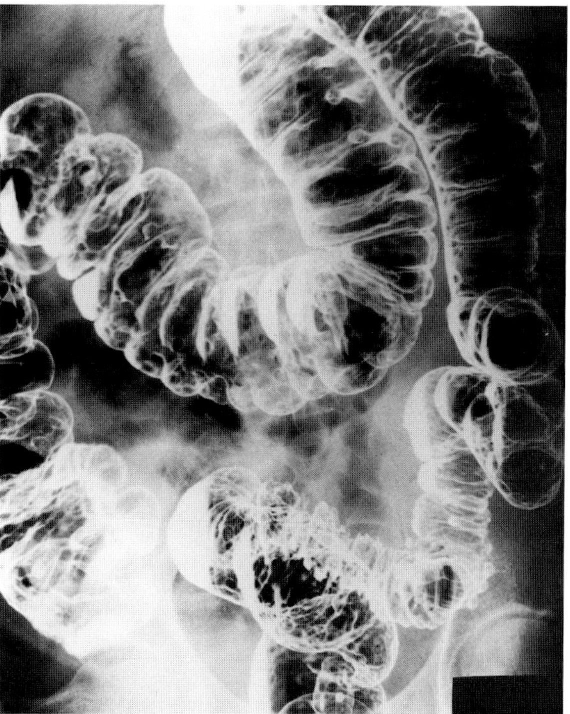

Fig. 4-21 Disseminated lymphoma. Numerous filling defects of variable sizes throughout the colon. Familial polyposis has a similar appearance.

aphthous ulcers in opportunistic colitis and early Crohn disease.

CROHN DISEASE

Crohn disease (granulomatous colitis) is the prototype for disease causing transmural inflammation of the intestines. The etiology and pathogenesis of Crohn disease are unknown. Granulomatous colitis and regional enteritis are other terms for Crohn disease, but are less specific; thus Crohn disease remains the preferred term. Epidemiologic data suggest that the disease is most common among people of European extraction, particularly Jewish people. The peak incidence of onset is between 15 and 30 years, and there appears to be some familial predisposition to the development of Crohn disease and ulcerative colitis.

Crohn disease may occur anywhere in the luminal GI tract from the mouth to the anus, unlike ulcerative colitis which is essentially confined to the colon. Histologically, the disease is characterized by transmural inflammation, especially by monocytes and histiocytes around lymphatic vessels, follicles, and Peyer patches. Discrete noncaseating granulomas are also found. The inflammatory process often extends into the mesentery and lymph nodes. Histologic abnormalities are often found in areas that are normal radiographically and endoscopically. Histologically, noncaseating granulomas are not a specific finding in Crohn disease. They may be found in many chronic inflammatory diseases and even in characteristic cases of Crohn disease based on clinical and radiographic criteria; they may be absent in up to 50 percent of patients.

Gross inspection in established disease shows rigidity and thickening of the bowel wall and mesentery, with increased fat and fibrous tissue "creeping" over the bowel wall. Angulation, stenosis, and fixation of bowel loops are common, with the mesenteric surface primarily involved. Although the descriptions of micro- and macroscopic findings of Crohn disease and ulcerative colitis sound very specific and distinct from each other, in about 20 percent of patients with only colon involvement it is impossible to make an unequivocal diagnosis of either entity. In such cases x-ray evaluation, especially of the terminal ileum and upper gastrointestinal tract (UGI) may be very helpful.

Anatomic distribution of the disease is very important. The small bowel is involved in 80 percent of patients with Crohn disease. Thirty percent of these have only small bowel involvement, whereas 50 percent have colon as well as small bowel involvement. A total of 70 percent of patients have colonic involvement and in 20 percent of those, only the colon is involved. Involvement of the entire colon (pancolitis) occurs in 25 percent of patients with colonic disease. Discontinuous areas of involvement, or skip lesions, are characteristic of Crohn disease; however, some data indicate that they may occur in as few as 25 percent of patients. Although *absence* of rectal disease strongly suggests Crohn disease as opposed to ulcerative colitis, it must be stressed that the rectum is involved in 25 to 50 percent of patients with colonic Crohn disease. Anal disease is common, and disease isolated to that area occurs in 1 to 2 percent of patients. Disease of the rectum, sigmoid, and the descending colon is more common in patients when the disease is limited to the colon. With ileal involvement, concurrent involvement of the cecum is most common.

Complications of Crohn disease are wide-ranging. Because the disease has a tendency to recur, particularly in proximity to operative sites, surgery is generally limited to treating the complications of Crohn disease. This is in contrast to ulcerative colitis where a total proctocolectomy is considered curative. Fistula formation is a very common and characteristic feature of Crohn disease, occurring in up to 50 percent of patients. Perianal and perirectal fistulas are particularly common. Fistulas may involve other organs of the gastrointestinal tract, urinary bladder, vagina, and skin.

Abdominal masses may be caused by inflammatory masses of thickened, matted bowel or there may be frank abscess formation. Because of the thickened bowel and walled-off abscess formation, free perforation in Crohn disease is very unusual.

Stricture formation is common and may lead to obstruction, although this complication is less common in the colon than in the small bowel.

The incidence of a carcinoma is higher in patients with Crohn disease than in the general population; however, it occurs only one-fourth as often as in patients with ulcerative colitis. Malignancy may develop in areas grossly uninvolved. Bypassed segments of small bowel appear to be at particular risk for the development of carcinoma.

Toxic megacolon occurs rarely in Crohn disease, but may occur with an acute presentation of the disease. Systemic complications of Crohn disease, especially when confined to the colon, are similar to those found in ulcerative colitis.

The contribution of radiologic studies is often invaluable, as the findings in established disease are often characteristic even with an unremarkable endoscopic evaluation. The double-contrast barium enema is the optimal examination for demonstrating superficial erosions (aphthous ulcers), which represent the earliest radiographic manifestation of the disease. Full-column studies may be preferable when the disease is complicated by sinus tract and fistula formation. Evaluation by computed tomography (CT) has proved exceptionally useful for demonstrating inflammatory masses and abscesses, both of which are frequent complications. Bowel wall thickness is evaluated more accurately by CT. A wall thickness greater than 10 mm suggests Crohn disease over ulcerative colitis; however, the bowel wall need not necessarily be that thick in Crohn disease, and it may be greater than 5 mm in ulcerative colitis. Hence, this is not a very reliable sign. Mesenteric fibrofatty changes, lymphadenopathy, and the extent of perirectal disease are also best evaluated by CT.

The earliest radiologic manifestation of Crohn disease, the aphthous-type ulcers, are small superficial erosions penetrating no deeper than the submucosa and surrounded by a lucent halo (Fig 4-22). These are found on a background of normal mucosa and are formed by necrosis of focal areas of lymphoid hyperplasia with a small amount of surrounding edema. Aphthous ulcers have been described as donut, target, or bull's-eye lesions. They may be the only radiographic findings in the early phase of the disease, or with a mild presentation. They may also be found in newly involved areas in a patient with active or well-established disease elsewhere. Aphthous ulcers may

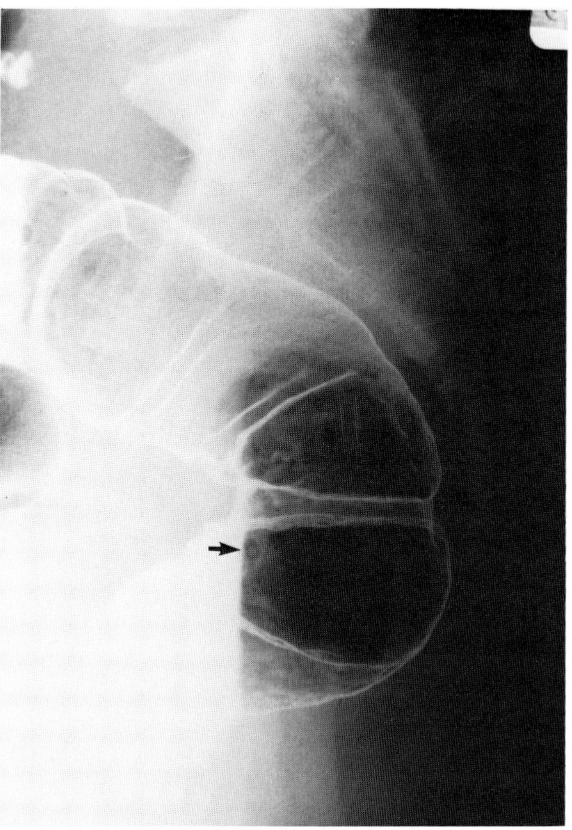

Fig. 4-22 Aphthous ulcers *(arrow)* in the rectum in a patient with Crohn disease. Background mucosa is normal. (Courtesy of Dr. AC Friedman.)

regress and occasionally heal without scarring; more often they progress to deep, more extensive areas of ulcerations. Sometimes aphthous ulcers persist for prolonged periods of time, either alone or with other manifestations of the disease.

With progression of disease, the well-established and characteristic features of Crohn disease predominate. Ulcerated regions become larger and deeper (Fig. 4-23). Typically the normal intervening mucosa is still identifiable, helping to distinguish Crohn disease from ulcerative colitis. Deep ulcers may appear identical to those of ulcerative colitis and have the configuration of a collar button, flask, or rosethorn. In the unusual case of severe pancolitis without disease elsewhere in the gastrointestinal tract, Crohn disease may be indistinguishable from ulcerative colitis, with deep confluent ulcerations.

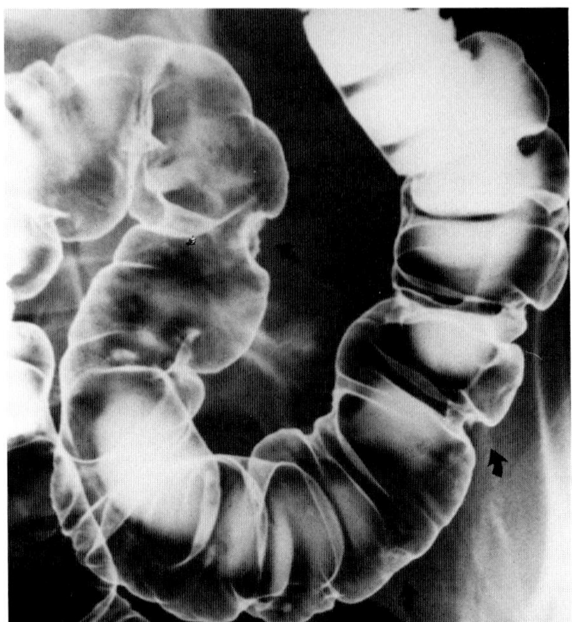

Fig. 4-23 Crohn disease. Scattered penetrating ulcers *(arrows)* with normal intervening mucosa found in same segment as aphthous ulcers.

Intervening areas of mucosa between the criss-crossing ulcers cause the cobblestoned appearance typically associated with Crohn disease (Fig. 4-24). Disease activity may regress, although the usual pattern is that of progression with scarring and the development of complications.

As bowel wall and mesenteric thickening progress and inflammatory masses develop, bowel loops become rigid and separate. This is often obvious in the small bowel but is also seen in the colon, especially in the relationships of the appendix, cecum, and sigmoid. Areas of the colon may be foreshortened and strictures and stenoses appear, leading to proximal obstruction. These strictures are generally not as smooth and tapered as seen with ulcerative colitis, and they have a much lower association with malignancy. Bowel retraction from thickened mesentery contributes to the typical asymmetry of the lesions. Asymmetric fibrosis with retraction of the mesenteric side of the bowel wall also leads to sacculation, another feature of Crohn disease.

Fistulas and abscesses are common complications of Crohn disease. These have a propensity to develop in the right lower-quadrant disease. Fistulas may occur between other viscera (Fig. 4-25), the genitourinary tract, and skin and muscle (psoas abscess). Perianal and perirectal fistulas are also common. Widening of the presacral space may occur as a result of fistulas and an inflammatory mass, but they may also be caused by narrowing of the area in chronic disease or the fat deposition associated with steroid therapy. Extraluminal complications of Crohn disease are often best demonstrated on CT examination (Fig. 4-26).

Polypoid lesions, including pseudopolyps, inflammatory, and postinflammatory polyps indistinguishable from those found in ulcerative colitis, are also found. These lesions have not been demonstrated to have malignant potential.

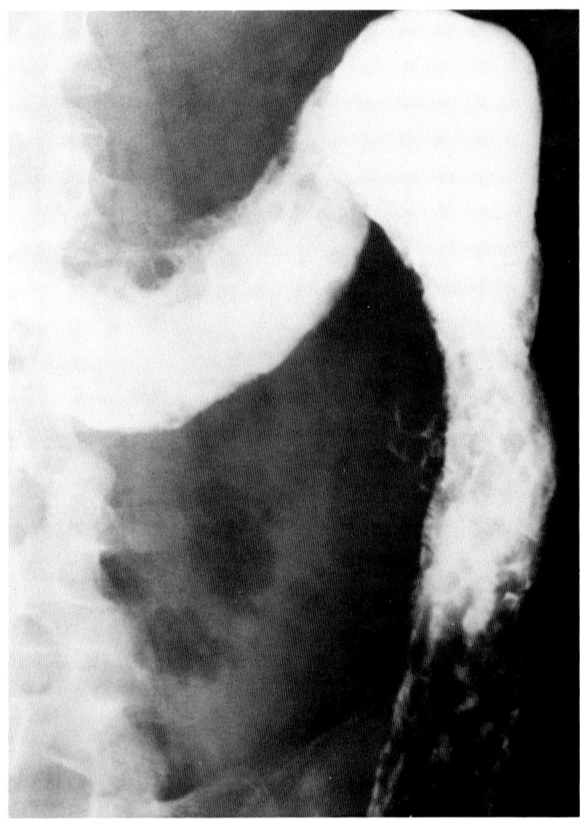

Fig. 4-24 Crohn disease. Advanced disease with "cobblestone" mucosa. Several small sinus tracts are also present.

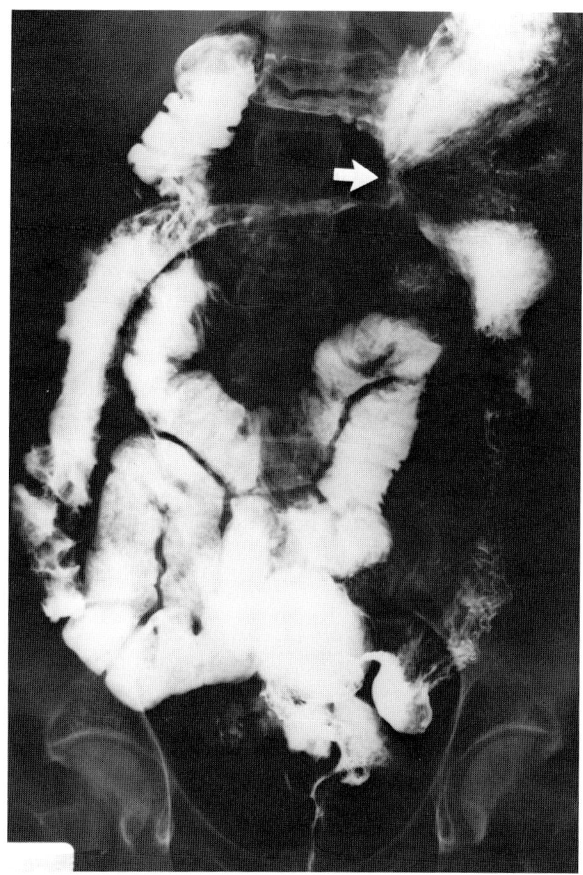

Fig. 4-25 Gastrocolic fistula *(arrow)* in patient with Crohn colitis.

Systemic associations with Crohn disease are wide-ranging and many are the same as those found in ulcerative colitis, including liver, bone, renal, skin, and hematologic disorders. Fistulas and abscess formation may be considered a manifestation rather than a complication of the disease, but these may lead to various complications, including renal obstruction (usually right ureter), anterior pararenal space abscesses, and inflammatory changes in the urinary bladder. Toxic megacolon occurs, but with a lesser frequency than with ulcerative colitis. Carcinomas also occur more commonly than in the general population, but again less often than in ulcerative colitis. Growth retardation is common in diseases presenting in childhood.

Differential diagnosis depends on the stage of the disease. Clinically and radiographically, the problem is generally to differentiate between ulcerative colitis and the colitis of Crohn disease. Infectious colitides must be ruled out in all cases. In the older population, the differential more often includes ischemic colitis and diverticulitis. Some investigators believe that in the older age group (over 50 years), most diagnoses of Crohn disease probably represent ischemic changes. Some of these patients have characteristic manifestations of Crohn disease with fistula formation, and other changes.

When the disease is manifested by aphthous ulcers, normal lymphoid follicles and innominate pits should be excluded. Of the pathologic conditions, the prime consideration is amebiasis. Bacterial (Yersinia) enterocolitis is also characterized by aphthous ulceration limited to the terminal ileum and proximal right colon.

Gonorrhea infection of the colon affects the rectum and sigmoid. Aphthous ulcers may be demonstrated on barium examination. There may also be considerable edema and spasm. Occasionally, rectal strictures may result from repeated infections.

Behcet syndrome, originally described as the association of oral and genital ulcers and occular inflammation, may also be associated with arthritis and inflammatory bowel disease. The colitis closely resembles Crohn disease in that aphthous ulcers or deeper, discrete ulcers with normal surrounding mucosa may be present. The lesions favor the right side of the colon. Bowel wall thickening and stricture formation are less dominant features and free perforation occurs more often. Because the etiology is unknown, this may be part of a large spectrum that includes inflammatory bowel disease and other arthritides, or it may be a distinct entity.

Deep ulcerations are found in many infectious colitides, including amebiasis, tuberculosis, histoplasmosis, shigellosis, salmonellosis, and others. In immunocompromised hosts, normally noninvasive organisms, including *Candida,* herpes, cryptosporidiosis, and cytomegalovirus, may be a cause of colitis.

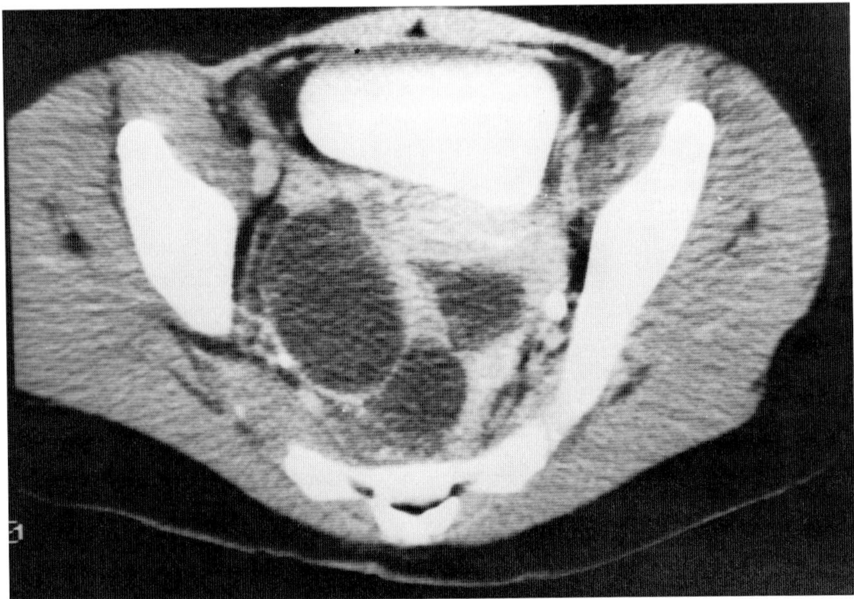

Fig. 4-26 Crohn disease. Large inflammatory mass in the pelvis.

The infection may vary in its seriousness and may be fatal.

Benign colonic ulcers are unusual, isolated ulcerations and are probably related to ischemic episodes. Ischemic colitis and acute radiation and other vasculitides may occasionally present with ulceration. Pseudomembranous colitis may mimic a colon severely ulcerated from any acute colitis.

The differential diagnosis for strictures includes ulcerative colitis, carcinoma, metastatic disease, lymphoma, amebiasis, tuberculosis, schistosomiasis, strongyloidiases, and lymphogranuloma venereum. Ischemia, radiation, and vasculitides also cause strictures. Rare causes include caustic colitis, pancreatitis, and endometriosis.

A constricted or coned cecum may be found in Crohn disease, tuberculosis and amebiasis, as well as with other chronic inflammation. Fistulas, often associated with stricture, are found characteristically in tuberculosis and actinomycosis, more often in the ileocecal area. Lymphogranuloma venereum always involves the rectum and may produce long strictures with extensive perirectal fistulas and abscesses.

Abscesses, fistulas, thickened bowel walls, and long, deep fissures parallel to the bowel lumen (double tracks) may be found in diverticulitis. It has been suggested that sinus tracts longer than 10 cm are more often associated with Crohn disease and short regions of involvement are more typical of diverticulitis, although this finding is nonspecific. The two diseases may coexist, and the differential may be difficult when the disease is confined to the left side of the colon. Pathologically, granuloma may be present in areas of chronic inflammation, further confusing the issue. Most often, other associated findings, including gastroduodenal, ileal or perianal disease, skip lesions, or extensive fistula formation will be present in Crohn disease. In contrast to Crohn disease, diverticula are rarely seen in the presence of ulcerative colitis.

ULCERATIVE COLITIS

Ulcerative colitis is an inflammatory disease of the colon of unknown etiology. Various studies indicate an incidence of about 5 per 100,000 population and a peak age of onset in the third decade of life. Some studies indicate a second peak in the fifth decade. Diarrhea and rectal bleeding are the most common presenting symptoms.

The disease primarily affects the mucosa; the submucosa in less involved. The pathophysiologic lesion is believed to be a sterile crypt abscess that involves the crypts of Lieberkun. Necrosis of the crypt epithelium and vascular engorgement of the intervening mucosa lead to the earliest visible changes.

Crypt abscesses are not unique to ulcerative colitis, and the diagnosis is made when a definable etiology for the signs and symptoms is not found. Several infectious colitides resemble ulcerative colitis clinically, pathologically, and radiologically. These include *Campylobacter, Shigella,* gonococcus, and *Entameba histolytica.* Toxic colitis, radiation colitis, and Crohn disease may also have crypt abscess formation. Although any of these entities may simulate it, idiopathic ulcerative colitis remains the prototype for all superficial colitides.

Ulcerative colitis may be associated with other systemic disorders. The pathologic basis is not well understood for any of these associations. Arthritis or arthalgias, predominantly affecting large joints, occur in about 25 percent of patients with ulcerative colitis. In addition, there is a higher incidence of ankylosing spondylitis and its variants, including isolated sacroileitis in patients with ulcerative colitis or their family members. This association is cited as support for an autoimmune etiology of ulerative colitis. Liver abnormalities occur in about 10 percent of patients with ulcerative colitis. The most striking of these radiologically is sclerosing cholangitis. Pericholangitis (which is in the spectrum of sclerosing cholangitis) and cholangiocarcinoma also are increased in incidence. Fatty infiltration or chronic active hepatitis are other liver disorders that occur with increased frequency. Dermatologic problems, most notably pyoderma gangrenosum and erythema nodosum, may complicate ulcerative colitis. Uveitis and episcleritis are the ocular conditions associated with ulcerative colitis. Various hematologic abnormalities, renal problems that include pyelonephritis as well as urolithiasis, and amyloidosis may complicate ulcerative colitis.

A characteristic of the disease is that it involves the colon only and is superficial, i.e., confined to mucosa

and submucosa in the uncomplicated state. The disease begins in the rectum and spreads continuously in a proximal fashion so that it may involve the entire colon. With universal colitis, the ileocecal valve gapes and backwash involvement of the terminal ileum occurs, the so-called reflux ulcerative ileitis.

Essential in the evaluation is assessment of the scout film for the possibility of toxic megacolon, the gravest complication of ulcerative colitis, before beginning a contrast study. The latter is contraindicated when toxic megacolon is a possibility. At this stage, because of its severity, the inflammation is transmural and may have a plain film appearance of edematous thick bowel wall with thumbprinting identical to ischemic changes (Fig. 4-27). Neuromuscular involvement leads to marked distension and thinning of the colon wall. Perforation can occur at either stage but is more frequent with a distended, thin-walled colon. The changes of toxic megacolon are usually most apparent in the transverse colon, possibly because its position is

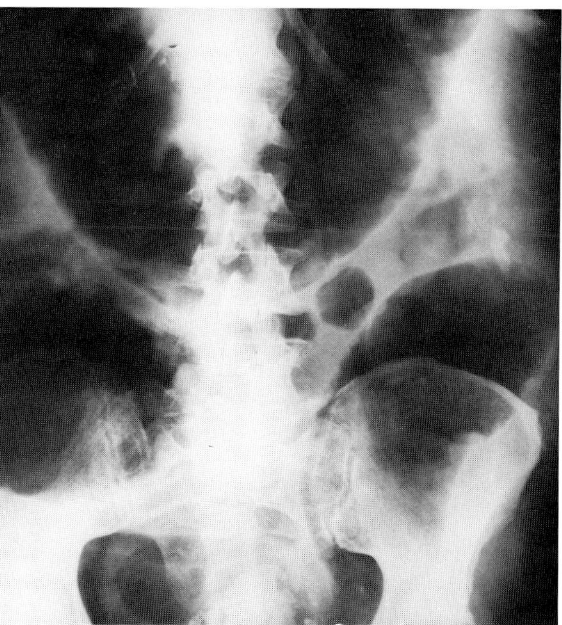

Fig. 4-27 Toxic megacolon in a patient with ulcerative colitis. The colon is diffusely dilated. Nodular soft tissue densities represent the en face appearance of submucosal edema and correspond to thumbprinting often seen along the bowel margins.

nondependent in the supine patient. Clinical toxicity and a change in lumen diameter are more important in the diagnosis of toxic megacolon than an absolute measurement of diameter. A transverse colon diameter greater than 5.5 cm and a cecum greater than 10 cm in diameter are usually considered abnormal. The entire colon may be of normal caliber but when it is gas-filled from cecum to rectum, a toxic megacolon should be suspected in a patient with known ulcerative colitis.

Plain radiographs are also useful in evaluating chronic disease. An air-filled foreshortened colon (lead pipe) of longstanding ulcerative colitis can be diagnosed on a plain film. The extent of active disease may be estimated because areas of active inflammation do not accumulate feces — e.g., a plain film in an unprepared patient with an empty left colon and with fecal debris

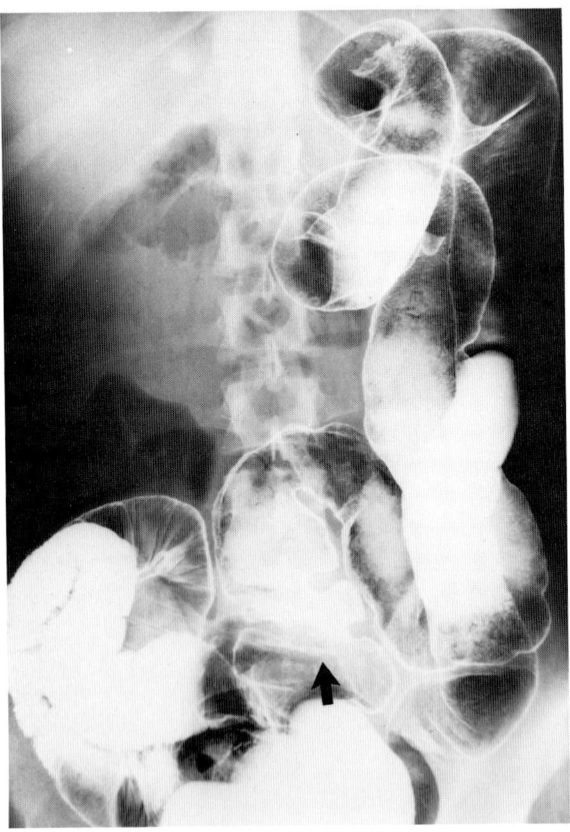

Fig. 4-28 The entire colon is left-sided. The ileocecal valve is marked with an arrow. Note diffuse mucosal granularity secondary to early ulcerative colitis.

on the right indicates left-sided disease. This is the basis of the instant enema, a useful technique in the follow-up of ulcerative colitis. Occasionally extensive inflammatory polyps, a manifestation of a healing phase of colitis, may appear as thumbprinting on plain film, mimicking toxic megacolon. Clinical correlation is essential.

The double-contrast enema is now uniformly accepted as the radiologic technique of choice for evaluating mucosal changes in any inflammatory bowel disease. Often, lesions are subtle and confined to the mucosa. Depending on clinical judgment, modifications may be necessary in patient preparation as well as in the proper timing of the examination during the course of a patient's attack. It should be stressed that the exam should not be done when there is risk of toxic megacolon or perforation. However, patients in remission may show little or no evidence of disease. It is, therefore, advisable to perform the barium enema during a relatively active, but not toxic phase of this disease rather than during a complete remission.

The earliest radiographic change of ulcerative colitis is that of uniform, fine mucosal granularity in the involved area (Fig. 4-28). There is also slight thickening and blurring of the mucosal line. These findings correspond to the endoscopic observation of an edematous, hyperemic mucosa. Fine stippling of the mucosal pattern, or a "grain of sand" appearance, corresponds to fine shallow ulcers in a friable mucosa (Fig. 4-29). These appear as fine serrations in profile and may be confused with filling of innominate grooves and pits seen occasionally in the normal patient. These are generally more regular and clearly defined against a background of normal mucosa.

As the disease increases in severity, ulceration becomes a more prominent feature and the mucosal pattern is more coarsely granular (Fig. 4-30). An even more coarsely granular mucosa, with little or no frank ulceration, is seen with chronic or inactive ulcerative colitis. At this stage, accompanying changes of shortening, straightening, and narrowing of the colon and rectum with loss of haustration and lead-pipe are often prominent features (Fig. 4-31).

The extent of ulceration correlates with the severity of the disease. Stippling of the finely granular mucosa

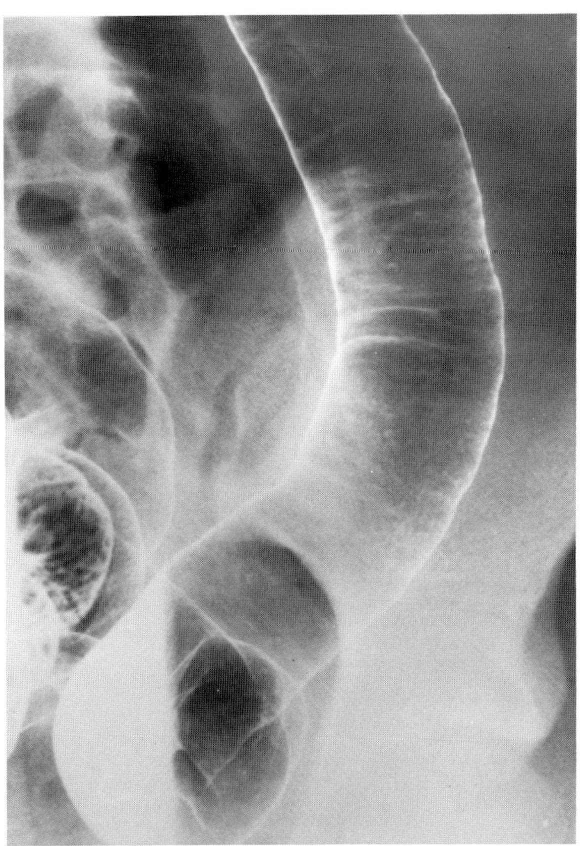

Fig. 4-29 Shallow ulcers in active ulcerative colitis.

Polypoid changes may be seen at all stages of inflammatory bowel disease of any etiology (Fig. 4-32). At each stage, the pathogenesis differs somewhat, but the radiologic findings overlap and are often not diagnostic. Thus, the terms pseudopolyp, inflammatory polyp, and postinflammatory polyp have been used interchangeably. With the presence of ulcerations, residual fragments of mucosa that are not actively ulcerated may assume a nodular or polypoid appearance. Thus, these mucosal remnants are often called pseudopolyps. However, since the entire mucosal surface is actively involved with inflammatory reaction in ulcerative colitis, histologically they are inflammatory polyps.

correlates with superficial ulceration of the friable mucosa. With increasing severity, the ulcers become deeper and often assume the characteristic shape of a flask, collar button, or T shape. This type of ulcer, although often found in ulcerative colitis, is not unique to this entity. The characteristic shape is caused by submucosal linear (longitudinal) extension of the ulcers with undermining of the mucosa. Nevertheless, the intervening mucosa is abnormal with a granular pattern. The submucosal ulceration may extend for a variable length. With the barium enema, the ulcers are apparent on profile as protrusions through the mucosal line. Pathologically, the ulcers are related to mucosal disruption secondary to crypt abscesses and are confined by the muscular layers (i.e., the disease is still not transmural). With very extensive ulceration and undermining of the mucosa, patches of mucosa may be sloughed and resemble the plaques of pseudomembranous colitis.

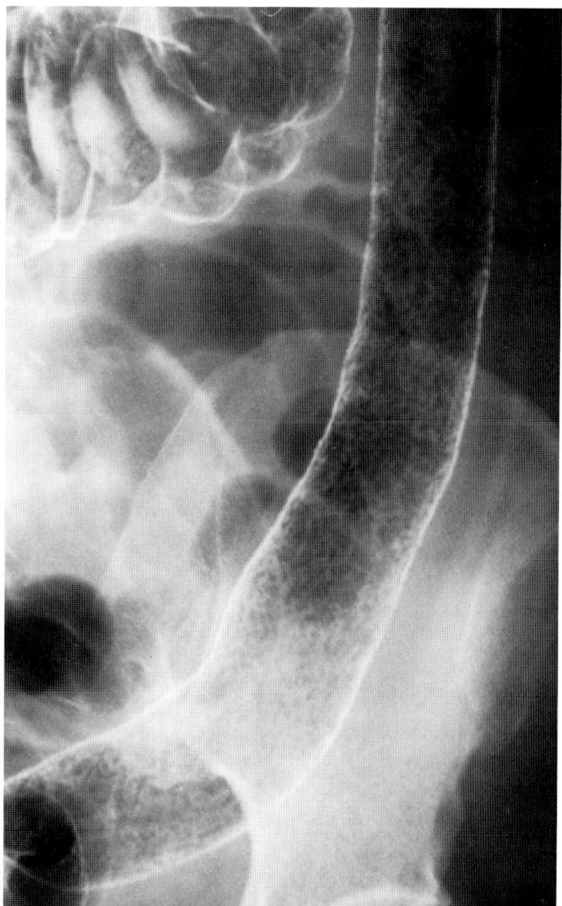

Fig. 4-30 Coarsely granular mucosa in chronic ulcerative colitis.

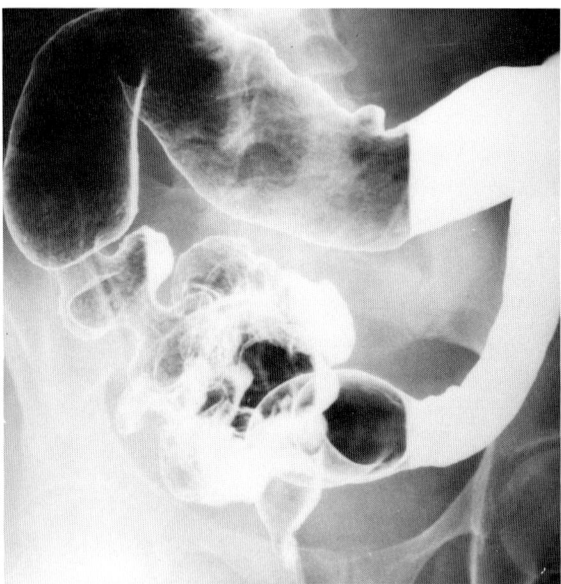

Fig. 4-31 Chronic ulcerative colitis. The entire colon is foreshortened with loss of haustral folds. The rectum is extremely narrow and rigid. The mucosa is very coarsely granular, consistent with inactive ulcerative colitis.

The mucosa of patients who have recovered from a bout of ulcerative colitis and no longer have active inflammation may show evidence of healing or regeneration. This leads to the visualization of polypoid filling defects on the barium enema. When these polyps are short and thin, they fit the description of filiform polyps, which are characteristic of regenerative mucosa (see Fig. 4-32B). These may be linear or branching and form mucosal bridges with both ends adherent to the mucosa. Any of the polypoid changes are seen in areas where there is, or has been active inflammation, but they occur only in about 15 percent of patients. They may be diffuse or segmental. They are more often multiple, but there may only be a scattered few or even a single sessile, nodular lesion. These cases may simulate a neoplastic polyp such as an adenoma, villous adenoma, or even a carcinoma, especially if the background mucosa appears to be normal. Diffuse nodularity may simulate thumbprinting on a plain film. Rarely, a mass of regenerative polyps may even obstruct the colon. Scattered filiform-type polyps may simulate small bits of adherent feces in a patient without prior colitis; excellent bowel preparation is required in these patients. It should be noted

that one of the polypoid changes in ulcerative colitis is neoplastic. The cobblestoned mucosa is a diffuse coarse nodularity usually associated with Crohn disease, but a similar appearance may also be seen in ulcerative colitis, or in other colitides.

Motility changes, especially spasm, widened haustral folds, and an abnormal mucosal fold pattern on a postevacuation film were changes stressed for the diagnosis of ulcerative colitis on single-contrast, barium enema studies. All of these changes, although certainly real, cannot evaluate early mucosal changes or small filiform polyps, and a double-contrast enema is the preferred technique.

In chronic end-stage ulcerative colitis, the colon becomes short and smooth with loss of haustrations and depression of the flexures. The lumen is narrow, tubular, and rigid, a configuration referred to as a lead pipe. Some of this appearance may be caused by fibrosis; however, most of the change is probably the result of hypertrophy of the muscularis mucosa and contraction of the mucosa by repeated reepithelization and granulation. Radiographically, at this stage it may be difficult to distinguish ulcerative colitis from other inflammatory bowel disorder.

Cathartic colon may simulate end-stage ulcerative colitis radiographically. However, this entity predominantly affects the right side of the colon, and although it is foreshortened and ahaustral, the colon is not rigid and areas of narrowing are not fixed.

Differentiating ulcerative colitis from the colitis of Crohn disease, which is a transmural disease, is not always clearcut. In about 15 percent of cases, they may be impossible to distinguish by any current means, including endoscopy or pathology. In 85 percent of patients differentiation between the two different inflammatory responses of the colon can be made with confidence. The distinguishing features are listed in Table 4-3.

The rectum and region of the ileocecal valve are the most critical areas in the colon regarding the distinction between ulcerative colitis and Crohn disease. In nearly every patient with ulcerative colitis, the rectum is involved. Patients with ulcerative colitis but without apparent rectal disease have frequently been

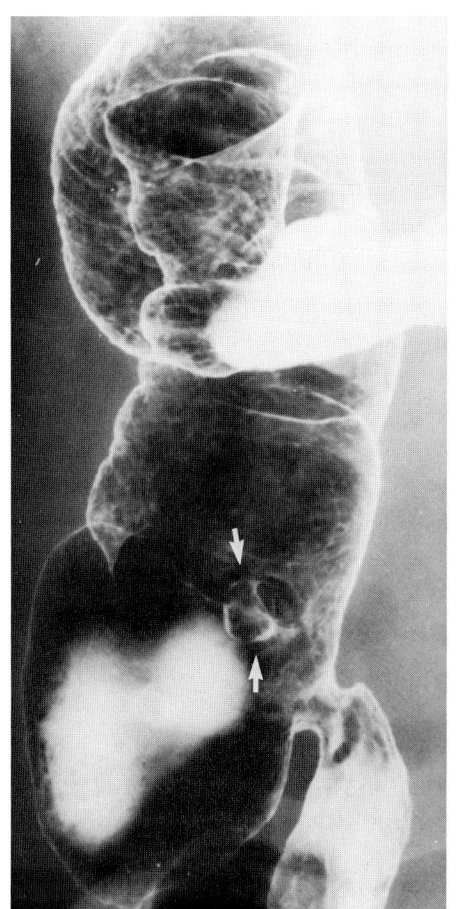
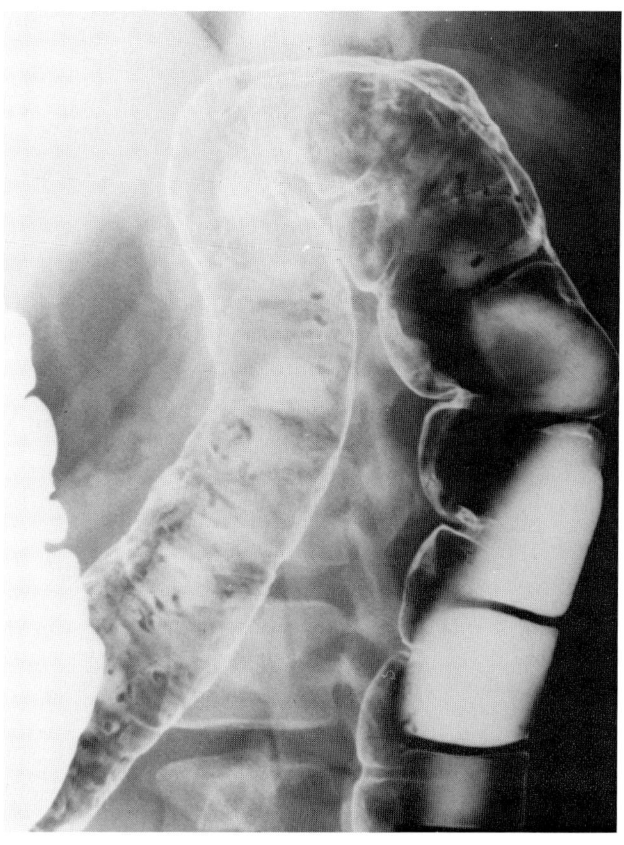

Fig. 4-32 **(A)** A polypoid filling defect *(arrows)* representing one of the many appearances of inflammatory polyps in a patient with ulcerative colitis. Note patulous ileocecal valve and "backwash" or reflux ulcerative ileitis. **(B)** Filiform polyps. Thin linear and branching filling defects found in the healing phase of inflammatory bowel disease in a patient with Crohn disease and in a patient with ulcerative colitis.

treated, especially with steroid enemas. The absence of rectal disease should strongly suggest Crohn disease, but the opposite is not true; 50 percent of patients with Crohn disease colitis have rectal involvement. Anal involvement and fistula formation on the other hand are characteristic of Crohn disease, and do not occur in ulcerative colitis, where the disease may be confined to the rectum or extend continuously to more proximal regions of the colon. As in other areas, rectal disease involves the entire mucosal surface, unlike Crohn disease which is patchy and segmental. With advanced inflammatory disease of any etiology, the rectum may become narrowed and nondistensible;

secondary widening of the presacral space is also observed but is an extremely nonspecific finding. Evaluation of the mucosal pattern and rectal distensibility are the important criteria in inflammation of the rectum.

Critical evaluation of the ileocecal valve and terminal ileum (TI) is essential. With ulcerative colitis, the ileocecal valve is either normal or gaping. In about 10 percent of cases there are changes in the terminal ileum. These changes are believed to be secondary to retrograde irritation of feces through an incompetent ileocecal valve. The TI may then be aperistaltic and

Table 4-3 Features Useful in Distinguishing Ulcerative Colitis from Crohn Disease

	Ulcerative Colitis	Crohn
Distribution	Confined to colon	May involve any area of GI tract
	Contiguous involvement from rectum proximally	Skip lesions
Rectal involvement	95%–100%	25%–50%
Anal involvement	No	Frequent fistulas and abscesses
Ileocecal valve	Gaping or normal	Narrow
Symmetry	Circumferential superficial	Eccenteric Transmural
Ulceration	Superficial	Deep or aphthoid
Background mucosa	Abnormal	Normal
Fistula	No	Frequent
Toxic megacolon	Infrequent	Rare
Pseudopolyps	Yes	Yes
Coexisting diverticula	Rare	May be present
Carcinoma	Significant increase after 8–10 years	Higher than general population, less than UC
Strictures	Yes	Yes
Surgery	Curative	May exacerbate disease

have a granular mucosa without discrete ulceration. This appearance, called backwash ileitis, contrasts with that of Crohn disease, where the TI is usually actively involved with narrowing, rigidity, and active ulceration. In cases where there is uncertainty about distinguishing the type of inflammatory bowel disease, it is often helpful to analyze the remainder of the GI tract since ulcerative colitis is confined to the mucosa, whereas Crohn disease may involve any part of the GI tract, from mouth to anus.

Complications of ulcerative colitis include toxic megacolon, development of strictures leading to obstructive symptoms, and predisposition to neoplastic change. Toxic megacolon may occur as an initial presentation of the disease or during subsequent exacerbation of ulcerative colitis in about 2 percent of cases. This is a grave complication of unknown etiology but probably involves extension of crypt abscesses into the muscularis, reflex neuromuscular changes, and possibly vascular changes as well. Its plain film findings have been described earlier.

Strictures develop in chronic disease in the actively involved bowel segments. These result from fibrosis or muscular hypertrophy, or they may be an "apparent" result of spasm. They are usually smooth and symmetric. Although the strictures are often benign, carcinomas in ulcerative colitis are often scirrhous and many feel that all strictures in this disease should be considered potentially malignant.

Development of malignancy in ulcerative colitis is often insidious; lesions are often scirrhous, multifocal, and may be indistinguishable from a benign stricture. Carcinoma is less often polypoid than in the general population and is more evenly distributed throughout the colon. It probably arises de novo in dysplastic mucosa, rather than in neoplastic polyps as most carcinomas probably develop.

Malignancy, in ulcerative colitis, develops with a frequency 5 to 30 times greater than in the average population and more often than in patients with Crohn disease. The risk of carcinoma increase significantly after a patient has had ulcerative colitis for more than 10 years, even if the disease is quiescent. Malignancy is more common in patients who develop symptoms during childhood and in those with pancolitis as opposed to those with disease limited to the rectum and sigmoid. Dysplastic changes in the mucosa have also been associated with a high incidence of malignant degeneration. Occasionally these may be suspected when patches of angular or faceted small nodules are seen on high quality radiographs from double-contrast barium enema studies in patients with inactive disease. Unfortunately, histologically detected dysplasia is often imperceptible both radiologically or endoscopically and requires random biopsies. Ulcerative colitis and its potential for malignant degeneration is believed to be cured by total proctocolectomy. An ileoanal anastomosis, stripping the anal mucosa but preserving the sphincter, is an alternative surgical procedure. With close clinical surveillance, definitive surgery may be postponed longer than in previous years.

The differential diagnosis of ulcerative colitis varies with the radiographic appearance at different stages of the disease.

An "end-stage" colon, which is foreshortened and ahaustral, may occur as a result of any longstanding colitis, and the specific etiology may be impossible to ascertain at this stage. Cathartic colitis is the other entity most likely to have a similar radiographic appearance.

The differential for polypoid change includes Crohn disease, where pseudopolyps or inflammatory polyps may appear identical to ulcerative colitis. Familial polyposis, which may simulate the extensive polypoid changes of ulcerative colitis, also has an increased incidence of malignancy; however, there is no inflammatory change. Malignant degeneration in polyposis syndromes usually occurs within existing polyps rather than infiltrating as is in ulcerative colitis. Patients with schistosomiasis may have multiple polypoid lesions as well as colonic narrowing and stricture formation. Occasionally, pseudopolyps, especially if single or few, may be mistaken for adenomatous polyps or even carcinomas. Colonic urticaria, generally related to edematous changes proximal to an obstruction, may also have a polypoid appearance. Strictures may be seen in Crohn disease, amebiasis, ischemic and radiation colitis, and schistosomiasis. Pseudostrictures may be seen in cathartic colon.

Manifestations of acute colitis, ranging from a finely granular mucosa to severe ulceration, may be seen in many infectious colitides. Most notably, these involve ameba, *Shigella, Campylobacter,* or *Salmonella.* Other infectious agents, not usually pathogenic in man, may cause acute colitis in immunocompromised patients. Crohn disease is usually segmental; aphthous ulcers are seen on a background of normal mucosa. However, in severe pancolitis, granulomatous findings may be indistinguishable from ulcerative colitis. Pseudomembranous colitis may also resemble severe ulcerative colitis. Findings are similar in ischemic colitis but there is more likely to be rectal sparing associated with extensive collateral circulation in that region. Gonorrhea, radiation colitis, traumatic colitis (proctitis), and colitis caused by caustic enemas are most likely to be limited to the rectum and sigmoid.

Toxic megacolon may also be caused by multiple etiologies. These include amebiasis, Chagas disease (Trypanosoma cruzi), ischemic and pseudomembranous colitis, Crohn disease, bacillary dysentery, colonic obstruction, and colonic ileus (pseudobstruction).

CATHARTIC COLON

Cathartic colon develops from chronic irritation of the colonic epithelium secondary to laxative abuse. Muscular activity is impaired or contractile force is insufficient to propel the colonic contents. The typical patient is a middle-aged female with a history of many years of constipation and chronic laxative use.

Contrast examination of the colon demonstrates a dilated colon with loss of haustral markings. Changes are more marked on the right side of the colon. The ileocecal valve is patent, and there may be secondary inflammatory changes in the terminal ileum. Overall, the colon remains distensible and pliable, but transient pseudostrictures may be seen. There may be overall shortening of the colon, but unlike ulcerative colitis the flexures remain in normal position. The rectum and sigmoid are relatively spared. The colonic mucosa is usually normal but may be somewhat granular because of chronic irritation (Fig. 4-33). The radiographic differential diagnosis is primarily that of burned-out ulcerative colitis. The significant characteristics of the two entities are listed in Table 4-4.

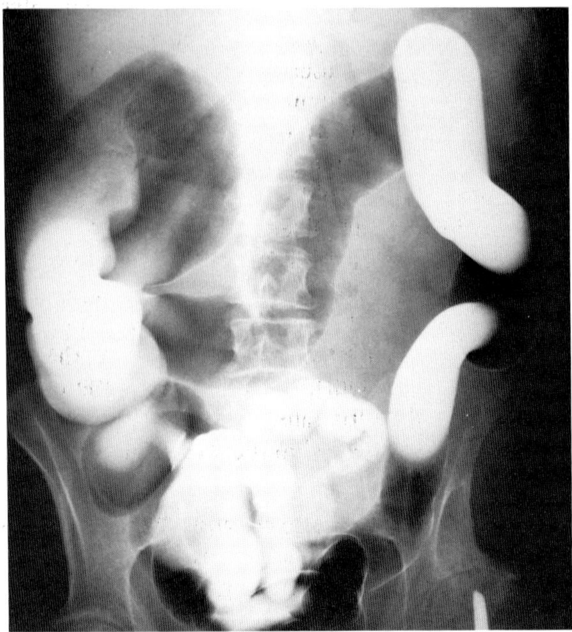

Fig. 4-33 Cathartic colon. The colon is smooth and ahaustral. Note normal position of flexures and massive reflux into distal ileum due to a gaping ileocecal valve.

ISCHEMIC COLITIS

Ischemic insult to the colon is caused by many underlying factors that manifest themselves with similar pathologic changes, all of which reflect impaired blood flow. Such changes may occur with venous obstruction; arterial occlusion, be it thrombotic or embolic; or with low flow states that result in hypoperfusion. Changes caused by radiation colitis or the vasculitides, which include systemic lupus erythematosus, polyarteritis nodosa, and allergic vasculitis, also reflect inadequate perfusion.

Clinically, acute ischemia is manifested by the abrupt onset of abdominal pain and tenderness, rectal bleeding ("cranberry" stool), and diarrhea. Bleeding and shock may be life-threatening. Chronic ischemia presents with milder symptoms. Patients in whom there should be a high suspicion of ischemic bowel disease include those over 50 years of age with a history of cardiovascular disease, including atherosclerosis, prosthetic valves, and vascular bypass, as well as any hypercoagulable state. The latter includes young women on birth control pills and patients with sickle cell disease.

Pathologically, the mucosa, being the most sensitive tissue layer, is affected earliest with hyperemia and superficial ulceration. Submucosal edema and hemorrhage may follow along with more extensive ulceration and mucosal sloughing. Superimposed bacterial invasion probably plays a role as well, but its course is variable. In some cases, the findings resolve completely. On the other hand, the acute episode may be severe enough to result in a toxic colon, peritonitis and perforation, and bowel infarctions. Late changes also include stricture formation. Skip areas may be present.

Classically, the sites of involvement have been the watershed areas of vascular supply, especially the splenic flexure where there may not be significant collateral circulation. However, various studies have found considerable variation in collateral blood supply; fewer cases of ischemia than expected have been found in the splenic flexure and a significant number in the rectum, which should have a generous collateral supply. Chronic ischemia may be expected to permit development of an extensive collateral blood supply.

Table 4-4 Differential Diagnosis of Cathartic Colon from Burned-Out Ulcerative Colitis

Ulcerative Colitis	Cathartic Colitis
More left side involvement	More right side involvement
Ulcerated mucosa	Smooth mucosa
Rigid bowel (lead pipe)	Distensible bowel
Short contracted colon	Short colon but normal position of flexure
Strictures	Inconstant pseudostrictures
Gaping ileocecal valve	Gaping ileocecal valve
Backwash ileitis	Backwash ileitis

Radiographic changes reflect the severity of the process. Plain films of the abdomen should be obtained as the initial study. In older, hospitalized patients, ischemia must be kept highly suspect since early changes are subtle and may be those of an ileus with mild diffuse bowel dilatation or an empty abdomen caused by spasm and bowel narrowing. Thumbprinting is a result of significant bowel wall thickening from submucosal edema, hemorrhage, or both. Plain films may mimic a mechanical obstruction. Ischemia may also develop either proximal to a true mechanical obstruction or within a closed loop obstruction. With severe ischemic insult, a toxic megacolon may occur. Pneumatosis manifested by linear collections of intramural air should suggest the presence of bowel necrosis. However, it should be remembered that other, less ominous causes of pneumatosis may also occur in patients with suspected ischemia. The presence of gas in the portal venous system of adults is nearly always associated with a grave prognosis.

In the acute stage of an ischemic event, angiography is often the most useful imaging modality as it may demonstrate emboli, plaques, or the narrowing and spasm associated with low flow states. Vasculitides, aneurysms, and other causes of pathology, including tumors, may also be seen.

Barium studies are most often useful in the subacute and chronic stages. The earliest changes are thickening of the bowel folds and wall associated with narowing and spasm. This is reflected as scalloping or thumbprinting of the bowel wall. Thumbprinting may cause multiple, nodular filling defects that may mimic multiple polyps. Ulceration may be superficial or deep, segmental, or generalized. Studies performed at least a month after an acute event may show a complete reversal of the abnormal findings (Fig. 4-34). In these cases, the ischemia is considered to be transient. If significant fibrosis occurs with healing, stricture formation ensues. Strictures tend to be

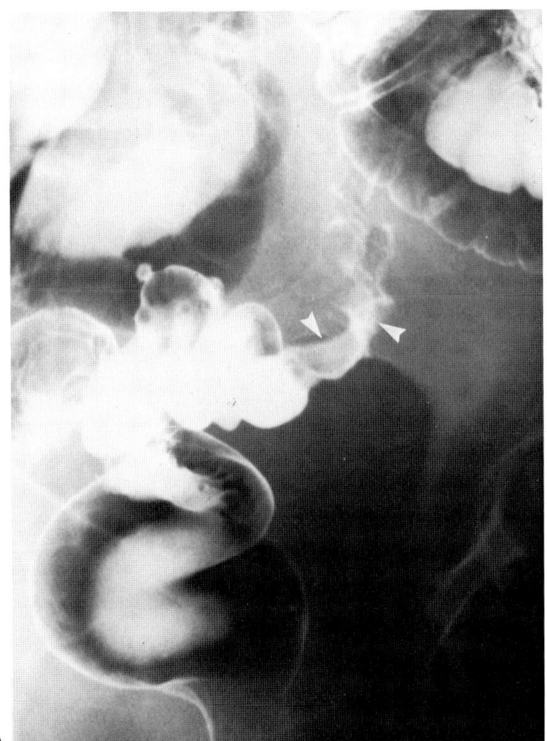

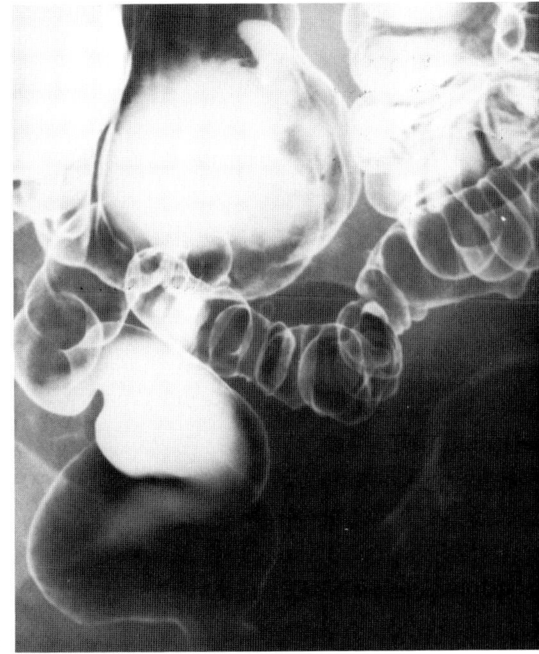

Fig. 4-34 Transient sigmoid ischemia. **(A)** Thumbprints *(arrowheads)* as well as spasm are present in the sigmoid. **(B)** Repeat barium enema after 1 month shows complete clearing of submucosal defects.

shorter than the area initially involved with ischemic changes. They may be long and smooth with tapering margins or asymmetric and sacculated. Pseudodiverticular formation resembling scleroderma has also been seen.

The radiographic changes on any given examination are likely to mimic those seen in either ulcerative colitis or Crohn disease. The clinical presentation and serial examinations are most helpful in distinguishing the entities, although there are some areas of overlap and controversy.

The differential diagnosis of ischemic disease is extensive. The rapid evolution of findings and the remission of symptoms over about a month suggest ischemia. That the rectum is spared and fistula and sinus tract formation are lacking are also suggestive. When colonic ischemia is diagnosed, a lesion distal to the ischemic segment, especially carcinoma, should be excluded.

DIFFERENTIAL DIAGNOSIS OF ISCHEMIC COLITIS

Crohn colitis

Ulcerative colitis

Infectious colitides

Vasculitis (similar pathogenesis)

Mural hemorrhage (anticoagulation, hemophilia, trauma, etc.)

Diverticular disease

Segmental extrinsic inflammation (e.g. pancreatitis)

Lymphoma

Polyposes (with extensive thumbprinting)

Scleroderma (sacculation)

INFECTIOUS COLITIS

Numerous infectious agents, including viruses, bacteria, fungi, protozoans, and worms are known to cause colitis. Most of these are of epidemiologic sig-

nificance in tropical climates or in immunocompromised hosts. Radiographic findings cover the spectrum described with ulcerative colitis and Crohn disease. Some of the organisms are much more likely to cause superficial reactions, as with ulcerative colitis, and others tend to be transmural, as with Crohn disease. Some have a clear predilection for specific areas of the bowel. All cases of colitis should include a complete workup to discover any possible infectious etiology. Where relevant, specific radiologic findings, which should increase suspicion of a particular agent, are emphasized.

Amebiasis

Amebic dysentery caused by *Entameba histolytica* is of particular importance because its distribution is worldwide and it has a wide range of radiographic and pathologic manifestations. The most common clinical presentation is bloody diarrhea with colicky abdominal pain. Infection is caused by the ingestion of protozoan cysts. Trophozoites released in the small bowel travel into the colon, where they release proteolytic enzymes and hyaluronidases that lyse the intestinal epithelium. The trophozoites also cause disease by burrowing into the mucosa, forming flask-shaped ulcers. Superinfection with bacteria is common. With heavy infestation, toxic megacolon and perforation may occur. The infection may resolve completely or it may progress and induce multiple systemic complications. The most serious complication is the migration of amebae to the liver, through the portal circulation where infectious cysts form. These may then rupture into the pleura and lungs, leading to widespread, often fatal disease.

Chronic manifestations of colonic disease include stricture formation, most often in the cecum; flexures; inflammatory polyposis; and, sometimes, localized abscesses, any of which may resemble idiopathic inflammatory bowel disease. The coned cecum, without involvement of the terminal ileum, is typical of amebiasis.

Amebomas, or mass lesions caused by infection and fibrosis, occur in the cecum or rectum and may be difficult to distinguish from carcinomas. They may also mimic diverticulitis when the mass is extraluminal and associated with narrowing of the lumen. Occasionally they obstruct the bowel.

During the acute phase of infestation there may be a diffuse colitis with superficial ulceration similar to that of ulcerative colitis. More often, deep flask- or collar-button-shaped ulcers are present; discontinuous, eccentric lesions in the cecum, rectosigmoid, and flexures, simulate those of Crohn disease. Unlike Crohn disease, however, the small bowel is rarely affected. With a fulminant infection, there may be severe widespread ulceration, wall thickening, and thumbprinting similar to those found with ischemic hemorrhage. Toxic megacolon and perforation may occur. Severe infection confined to the cecum and appendix may be considered a form of typhlitis.

Tuberculosis

Intestinal tuberculosis is uncommon in North America but is still common in Asia and Africa. Patients at high risk for tuberculosis in North America are intravenous drug abusers, the immunocompromised, and those with chronic debilitating disease. In Africa, annular lesions are more likely to be tuberculosis than carcinoma of the colon. The disease is caused by infection with acid-fast mycobacterium — primary intestinal tuberculosis from milk infected with *M. bovis*. Intestinal tuberculosis may also be caused by hematogenous and lymphatic spread, usually from primary pulmonary disease. Only about 50 percent of patients with intestinal tuberculosis have radiographically evident pulmonary disease. Intestinal tuberculosis causes a hypertrophic, ulcerative, or mixed type lesion. Small bowel mesenteric involvement is common.

Involvement of the ileocecal region occurs in 80 to 90 percent of patients with intestinal tuberculosis, but diffuse colitis is a distinctly rare entity. The clinical and radiologic features closely resemble Crohn disease. In the ileocecal region, there may be edema and ulceration early in the course of the disease. The cecum may be contracted and cone-shaped in the chronic state. The terminal ileum is narrow (Stierlin sign) in contradistinction to amebiasis, where the terminal ileum is usually normal. The ileocecal valve itself may be fixed in a gaping position with a triangular deformity and narrowing of the cecum (Fleischner sign).

The hypertrophic form of tuberculosis causes abdominal masses, bowel stenoses, and strictures that may cause obstruction. The strictures may involve skip areas. Diseases isolated to areas of colon other than the ileocecal region are rare. Fistula formation may occur, but free perforation is rare. Actinomycosis and blastomycosis (Brazilian) are other infections with a predilection to extensive fistula formation in the right lower quadrant. Lymphoma and Crohn disease should also be considered in the differential diagnosis of hypertrophic tuberculosis.

Shigellosis

Bacterial dysentery caused by shigellosis may clinically involve the central nervous system and is associated with acute, severe diarrhea. The bacterial pathogen is either *Shigella sonnei* or *S. flexneri*. Radiographic findings usually demonstrate superficial ulceration of the colon, which is most severe in the rectosigmoid and similar to ulcerative colitis in this respect.

Salmonella

Dysentery caused by *Salmonella* usually results from food poisoning. Findings are generally confined to the colon. The mucosa is inflamed and edematous, similar to ulcerative colitis, but the right side of the colon is more commonly involved. Barium studies are rarely performed because the disease is acute and self-limited. There may also be associated lymphoid hyperplasia. Other species of *Salmonella* (*S. typhi* and *S. paratyphi*) involve the small bowel. *S. typhi* and *S. paratyphi* (typhoid and paratyphoid fevers) are systemic infections. Lymphoid hyperplasia and ulceration may be found in the ascending colon and terminal ileum.

Campylobacter

Campylobacter fetus jejuni is a recently recognized but common cause of infectious colitis. It presents with acute diarrhea, abdominal pain, and fever. The mucosa is inflamed with bloody exudate; radiographically it is indistinguishable from acute ulcerative colitis. *Campylobacter* colitis is usually self-limited and heals completely.

Lymphogranuloma Venereum

This venereal disease, a chlamydial infection, causes a severe vesicular and ulcerative proctitis. It may progress to cause pelvic, perineal, and anorectal abscesses as well as fistulas associated with severe femoral and inguinal adenopathy. Considerable fibrosis accompanies healing and stenosis; stricture formation is characteristic of the late stage of the disease.

Radiographically, rectal strictures are most characteristic. They begin just above the anus and are of variable length (up to 25 cm). The strictures may be very severe and resemble strings or tubes (Fig. 4-35). Widening of the presacral space is also common. During the acute phase of the disease, multiple deep ulcerations are demonstrated in the rectum. Sinus tracks, fistulas, and abscess cavities may also be filled on contrast examination.

Differential diagnosis includes Crohn proctitis, radiation, scirrhous carcinoma, syphilis, and metastases.

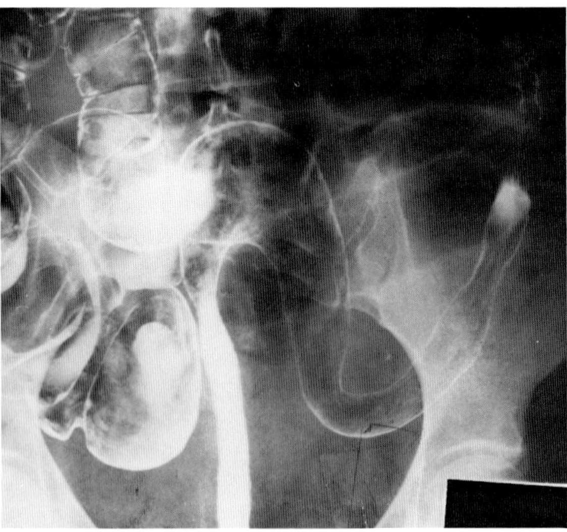

Fig. 4-35 Lymphogranuloma venereum. Fibrotic stage of the disease with long smooth stricture of the rectum and sigmoid. This patient did not have a fistula or abscess at this time.

Gonococcus infection causes ulcerative changes that are usually confined to the rectum. Radiographically, the appearance may be indistinguishable from idiopathic ulcerative proctitis.

Viral Colitis

Viral colitides are opportunistic infections caused by viruses and are prone to occur in patients with acquired immunodeficiency syndrome (AIDS), transplants, and other immunocompromised hosts. Herpes and cytomegalovirus may manifest radiographically with aphthous-type lesions or deep penetrating ulcers similar to those of Crohn disease but with a tendency to perforate. It may also manifest as thickening of the bowel wall and focal spasm, much like ischemia.

Yersinia Enterocolitis

Yersinia causes smooth, nodular lesions owing to lymphoid hyperplasia. These are most often confined to the terminal ileum but may extend into the ascending colon. Ulceration simulating Crohn disease may occur. *Yersinia* is probably responsible for many cases previously diagnosed as spontaneously resolving Crohn disease.

Strongyloides stercoralis

S. stercoralis is similar to hookworm. Infection occurs by skin penetration. It usually affects the duodenum and jejunum. The colon may be ulcerated, mimicking ulcerative colitis. Strictures occasionally are found.

Anisakiasis

This ascaris-like nematode is acquired from the ingestion of raw fish, and is found mainly in Japan. Infection results in thickening of the bowel wall of the cecum and terminal ileum.

Oesophagostomum

This nematode is usually found in monkeys and apes. Larvae penetrate the colonic wall. Transmural nodular lesions, fibrosis, and inflammation may be found in the colon, extending into pericolonic tissue. The lesions may ulcerate to form abscesses.

Trichiuris trichiura (Whipworm)

Whipworm is a common infection, which may cause severe chronic diarrhea. It may be found incidentally on barium study. The worms may be identified as small coils or wavy lines associated with an edematous mucosa. Rectal prolapse may also occur.

Schistosomiasis (Bilharhziasis)

Schistosomiasis is caused by infection wth blood flukes of the species *Schistosoma*. The colon is the most commonly affected region of the luminal GI tract. Ova are deposited in the inferior mesenteric vein, hence the rectum, sigmoid, and descending colon are usually involved.

The early changes on a double-contrast barium enema may be that of an edematous mucosa. Fine ulcerations may create a granular mucosal pattern. Heavy infestations cause a granulomatous reaction that leads to multiple polypoid defects. These are occasionally large enough to cause colonic obstruction. Fibrotic strictures may result from the healing process. Extrinsic colonic impressions from an enlarged liver and spleen occur as a result of portal hypertension associated with schistosomiasis.

Chagas Disease

This disease, found in Central and South America, is caused by *Trypanosoma cruzi*. The protozoan destroys ganglion cells. Cardiomyopathy is the most serious manifestation of the disease. The colon and esophagus are also commonly involved, causing megacolon and megaesophagus. The colon is markedly distended, often with chronic fecal impactions. The findings are identical to Hirschsprung disease. These patients are predisposed to the development of volvulus.

NECROTIZING ENTEROCOLITIS

Necrotizing enterocolitis is an entity found in neonates, especially premature babies, and presents as bloody diarrhea. The etiology is unknown. Breast feeding appears to afford some protection against its development. The small bowel is involved preferentially; however, the colon is often affected as well. Patients are followed with plain films; contrast studies are rarely, if ever, performed.

Early radiographic findings may be subtle distension of bowel. The bowel wall may become scalloped and hazy, and bowel loops may separate. The development of intramural, usually linear collections of gas parallel to the bowel lumen (pneumatosis intestinalis) is characteristic of the disease. Necrotizing enterocolitis may be complicated by the development of portal venous gas, bowel perforation, and rarely stricture formation.

RADIATION COLITIS

The effects of radiation in the colon are usually confined to the rectum and sigmoid and occur secondary to pelvic irradiation. Treatment of gynecologic malignancies with internal and external radiation lead to the most severe reactions. With current dosage regimens, it is much more common to see chronic rather than acute radiation changes. With acute radiation damage, the appearance of the rectum is indistinguishable from ulcerative proctitis or proctosigmoiditis with a diffusely granular mucosa. Thickening of the bowel wall may be present. These changes result from an endarteritis and epithelial damage similar to that induced by ischemia.

Chronic radiation changes manifest about a year after therapy, although presentation may be delayed for many years (6 months to 12 years). Acute radiation colitis is not a necessary precursor for chronic radiation damage. The pathogenesis is similar to ischemia; however, changes in the field of radiation outside the bowel itself, modify the appearance. Considerable fibrosis leads to a narrow, rigid, featureless bowel segment. The presacral space is widened and the rectosigmoid may be elevated out of the pelvis. Adhesions may form and a fibrotic reaction outside of the bowel may cause an extrinsic impression. This is less apparent than with recurrent tumor. Focal areas of ulceration may occur and result in fistula formation. Ulceration and subsequent healing may lead to the formation of pseudopolyps and postinflammatory polyps.

The differential diagnosis is usually not difficult with the appropriate clinical history. However, it may be difficult to exclude recurrent malignancy or a new colonic primary. The radiographic differential is given below. Note that although the pathogenesis is similar to ischemic colitis, the rectum is usually spared in the latter entity.

DIFFERENTIAL DIAGNOSIS OF RADIATION COLITIS

Acute
    Ulcerative proctitis
    Infectious proctitis (gonorrhea)
    Traumatic proctitis
Chronic
    Stricture formation and narrowed rectum
        Ulcerative or other "burned out" colitis
        Scirrhous carcinoma
        Recurrence or extension of the tumor
        Lymphogranuloma venereum (LGV)
        Prostatic disease
        Lymphoma
        Endometriosis
        Pelvic lipomatosis
        Amyloidosis
    Fistula formation and other complications
        Crohn disease
        Lymphogranuloma venereum
        Perforated carcinoma
        Diverticulitis

PSEUDOMEMBRANOUS COLITIS

Pseudomembranous (postantibiotic) colitis is associated with a severe watery diarrhea that develops either during or within 6 weeks after antibiotic treatment. In the 1970s clindamycin was the most frequently implicated antibiotic. However, this condition has been ascribed to many other antibiotics including tetracycline, ampicillin, chloramphenicol, and the cephalosporins as well as other broad-spectrum penicillins. Cytotoxin and enterotoxin, formed from an overgrowth of the gram-positive rod *Clostridium difficile,* is believed to cause pseudomembranous colitis. The most accurate diagnostic procedure is a stool assay for *C. difficile* cytotoxin. Presenting symptoms may range from mild to fulminant diarrhea, which usually resolves spontaneously or with vancomycin therapy. Most patients have no underlying primary colon disease. Cancer chemotherapy, uremia, and other conditions may predispose to the development of pseudomembranous colitis. The colon is almost invariably affected. Rarely is the small bowel involved.

Endoscopically, the most characteristic feature is the pseudomembrane — focally adherent yellow or white plaques with intervening hyperemic mucosa. The plaques represent sloughed areas of mucosa. The findings may be considerably more subtle and resemble early ulcerative colitis with friable, granular, or swollen mucosa.

On plain radiographs of the abdomen, the bowel wall may appear thickened or thumbprinted. With severe disease, toxic megacolon and perforation may occur. Peritoneal irritation may cause a diffuse ileus. Later in the course of the disease, the colon may appear rigid and tubelike; occasionally strictures develop.

Barium enemas are performed much less often because the patient's clinical history and sigmoidoscopic findings are characteristic. The entire colon may be involved. The bowel wall is thickened and the mucosal pattern may appear shaggy and irregular, caused by a combination of elevated plaques, ulcers, and edema. The radiographic differential diagnosis includes ischemic, acute infectious, ulcerative and granulomatous colitides.

DIVERTICULAR DISEASE

Diverticular disease of the colon is a common, acquired condition in Western countries. The incidence and prevalence of the condition increases markedly with advancing age, being a rarity before age 40 and affecting over half of the individuals over 60 years of age. The condition has also become more prevalent since the beginning of the twentieth century. The most popular theory regarding the etiology of the diverticular disease is based on the increasing use of refined carbohydrates in the Western diet; a diet high in crude fiber is believed to be protective.

Diverticular disease encompasses a spectrum of conditions, ranging from muscular abnormalities of the colonic wall through acute inflammation and its complications. The underlying pathogenesis is believed to relate to a motor abnormality, creating a greater than normal pressure gradient between the lumen of the colon and the peritoneal cavity. The abnormal contractions cause segmentation of the bowel. The motor disorder may also result in hypertrophy of the circular muscle of the colon wall (sometimes called prediverticular disease or myochosis).

Herniation of the colonic mucosa and muscularis mucosal layers through points of diminished resistance in the bowel wall form the small saccules known as diverticula. Pathologically, these are really pseudodiverticula since they do not include all layers of the bowel wall. Diverticulosis refers to the presence of diverticula with or without apparent muscular hypertrophy. The term diverticulitis is confined to the presence of active inflammation of one or more diverticula. The inflammation causes micro- or macroperforations of the affected diverticula with pericolic abscess formation. Sometimes this may be complicated by fistula formation, obstruction, or peritonitis.

Diverticula form in two parallel rows between the bands of longitudinal muscle (taenia). Arterial blood reaches the colon via the mesentery. The small arteries divide as they approach the mesenteric taenia and run along the outside of the colon. Nutrient arteries penetrate the circular muscle into the submucosa in two rows that lie between the mesenteric taenia and the two antimesenteric taeniae. Thus, pathologic specimens demonstrate diverticula in two parallel bands. This distribution may be difficult to appreciate on barium studies. A few small diverticula may form in the region between the two antimesenteric taeniae.

The sigmoid colon is involved in 90 to 95 percent of cases. Proximal colonic involvement occurs in about 20 percent of patients and is usually associated with the presence of sigmoid diverticula. Diverticulosis is confined to the cecum and ascending colon in fewer than 10 percent of cases. Most right-sided diverticular are, as in the rest of the colon, acquired pseudodiverticula. Occasionally, isolated diverticula may be congenital, a true diverticulum. Rectal diverticula are very rare because the rectum is completely invested by longitudinal muscles. Another rare entity is an isolated giant sigmoid diverticulum, a variant that may be formed by a ball-valve mechanism, resulting in unusual distension of the diverticulum.

Diverticulitis, the most common complication of diverticulosis, occurs in about 15 percent of patients. Clinically, it usually presents with pain (most often in the left lower quadrant), fever, and leukocytosis. Symptoms result from extension of the inflammatory process beyond the lumen of the diverticulum (peridiverticulitis). Other presentations may relate to abscess formation, obstruction, fistulas, or peritonitis caused by diverticulitis. Although diverticulitis almost always occurs in the sigmoid, any area of the colon, including the cecum and even the appendix, may be involved.

Diverticular disease is the most common cause of severe rectal bleeding. Diverticular hemorrhage occurs most often with no evidence of frank diverticulitis. Rather, it results from erosion into the wall of the small artery, at the dome of the diverticulum, secondary to the irritating action of the fecal stream or inspissated feces. Significant bleeding occurs most often with right-sided diverticula. These are larger and have wider necks than left-sided diverticula. Spasm of thickened muscle in the sigmoid may also decrease the incidence of significant bleeding in this segment, whereas the muscle wall is less thick on the right side of the colon. Right-sided hemorrhage is best diagnosed by angiography and radionuclide scintigraphy. It should be differentiated from angiodysplasia, which are tiny acquired vascular malformations that cannot be diagnosed by barium studies.

Uncomplicated diverticular disease is often detected incidentally on plain films or by abdominal CT. Thickening of the bowel wall of the sigmoid is most often associated with diverticular disease. Multiple diverticula may cause a mottled appearance that can mimic debris in the colon or even an abscess.

The barium enema is the standard method for evaluating diverticular disease. The contrast enema will, in most cases, demonstrate both the muscular abnormality and the diverticula. The muscular abnormality is manifested as thickening of the bowel wall with shortening, lack of distensibility, and mucosal redundancy. The changes on contrast examination have been likened to a concertina or accordion. Thickened muscle interdigitated between the barium-coated lumen may also cause a sawtoothed or even thumb-printed appearance.

The saccular appearance of the diverticula varies on the barium examination, depending on position. When they are viewed in profile, they are usually smooth, round, or oval projections from the bowel wall and may be filled with barium or air. Occasionally they may be irregular in shape, contain filling defects (inspissated feces), or even have small protrusions. Some irregularly shaped diverticula may result from prior episodes of diverticulitis. Diverticula seen en face may be filled with barium or air and appear as filling defects in some projections.

Differentiating diverticula from polyps is a matter of some importance. Both entities occur in the same population and are often similar in size. Although it is sometimes impossible to exclude the presence of polyps when massed diverticula or extreme distortion of the sigmoid is associated with muscular abnormality, several points should be helpful in determining whether polyps are present (Fig. 4-36). Since polyps are solid lesions, barium cannot collect within them. Demonstration of the barium meniscus fading toward the center of a lesion occurs in a diverticulum, but not in a polyp. Barium fades away from a polypoid lesion. Extra fluoroscopic views of the suspected lesion in profile will demonstrate a diverticulum protruding outside the expected lumen of the bowel. The presence of a polyp may be confirmed by demonstrating a stalk. Some people favor a biphasic examination; that is, a full-column examination of the sigmoid with dilute barium, after the double-contrast examination, to accentuate the presence of polyps as filling defects (see the section Biphasic Barium Enema).

With a classic clincial presentation of acute diverticulitis, barium enemas are usually not performed immediately but are reserved for the subacute phase of the disease. If the diagnosis is questionable, the barium enema may be requested to diagnose acute diverticulitis. Free intraperitoneal perforation is very rare in diverticulitis, since the perforation is generally rapidly walled-off by adhesions and inflammatory tissue. However, a horizontal beam (left lateral decubitus) or an upright radiograph should be obtained before the examination. If there is a question of free perforation,

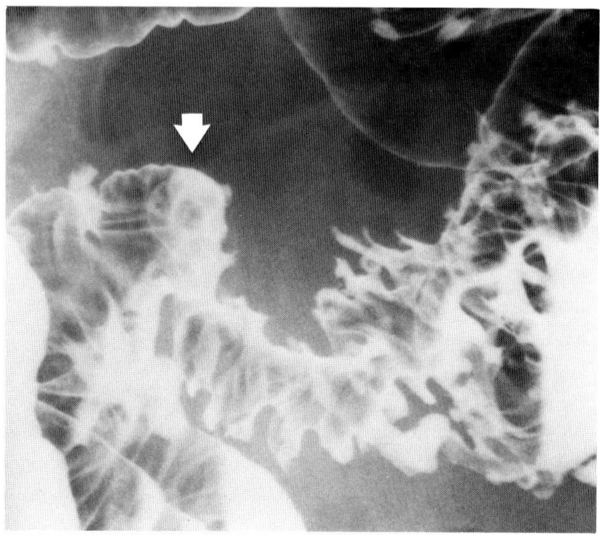

Fig. 4-36 Sigmoid diverticulitis. An inflammatory mass on the mesenteric surface is present. There is narrowing of the lumen and distortion of multiple diverticula. Concurrent polyps are common but difficult to detect in the presence of multiple diverticula. This polyp *(arrowhead)* was overlooked on the initial evaluation.

use of a water-soluble contrast agent may be preferable; however, subtle areas of extravasation may be missed with the inferior contrast of water-soluble agents compared with barium. A contrast examination in the presence of acute diverticulitis may be performed without patient preparation. The colon need then be filled with thin barium, only through the sigmoid, to define the area in question and a complete examination deferred for another time. On those occasions in which a double-contrast examination demonstrates acute diverticulitis — either suspected or unsuspected — postevacuation films may be especially helpful in demonstrating small perforations or tracks.

To make the specific diagnosis of diverticulitis on a barium examination, extravasation from the tip of a diverticulum should be demonstrated. The amount may vary from a microperforation to filling of a large abscess cavity. Demonstration of a pericolic mass is a slightly less specific but more common sign of diverticulitis caused by a pericolic abscess. This is demonstrated as an extraluminal, extrinsic mass impression on the bowel. The mucosal folds should be preserved.

They are sometimes difficult to demonstrate, owing to associated spasm and edema. Adjacent deformed and attenuated diverticula may drape over the mass. The pericolic abscess may contain pockets of gas that may or may not communicate with the bowel lumen. CT may demonstrate the pericolic abscess much better than a barium enema, especially if there is no significant mass effect on the bowel (Fig. 4-37). Diverticulitis may also occur in a region devoid of other diverticula. The important radiographic findings of diverticulitis are listed below.

X-RAY FINDINGS OF DIVERTICULITIS

1. Extravasation
2. Tracking
3. Pericolic mass
4. Stenosis
5. Fistula
6. Ileus
7. Small or large bowel obstruction
8. Free intraperitoneal air
9. Unilateral or anal obstruction

Narrowing of the lumen by spasm and inflammation may be seen but is not specific for diverticulitis. Other nonspecific changes include diffuse or focal ileus, small or large bowel obstruction, and free intraperitoneal and extraperitoneal perforation. Obstruction of the left ureter from sigmoid diverticulitis and psoas abscesses are examples of diverticulitis involving organs outside the bowel. Other conditions that may produce stenotic segments in the bowel include ischemic colitis, Crohn disease, and infectious colitis.

Fistulas are a complication of diverticulitis and result from dissection of an abscess through tissue planes to adjacent organs. CT is informative in demonstrating fistulas. The bladder is the site most commonly affected by the formation of a colovesical fistula. The Bourne test — i.e., the examination of urine for barium sediments — is helpful when the barium enema examination is inconclusive. The vagina, small bowel, and skin are also sites of fistulas.

Most episodes of diverticulitis resolve completely. Sometimes, strictures may persist and cause obstructive symptoms that require surgical intervention.

The most important considerations in the differential diagnosis of diverticular disease are listed below. The

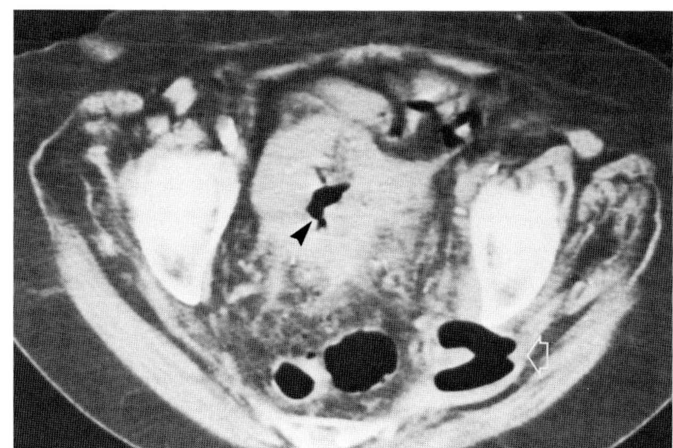
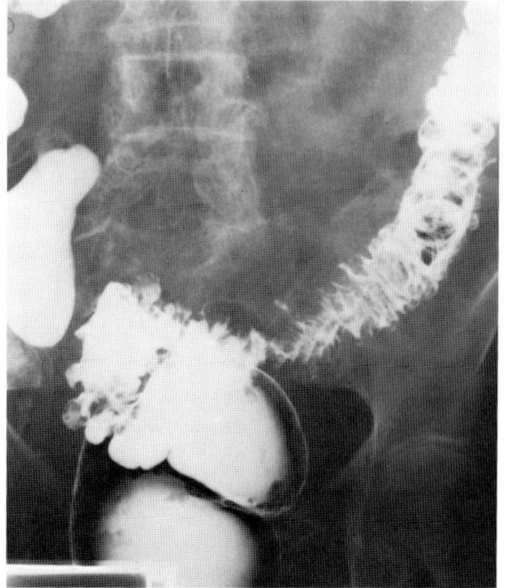

Fig. 4-37 CT in diverticulitis. **(A)** Pyometria suggested by gas *(arrowhead)* in uterus and abscess *(arrow)* adjacent to the left hip are well demonstrated by CT. **(B)** The barium enema, although diagnostic of diverticulitis, does not reflect the extent of the inflammatory process.

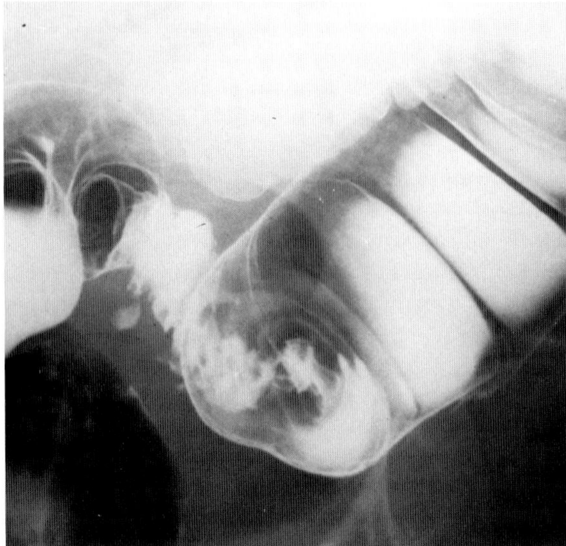

Fig. 4-38 Sigmoid diverticulitis indicated by an area of narrowing with intact mucosal folds. Compare to Figure 4-18, sigmoid narrowing secondary to carcinoma in an area of diverticulosis.

incidence of diverticular disease, polyps, carcinomas, and ischemia increase with advancing age in the Western population; these entities may coexist or mimic each other. Contained perforation of a sigmoid carcinoma is the most common significant pathologic entity to coexist with diverticular disease and may be impossible to distinguish from diverticulitis. Restudying patients with such a questionable lesion after a course of antibiotics may clarify the diagnosis. Rarely, the diagnosis can only be made by the pathologist. The narrowed segment, secondary to spasm in diverticulitis, should be differentiated from an annular carcinoma. In diverticulitis, the margins of the narrowed segment are tapered; thick mucosal folds are seen in the area of narrowing (Fig. 4-38). An annular carcinoma has abrupt shelflike margins; destruction of the mucosa is apparent.

DIFFERENTIAL DIAGNOSIS OF DIVERTICULAR DISEASE

Diverticula
   polyps
   scleroderma

Muscle thickening
   ischemia
   Crohn disease
   metastases
Diverticulitis
   primary colon carcinoma
   metastasis
   Crohn disease
   radiation colitis
   ischemic colitis
   diverticulosis

Metastatic disease and endometriosis may cause mass effects and a serosal reaction similar to that of a pericolic abscess (Fig. 4-39). Endometriosis usually affects women younger than those affected by diverticulitis.

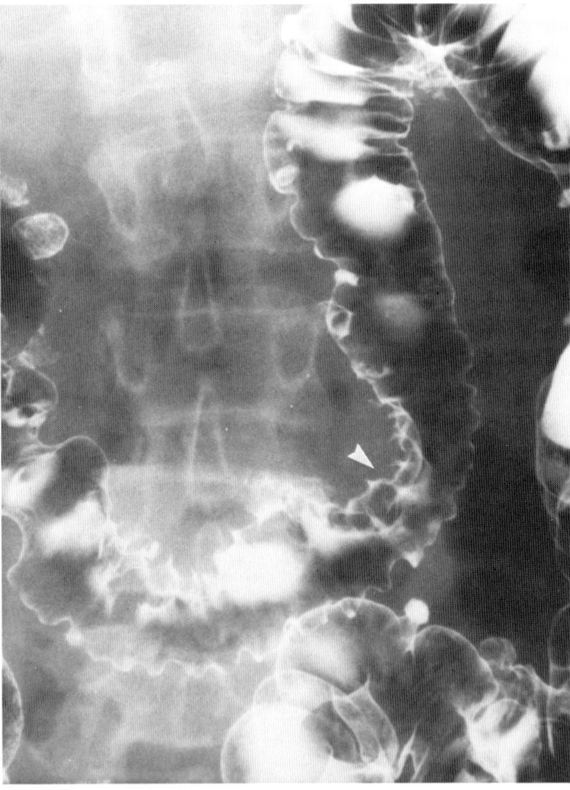

Fig. 4-39 Transverse colon diverticulitis. The abscess *(arrowhead)* secondary to a ruptured transverse colon diverticulum would be difficult to differentiate from metastatic disease. Diverticulitis in this segment is even rarer than cecal diverticulitis. (Courtesy of Dr. M Davis.)

Ischemic colitis may also cause edema, spasm, and thickening of the bowel wall; like diverticulitis, it is often a focal lesion. Crohn disease occurs with some frequency in the 50- to 60-year-old group. Thickened bowel and long longitudinal tracks may coexist with and/or mimic diverticulitis.

Ulcerative colitis may also coexist with diverticular disease; however, many investigators feel that the mucosal scarring of ulcerative colitis may make preexisting diverticula disappear. Uncomplicated diverticulosis or resolved diverticulitis may also be difficult to distinguish from active diverticulitis.

Scleroderma may be considered in the differential diagnosis of diverticulosis. Wide-mouthed diverticula form as the muscular atrophy of scleroderma progresses. These large, wide sacculations are easily distinguished from ordinary diverticula.

OBSTRUCTION

Twenty percent of intestinal obstructions are colonic but the vast majority occur in the small bowel. Carcinomas, predominantly in the sigmoid, account for most colonic obstructions (65 percent). Diverticulitis accounts for about 20 percent of obstructions. Volvulus (5 percent) occurs in intraperitoneal segments of colon. The sigmoid, cecum, and transverse colon are affected in decreasing order. Rarely, two separate loops of bowel can twist around each other to form an intestinal knot, or compound volvulus. Redundant loops of bowel, elongated mesentery, and colonic distension predispose to the development of a volvulus. Less frequent causes of colonic obstruction include incarcerated hernias, intussusception, abscess, metastases or extension of pelvic tumor, and foreign bodies.

Clinically, patients usually present with colicky pain, distension, and constipation. High-pitched bowel sounds are found on physical examination. Mechanical obstruction of the colon is frequently a surgical emergency and requires a prompt and efficient evaluation.

Plain-film radiography plays a major role in diagnosis. Lumen diameters over 7 cm in the transverse colon and 10 cm in the cecum are considered to be at high risk for perforation, if they are not caused by chronic conditions (e.g., as in psychotics, chronic constipation, and others). Evaluation for colonic obstruction should include positions favoring the collection of air in distal bowel segments in addition to supine and erect radiographs. Right-lateral and prone positions, with a vertical or horizontal beam, are used to detect air in the left side of the colon and rectum. The absence of air in the rectum suggests a colonic obstruction. The left-lateral decubitus radiograph is helpful in evaluating the ascending colon and cecum.

The presence of an air-fluid level beyond the hepatic flexure in the absence of diarrhea or recent enemas is another sign of colonic obstruction. A soft tissue mass may be another helpful finding on plain radiographs.

Sigmoid and cecal volvulus have characteristic findings on plain films. In sigmoid volvulus, the most common, the sigmoid twists on its mesentery, causing an essentially blind loop (Fig. 4-40). This undergoes massive dilatation and projects up from the pelvis toward the right upper quadrant. At the base of the volvulus, the adjacent walls of the two arms of the twisted segment may be detected. On erect or decubitus radiographs, two separate air-fluid levels are seen.

Volvulus of the cecum causes obstruction of the cecum and a variable amount of ascending colon. The dilated cecum rotates toward the midabdomen and left upper quadrant (Fig. 4-41). Cecal volvulus may be accompanied by considerable small bowel distension if the colon decompresses through the ileocecal valve. A single, long air-fluid level is seen on erect or decubitus radiographs. Distension of the cecum (cecal ileus) may also occur with a cecal bascule. In this condition a mobile cecum may be folded across the more distal ascending colon rather than twisted around the mesentery. The distension in a bascule is relieved by positional variation and is usually asymptomatic.

In cases of suspected colonic obstruction, a single-contrast barium enema is performed as an emergency study on an unprepared patient to confirm the diagnosis. The presence of a toxic megacolon or free intraperitoneal air are the only contraindications to barium study. Water-soluble contrast may be instilled up to the point of obstruction, if impending perforation

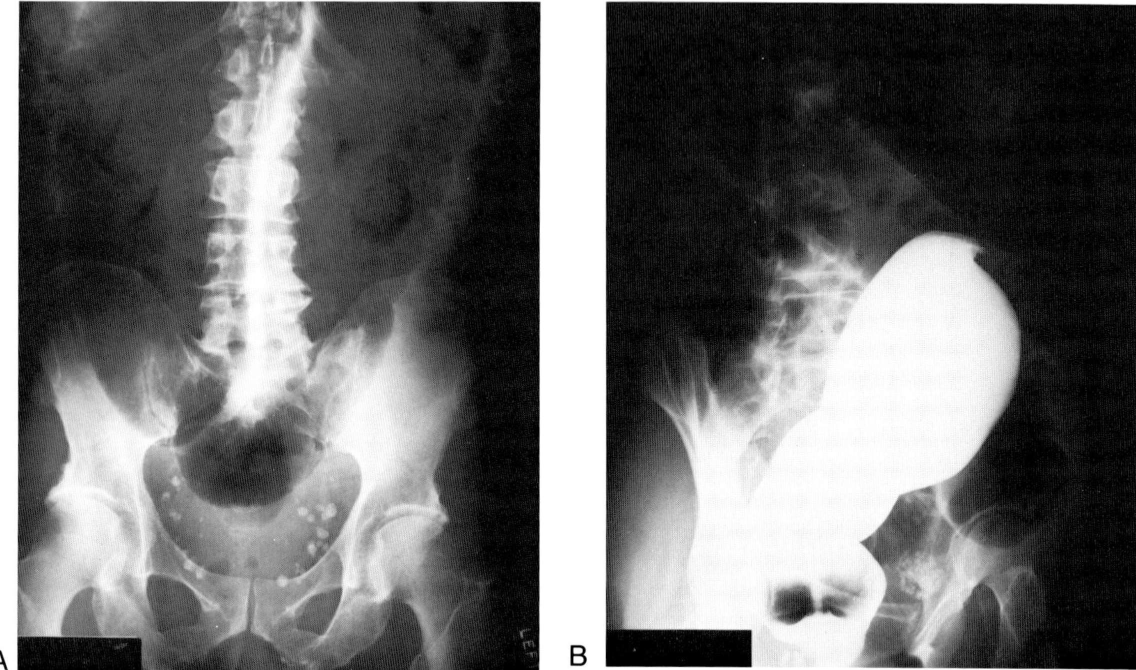

Fig. 4-40 Sigmoid volvulus. **(A)** Supine film of the abdomen showing two parallel dilated loops of bowel rising out of the pelvis. The dense vertical stripe separating the loops (overlying the spine) represents apposed bowel walls and twisted mesentery. **(B)** The contrast column ends abruptly in a ''beak'' at the point where the bowel is twisted. Barium should not be forced proximal to the obstruction.

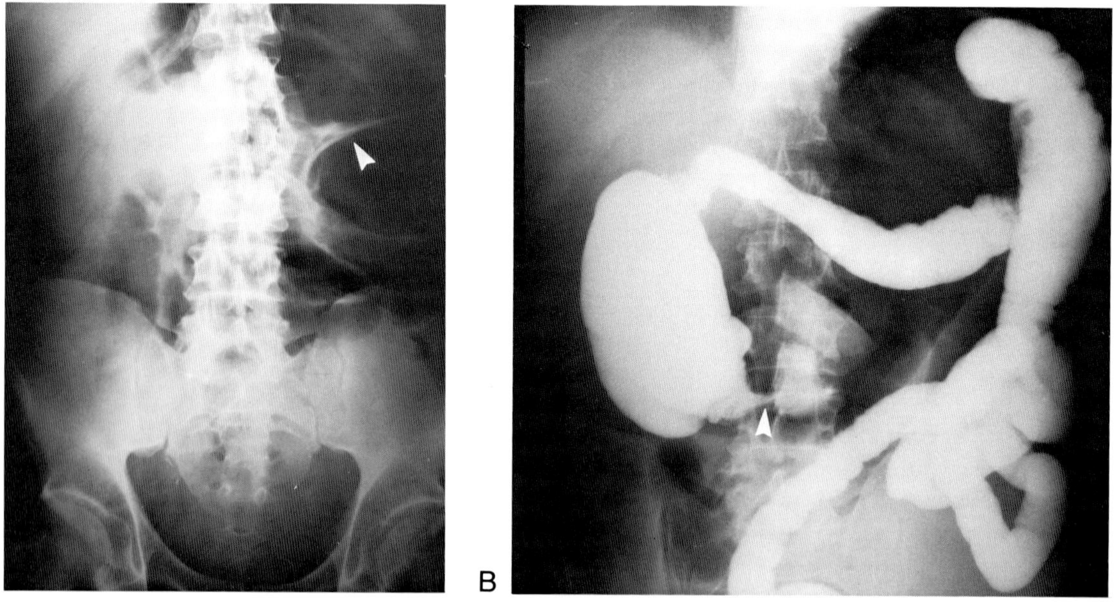

Fig. 4-41 Cecal volvulus. **(A)** Supine radiograph shows dilated cecum in the left upper quadrant. The ileocecal valve can be identified *(arrowhead)*. **(B)** The point of twist is demonstrated by the barium enema *(arrowhead)*.

is a concern. Barium is introduced at low pressure, under fluoroscopic control, until the point of obstruction is identified and, if possible, defined.

Obstructing carcinomas are identified by an abrupt shelflike termination of the barium column. Nodular filling defects often protrude into the edge of the barium. A trickle of barium may pass through the nearly obstructed lumen and define the length of the lesion. Obstruction by acute diverticulitis may show extravasation into the pericolonic abscess. Frequently, no barium can be demonstrated outside the lumen, and the column may have an irregular termination indistinguishable from a carcinoma. If the obstruction is associated with chronic or healed diverticulitis, the cause is usually a fibrotic stricture. In the case of a volvulus, the barium ends in a smooth, tapered beak at the point the bowel twists. If the obstruction is incomplete, some barium may flow into the dilated proximal loop.

Intussusceptions have a characteristic coiled-spring appearance where the invaginated segment, the intussusceptum, is pushed through the surrounding bowel, the intussuscipiens. In adults, the lead point of an intussusception is almost always from a mass lesion. Children under 2 years of age account for 85 percent of all cases of intussusception, nearly all of which are of the ileocolic type and idiopathic. Most can be reduced by a carefully monitored barium enema, whereas those in adults cannot.

PSEUDOOBSTRUCTION

Colonic pseudoobstruction (Ogilve syndrome or colonic ileus) usually refers to acute dilatation of the colon without evidence of mechanical obstruction. Although classic toxic megacolon is not present, cecal perforation may occur with pseudoobstruction and thus be life-threatening. Pseudoobstructions usually develop in elderly patients who have undergone recent surgery or who have major systemic abnormalities.

Plain films of the abdomen demonstrate distension of the colon without accompanying small bowel distension. The wall of the colon remains thin. The changes are most prominent in the transverse colon and

cecum. Sometimes distension is confined to the cecum, which may be deviated toward the patient's left. With proper positioning (left lateral or right decubitus), air can generally be demonstrated in the rectum. A contrast examination may be done to rule out mechanical obstruction in equivocal cases. Pseudoobstructions may be reduced colonoscopically or by a cecostomy.

The differential diagnosis of colonic pseudoobstruction includes mechanical obstruction, sigmoid or cecal volvulus, mesenteric vascular disease, and toxic megacolon.

MEGACOLON

Megacolon is a descriptive term for an abnormally distended colon. The condition may be acute or chronic and either of minimal clinical significance or life-threatening.

Toxic megacolon occurs as a complication of inflammatory conditions such as ulcerative colitis, ischemic colitis, Crohn disease, amebiasis, and shigellosis. It is a grave condition predisposing to bowel perforation. If toxic megacolon is suspected, contrast examinations are contraindicated. Plain abdominal radiographs demonstrate an enlarged, thin-walled colon. The changes are usually most visible in the transverse colon because it is anterior in the abdomen and air will collect in it. Sometimes toxic colons may have thickened bowel walls with nodular soft-tissue compressions (thumbprinting) visible on plain films.

Acutely developing colonic distension, which does not fit the classic description of toxic megacolon, may also lead to perforation and be every bit as life-threatening as toxic colon. Such colonic distension may occur as a result of obstruction, the most common cause of which is a sigmoid carcinoma. Nonobstructive conditions such as abdominal or extraabdominal surgery, electrolyte abnormalities, shock, sepsis, and other causes of colonic ileus or pseudoobstruction may result in megacolon and perforation.

Chronic megacolon occurs with various conditions and is unlikely to lead to perforation. Congenital megacolon is a synonym for Hirschsprung disease.

The identical pathogenesis—i.e., destruction of the myenteric plexus—is acquired in Chagas disease. Chronic constipation of any etiology may also cause a chronic megacolon. A list of multiple causes of chronic colon dilatation is given below. Patients with a chronic megacolon are predisposed to the development of volvulus.

SOME CAUSES OF CHRONIC MEGACOLON

Hirschsprung disease (congenital megacolon)

Chagas disease

Psychogenic

Neurologic and muscular
    Parkinson disease
    diabetic neuropathy
    mystonic dystrophy
    scleroderma
    amyloidosis
    pseudoobstruction
Metabolic
    hypothyroid
    electrolyte imbalances
    porphyria
    narcotic abuse

Amyloid

Amyloidosis is an unusual systemic disorder arising from the deposition of abnormal protein-polysaccharide around blood vessels, muscle layers of the intestines, and mucous membranes. The disorder may be idiopathic or secondary to many chronic conditions. Tissue damage occurs by infiltration or ischemia. Histologic staining for amyloid provides the definitive diagnosis.

Radiographically, there are many manifestations of amyloidosis; also, it may mimic many other conditions. Many of the changes observed resemble chronic ulcerative colitis and ischemia. The bowel wall or mucosal folds may be thickened and contain multiple, nodular polypoid lesions. Infiltration may lead to a narrow rigid bowel and loss of haustral markings. Alternatively, neuromuscular involvement may cause

a diffusely dilated, thin-walled colon (megacolon). Occasionally the mucosa may be ulcerated.

SCLERODERMA

Scleroderma (progressive systemic sclerosis) is a collagen-vascular disease of unknown etiology. A predominant feature is the replacement of muscle with collagen and other connective tissue. In the GI tract, the esophagus and small bowel are most often involved. The colon as well as the small bowel may show diffuse dilatation and functional pseudoobstruction. Pneumatosis intestinalis may also be found. In addition to colonic distension, barium enema may

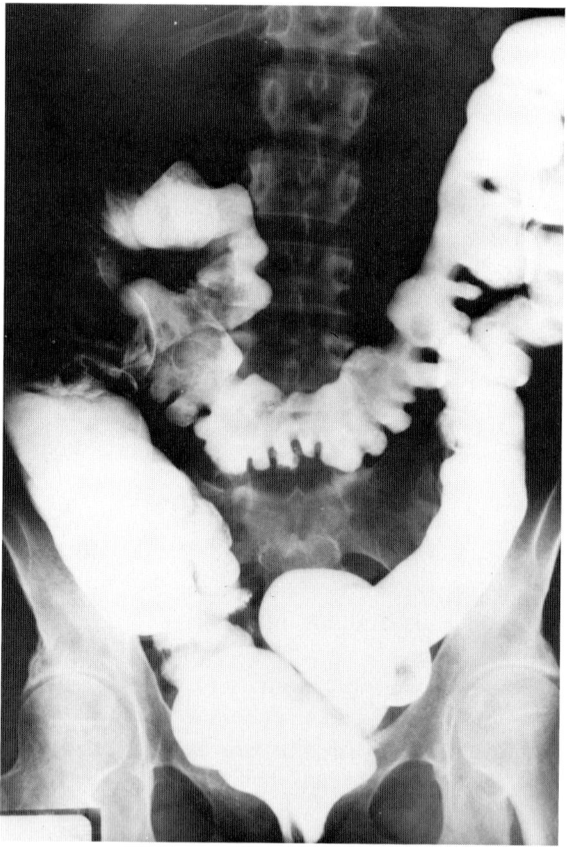

Fig. 4-42 Scleroderma. Large sacculations or wide-mouthed diverticula on the antimesenteric surface of the colon characteristic of scleroderma. The colon may also be dilated and atonic.

reveal large asymmetric sacculations (wide-mouth diverticula). These are haustra distorted by the loss of normal musculature (Fig. 4-42).

ENDOMETRIOSIS

Endometriosis results from the presence of extrauterine endometrial tissue. Several theories exist as to its pathogenesis. These include (1) the retrograde flow of endometrial cells through the fallopian tubes and subsequent implantation on serosal surfaces, (2) metaplastic change of multipotential mesothelial cells, and (3) lymphatic or hematologic dissemination.

The condition usually affects the reproductive organs in contiguity with the uterus, but on occasion it involves the colon, small bowel, urinary bladder, and may even have remote implants, e.g., pleura. Intestinal involvement is most often in the pelvis; the rectosigmoid is involved in 25 percent of these cases. The appendix, cecum, and ileum may also be involved.

Findings on barium examination are generally those of a serosal implant and include stretching or spiculation of the mucosal folds (see Fig. 4-14). En face, the mucosa appears crinkled or crenulated—closely simulating a metastatic lesion. Endometrial implants may invade the mucosa or have a polypoid appearance. These lesions may cause rectal bleeding during menstruation. Endometriosis may also incite a fibrotic response, resulting in stricture and adhesion formation that may occasionally cause bowel obstruction.

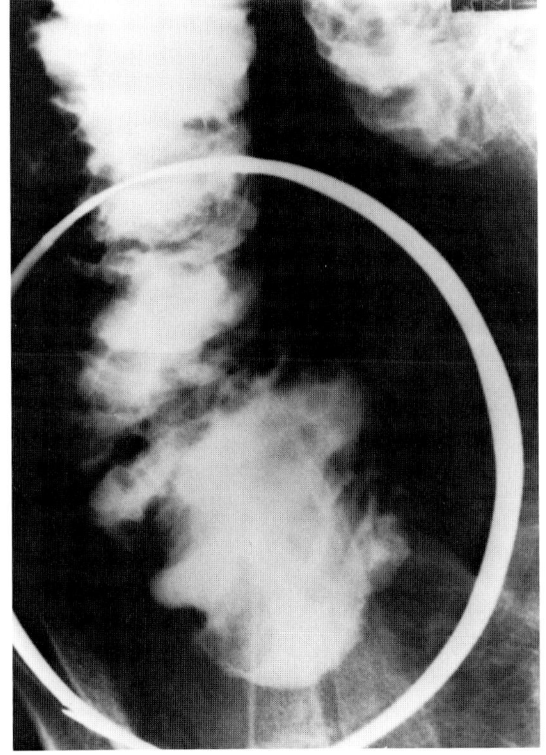
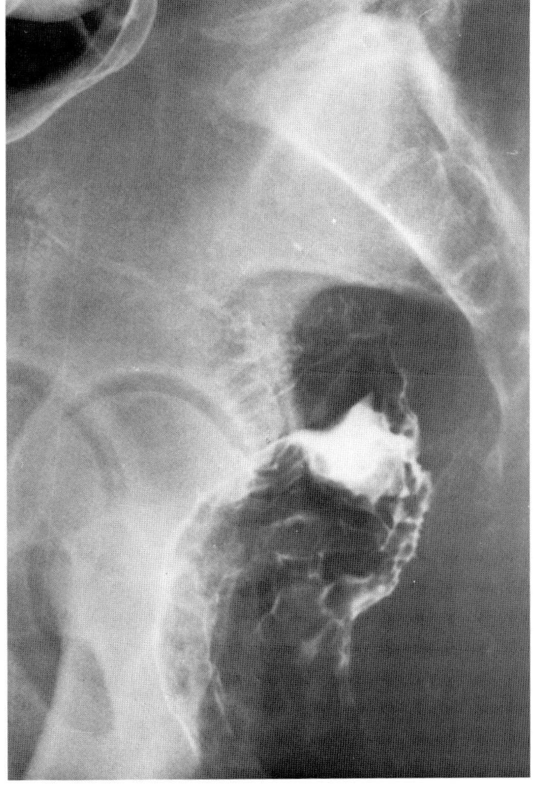

Fig. 4-43 Varices of colon in a patient with portal hypertension. This represents an unusual finding in portal hypertension. **(A)** There is spasm in the ascending colon with multiple nodular and serpiginous filling defects. **(B)** Appearance of rectal varices on double contrast study in another patient. Note spasm of distal sigmoid.

The differential diagnosis of endometriosis includes metastases, carcinoma, diverticulitis, chronic inflammatory disease, carcinoid, polyp, and pelvic tumor.

VASCULAR ABNORMALITIES

Hemorrhoids are the most common vascular abnormality of the colon. The internal hemorrhoidal veins are found at the anorectal junction. When they are enlarged, they may be seen on barium-enema radiographs after the enema tip is removed. They appear as submucosal nodules or serpiginous filling defects, extending for up to several centimeters from the anorectal junction. They may resemble smooth rectal polyps and occasionally a plaquelike carcinoma.

Varices elsewhere in the colon, although rare, may occur idiopathically as a result of portal hypertension and mesenteric venous obstruction. They may be seen endoscopically or on barium examination, but angiography may be the definitive procedure (Fig. 4-43).

Hemangiomas may occur as isolated lesions, usually in the rectum, and as multiple lesions in the colon or as part of a system angiomatosis. If they are small, they will be imperceptible on barium examination radiographs. Large lesions may appear as mass lesions; these are usually pliable submucosal masses. The presence of phleboliths may be most helpful in distinguishing hemangiomas from other neoplasms.

Angiodysplasia has been identified as a source of chronic or acute GI bleeding in elderly people. There may be an increased incidence in patients with prosthetic aortic valves. The etiology of these acquired lesions is not clear. They are undetected on barium examination but are diagnosed by superior mesenteric arteriography in acutely bleeding patients. Characteristic clusters of small arteries may be identified. Injection of resected specimens best demonstrates the morphology of the lesion.

COLITIS CYSTICA PROFUNDA

Colitis cystica profunda may be a complication of bacillary dysentery or chronic inflammation. It is be-lieved to develop from persistent regenerated islands of epithelial tissue in the submucosa with the formation of mucus retention cysts. Multiple cysts, up to 5 mm in diameter, are found in the rectosigmoid. Single lesions are rare, as is involvement proximal to the sigmoid.

On contrast examination, they appear as multiple filling defects that suggest polyps. Occasionally, scalloping of the wall resembles ischemia or pneumatosis coli. Barium trapped between folds may occasionally simulate ulceration.

PNEUMATOSIS COLI

Pneumatosis intestinalis describes the radiographic finding of air within the bowel wall. The collections may be linear or ovoid (pneumatosis intestinalis cystoides), and may extend into the mesentery or other adjacent structures.

Various theories proposed for the etiology of pneumatosis include (1) mechanical disruption of the mucosa, (2) bacterial invasion and subsequent mucosal necrosis, and (3) trapping of absorbed gas in the bowel wall. The condition may or may not be of clinical importance. If it is the result of ischemia, necrosis, obstruction, or infection, it may be life-threatening. However, it may also be an incidental finding in patients with obstructive lung disease, connective tissue disorders, and jejunoileal bypasses. Asymptomatic pneumoperitoneum may also be found in these patients.

Plain radiographs may show linear or oval lucencies around the colonic wall. A mottled appearance, similar to that seen with abscesses or retained stool, may be found. If there is no suggestion of a life-threatening process or perforation, barium examination may be performed. The gas collections may then be identified outside the bowel lumen. If the air density is not appreciated, scalloping of the bowel wall may mimic ischemia, lymphoma, or multiple polyps.

Some of the many conditions associated with pneumatosis are listed here.

CONDITIONS ASSOCIATED WITH PNEUMATOSIS INTESTINAL COLI

Peptic ulcer disease

Obstruction

Mesenteric vascular disease

NEC

Caustic ingestion

Lymphoma

Postsurgical anastomosis

Jejunoileal bypass

Scleroderma

Diabetic enteropathy

Trauma

Diverticulitis

SOLITARY RECTAL ULCER SYNDROME

The solitary rectal ulcer syndrome (SRUS) is caused by muscular discoordination during defecation. It occurs mainly in young adults and presents with rectal bleeding. The term SRUS is somewhat misleading because patients may have no demonstrable ulcers or they may have multiple ulcers. Barium enema may demonstrate diffuse edema, thickening of the valves of Houston, ulcers (usually in the anterior wall), or stricture.

ILEOCECAL REGION

The region of the bowel from the appendix to the ileocecal valve may be affected by conditions unique to that region as well as to the entire spectrum of colonic pathology. The cecum is the blind proximal pouch of ascending colon that extends distally to the level of the first prominent haustral fold. The ileocecal valve is situated on its medial or posteromedial aspect. The appendix arises as an outpouching from the tip of the cecum, at the origin of the three strips of longitudinal muscle or taeniae. The appendix and

ileocecal valve are always on the same side of the cecum, appearing on the medial surface in 85 percent of cases. A laterally or posteriorly placed ileocecal valve and appendix occurs in less than 10 percent of cases; anterior placement is very rare.

Since the ileocecal valve is bilobed, the terminal ileum enters the colon between the lips of the valve, forming a beaklike configuration. In profile, the medial aspect of the cecal folds tapers-out to form the labia. The valve may also appear somewhat papillary. En face, it appears as a rosette or as an ovoid lucency, sometimes with radiating folds. The size of the valve changes with varying distension of the cecum. Also, the valve or terminal ileum may prolapse into the medial portion of the cecum. The appearance and location of the valves usually do not present a diagnostic problem. However, a polypoid lesion should be suspected if the valve does not arise from the same side as the appendix.

Alterations in the ileocecal valve occur in a variety of conditions. The most common is fatty infiltration or lipomatosis, which is caused by unencapsulated infiltration of the submucosa with fat. It results in symmetric enlargement of the valve, which remains soft and pliable. This finding is more frequent in women and is of no clinical significance, although it may occasionally simulate an inflammatory or neoplastic lesion. Edema of the valve secondary to an intussusception or inflammation may also cause symmetric enlargement.

Neoplasms Involving the Ileocecal Region

True lipomas, which are encapsulated benign neoplasms, have an incidence second to adenomas in the colon. A preponderance of these lesions is found around the ileocecal junction. Most arise in the submucosa and may form a pseudopedicle to appear stalked. They are soft, pliable, and characteristically change configuration with any change in position or compression. CT is confirmatory.

Other neoplastic lesions may also involve the valve. Adenomatous polyps rarely arise on the valves, but they may be found in the cecum. Carcinomas of the cecum frequently involve the valve but rarely arise in it. Carcinoid tumors may arise in the valve, where their appearance may vary from merely slight prominence of the valve to frank large ulcerated polypoid lesions that mimic carcinoma. Lymphomas involving the valve are usually associated with involvement of the terminal ileum.

Neoplasms in the cecum are of the same histologic types as elsewhere in the colon, but several features of importance are related to their location. Because of its larger diameter compared with that of the distal colon, adenocarcinomas of the cecum are more likely to be large polypoid lesions and are less likely to obstruct. However, intussusceptions, with the polyps as a lead point, may occur and may cause obstruction. In contrast to lymphomas, carcinomas are much less likely to involve the terminal ileum; however, this observation should not be used to rule out either tumor.

Distal obstructions may cause a curious urticaria-like pattern in the cecum, with multiple small, smooth, and somewhat angular filling defects appearing. However, these defects are probably associated with submucosal edema and may be related to chronic ischemia. A few cases of true colonic urticaria associated with allergic responses have also been documented. In response to distal obstruction, the cecum, which is thin-walled compared to the rest of the colon, may distend and perforate. Diastasis of the muscular layers may also occur.

Hodgkin and non-Hodgkin lymphomas often involve the distal ileum. Hodgkin disease causes a marked desmoplastic reaction that may lead to considerable distortion of the ileocecal region and luminal narrowing, making it indistinguishable from Crohn disease. Aggressive carcinoids that may incite fibrogenesis also favor the distal ileum. When this occurs, deformity of the ileocecal region often results. Other neoplastic and inflammatory lesions of the mesentery may also distort the ileocecal region. In many ways, endometriosis behaves like metastatic disease. In the cecum, it tends to form a smooth mural mass that resembles a mucocele or appendiceal abscess. It may also cause polypoid mucosal lesions that mimic carcinoma and like any other polypoid cecal or ileal mass, endometriosis can lead to intussusception.

Inflammatory Conditions Involving the Ileocecal Region

The appearance of the ileocecal valve and cecum is frequently of particular importance in the diagnosis of a specific inflammatory process. In ulcerative colitis the valve is normal, gaping, and its labia may be atrophied. The terminal ileum is not involved, except for the occasional occurrence of backwash ileitis. Cathartic colitis may involve the ileocecal region in an identical manner. With Crohn disease, the cecum and terminal ileum are usually involved; the latter is ulcerated, cobblestoned, or severely narrowed, forming the string sign. The ostium of the valve is narrowed, although fatty hypertrophy of the labia may be evident. Fistulas and inflammatory masses are also common, involving the ileocecal region in Crohn disease but not in ulcerative colitis.

Amebiasis and tuberculosis are infectious processes that classically involve the ileocecal region. Both may lead to scarring and narrowing of the cecum. Amebiasis classically spares the terminal ileum with a normal or gaping ileocecal valve. In contrast, the terminal ileum is significantly involved in tuberculosis; the labia of the valve are thickened, distorted, and may resemble an inverted umbrella. Fistula formation is also relatively common in tuberculosis. Actinomycosis, histoplasmosis, and blastomycosis may produce similar changes in the ileocecal region.

Typhlitis—a word derived from the Greek *typhlon,* meaning cecum—is an unusual inflammatory change confined to the cecum. Originally, the term probably included appendicitis as well, but at present it is used primarily for changes seen in patients being treated for leukemia, whose cecums have been distorted by infiltration, bleeding, nonneoplastic inflammation, or infection of ischemic changes. On plain radiographs, gas may be absent from the cecum or a focal right-lower quadrant ileus may be evident. The changes seen with barium enema radiography are generally those of infiltration—i.e., thick walls and thumbprinting. Ulceration and perforation may occur, and this complication is likely to be fatal in already compromised patients.

APPENDIX

Considering its limited function, if any, the vermiform appendix is involved in a considerable amount of gastrointestinal pathology.

Acute Appendicitis

Inflammation is the most common lesion of the appendix and, in fact, is the most common cause of emergency abdominal surgery. Although the characteristic clinical presentation of appendicitis includes tenderness at the McBurney point, which is 2 inches medial to the right anterior superior iliac spine, a wide variety of atypical presentations have been observed. In these cases, in particular, radiographic procedures are useful.

The position of the appendix varies widely and corresponds to the embryologic development of the bowel. Any abnormal rotation or descent of the cecum, retention of mesentery on the ascending colon, length and position of the appendix, as well as other factors may alter the site of the appendix. Embryologically, the appendix arises as a conical projection from the base of the cecum. The wide mouth of the juvenile configuration accounts for the infrequency of appendicitis in neonates and in persons in whom this configuration is retained. With development, there is preferential lengthening of the taenia omentalis (which is on the lateral border of the ascending colon) relative to the medially placed mesocolic taenia. The appendix, which narrows and elongates at the same time, moves medially. The most common location of the appendix is the medial wall of the cecum, about 3 cm below the ileocecal valve. Its congenital absence or duplication is very rare; however, variations in shape as well as diverticular formation do occur. In most cases, the appendix is not fixed but moves freely with changes in position and distension. It may be intra- or retroperitoneal. Its location may be retrocecal or anterior to the cecum, subcecal, pelvic or retroileal, and is influenced by the position of the ascending colon. The variable location and length of the appendix ac-

count for the wide spectrum of signs and symptoms associated with appendiceal disease.

The pathogenesis of appendicitis is believed to be related to obstruction of the lumen of the appendix, usually caused by fecal residue that may calcify, forming fecaliths or appendicoliths. Foreign bodies, tumors, or parasites may also obstruct the appendix and become the inciting cause of appendicitis. It has been suggested that barium retained in the appendix has caused appendicitis but the association is infrequent and has been shown to be incidental. Acute appendicitis results from ischemia of the obstructed appendix, which then becomes infected and may undergo necrosis and perforate. A list of some important entities in the differential diagnosis of appendicitis is given below.

DIFFERENTIAL DIAGNOSIS OF ACUTE APPENDICITIS

Crohn disease

Yersinia enterocolitis and other causes of gastroenteritis

Gyneocologic disorders, especially pelvic inflammatory disease and ectopic pregnancy

Meckel diverticulitis

Diverticulitis

Carcinoma

Cholecystitis

Pyelonephritis

Ureteral calculi

In typical cases, plain abdominal radiographs may be helpful, although they are entirely normal in about half the patients with acute appendicitis. The presence of a calculus in the right lower quadrant of a patient with symptoms is the most significant radiographic sign. It may be seen in up to one-third of such patients, although some report its incidence is considerably lower. Sometimes appendicoliths are seen incidentally in asymptomatic patients. Many surgeons believe this is a significant finding in that this group of patients has an increased risk of appendicitis and should have prophylactic appendectomies. Other plain radiographic signs of appendicitis include an air-fluid level in the cecum or distal ileum, a soft tissue mass in the right lower quadrant, and ileus which may be diffuse or confined to the right lower quadrant. Lumbar scoliosis secondary to splinting and obliteration of the psoas margin or flank stripe may also be seen. The presence of gas in the appendix is rarely significant, unless it is associated with an appendicolith. It may be seen in normal patients, especially with a retrocecal appendix.

Complications

The complications of appendicitis are secondary to necrosis and perforation with subsequent inflammation and abscess formation. Free perforation with pneumoperitoneum is rare because the perforation is confined by the inflammatory process, the development of adhesions, and the paucity of air in the appendix. A soft tissue mass, displacement of bowel, and a mottled air pattern should suggest abscess formation. Small bowel obstructions are not infrequent complications of periappendiceal inflammation. Plain radiographs are also useful in distinguishing other etiologies of symptoms, including cholelithiasis or ureterolithiasis, perforation of a viscus, and other entities considered in the clinical differential.

Barium examinations should be performed in atypical or equivocal presentations of appendicitis. Ultrasound and CT may also be used, especially to define appendiceal perforation with periappendiceal inflammation or abscess (Fig. 4-6). In young patients, a single-contrast barium enema is the method of choice to exclude acute appendicitis. In older patients in whom other lesions are much more likely, a double-contrast examination is much more useful, if the study can be performed electively. Complete filling of the appendix in the barium study virtually eliminates the possibility of acute appendicitis, although incomplete filling does not exclude the diagnosis. Unfortunately, the appendix does not fill in about 15 percent of normal patients; incomplete filling occurs more often. Partial filling of an irregular or shaggy-appearing appendix suggests appendicitis. Demonstrating the position of the cecum and appendix is useful in atypical presentations. For example, a long retrocecal appendix may mimic acute cholecystitis, a pelvic appendix situation

in the cul-de-sac may mimic pelvic inflammatory disease, and a mobile cecum may cause left-upper quadrant symptoms.

Perforation of the appendix may lead to changes that cause mass impression on the base or wall of the cecum or on adjacent structures, such as the sigmoid, rectum, and terminal ileum. Acute appendicitis can also cause inflammatory changes in affected bowel; infiltration, thickening, and spiculation of folds along with deformity secondary to mass effect or inflammatory adhesions.

A smooth impression at the base of the cecum may be caused by a wide variety of conditions. Defects from inverted appendiceal stumps are usually small and associated with prior appendectomies. If a study is done shortly after an appendectomy, the defect may be quite large, owing to edema, and simulate a more significant appendiceal or cecal lesion.

Another cause of smooth mass at the base of the cecum is appendiceal intussusception. This has been reported in patients with vague symptoms and even in those with acute obstruction. It is manifested as a coil-spring defect in the cecum at the expected location of the appendix on barium enemas. Transient intussusceptions probably occur much more frequently than was previously believed and are not generally associated with symptoms. They often reduce spontaneously during the procedure. Occasionally the appendix may be completely inverted within the cecum.

Neoplasms Involving the Appendix

Benign and malignant tumors, including mucoceles, cystadenomas and cystadenocarcinomas, adenomas, and adenocarcinomas may all cause similar defects at the base of the cecum (Fig. 4-44). Carcinoids, although the most common neoplasms of the appendix, are almost always small, are found incidentally at surgery, and are almost never malignant. Mucoceles are mass lesions that may range considerably in size. Their pathogenesis may be due to obstruction of the base of the appendix and filling of the lumen with mucus, or it may be a primary process of excessive mucus secretion, as may occur with a cystadenoma or cystadenocarcinoma. Occasionally, globules

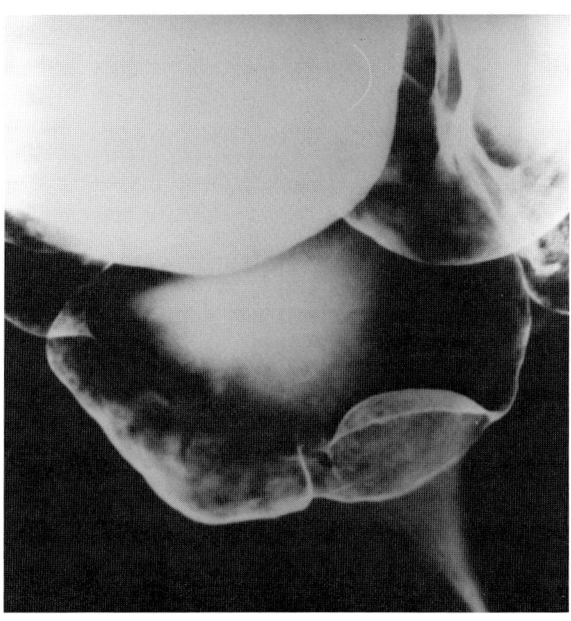

Fig. 4-44 Smooth impression on the base of the cecum. This was due to a mucinous cystadenoma of the appendix. The appearance is identical to a mucocele of the appendix.

of mucus may calcify and lead to a condition known as myxoglobulosis of the appendix. Rupture of a mucocele, another rare complication, leads to pseudomyxoma peritonei, with multiple peritoneal implants of mucoid material and ascites. The pathogenesis of this condition is uncertain, but it may exhibit aggressive neoplastic-like behavior with extension of the implants, ascites, and recurrent bowel obstructions.

In patients with Crohn disease involving the terminal ileum and cecum, the appendix is also frequently involved. It may exhibit a cobblestone or ulcerated mucosa or be fixed within an inflammatory mass. Fistulas involving the appendix may occur with Crohn disease as well as with infections such as tuberculosis and actinomycosis, which have a predisposition to the right lower quadrant. Fistula formation with uncomplicated appendicitis is unusual.

EXTRINSIC DEFORMATIONS OF THE COLON

Inflammatory processes, neoplasms, and nonneoplastic mass lesions of adjacent organs or spaces may cause extrinsic involvement of the colon or rectum. Because of its long course through the abdomen, processes primary to many organs may be contiguous with the colon or rectum. The gallbladder, kidneys, pancreas, stomach, liver, and spleen may extend to involve portions of the colon. Processes affecting the bladder, prostate, uterus, and ovaries may involve the rectum or sigmoid. Extension of processes from contiguous or noncontiguous organs, which spread through the peritoneum or along peritoneal reflections or fascial planes, may also cause extrinsic involvement. Appendiceal lesions are discussed separately.

Whatever the organ or origin, the specific pathologic process involved determines the nature of colonic involvement. The primary organ of involvement may often be deduced on barium examination by the specific site of involvement. CT examination often helps to elucidate the source and extent of the pathologic process. Barium examinations yield more specific information concerning actual infiltration of the bowel.

Smooth, obtuse impressions on a portion of the colon may be caused normally — e.g., by the right lobe of the liver, gallbladder, right kidney, and uterus. Enlarged organs, or smooth encapsulated masses cause a similar impression. Examples are hydrops of the gallbladder, enlarged urinary bladder secondary to retention, hydronephrosis, renal cysts, pancreatic pseudocysts, and noninvasive neoplasms, including uterine fibroids and dermoids. Impingement on the colon may occasionally be great enough to cause significant narrowing or even obstruction of the lumen.

Pelvic lipomatosis, an asymptomatic condition in which there is extensive nonneoplastic fatty and fibrous proliferation in the pelvis is an unusual example of extrinsic impression on the rectum and sigmoid. This is more often associated with contour abnormalities of the urinary bladder, but it may also affect the rectum. Pelvic lipomatosis may appear as a pelvic mass impressing the anterior wall of the rectosigmoid, or it may cause narrowing of the rectum and sigmoid, elevation of the sigmoid, and widening of the presacral space. On plain radiographs the pelvic mass may be lucent, suggesting fat. CT scanning is definitive.

Findings in inflammatory and neoplastic involvement of the colon overlap, but there are often distinguishing clues. With most types of secondary involvement by malignancy, the colonic wall is involved first and the mucosa is spared until very late in the course. With metastatic disease, the lesions tend to be more discrete and numerous. Many separate areas of involvement usually occur. In addition, a well-formed mass favors malignancy. The bowel wall in the segment with neoplastic or inflammatory involvement may be thickened, fixed, and/or have spiculated folds. The involved bowel folds become distorted and hazy.

If there is circumferential involvement, it may be difficult or impossible to distinguish a primary colonic malignancy. Metastases spread through the bloodstream are mucosal lesions that may be ulcerated. Melanoma, bronchogenic carcinoma, and carcinoma of the breast are likely sources of such lesions.

Intraperitoneal seeding of metastatic disease has a predisposition to affect dependent areas of the abdomen. The most commonly affected region is the cul-de-sac, which is the rectouterine pouch of Douglas in the female and the rectovesical pouch in the male (Fig. 4-45). The medial wall of the cecum and terminal ileum is the next most common area of involvement since they are found at the most dependent portion of the small bowel mesentery. The superior aspect of the sigmoid and the right paracolic gutter are also often involved.

Inflammatory processes may also cause spasm, edema and thickening, as well as spiculation of folds in an affected area. Generally, discrete masses are not as prominent a finding as with metastatic disease. Multiple areas of involvement are not as common with inflammation. The affected region is usually contiguous with the site of inflammation. Sometimes the infection is spread intraperitoneally, tracking down the mesentery and up along the lateral gutters. The findings may then be indistinguishable from metastases.

Fistula formation may occur with either neoplasms or inflammatory changes. Gastrocolic fistulas, from the greater curvature of the stomach to the transverse colon, occur with primary malignancies of the stomach or colon, Crohn disease, perforation of a peptic ulcer, or postoperative abscess.

Duodenocolic fistulas are rare and result from peptic ulcer or Crohn disease. With cholecystitis, fistulas are more likely to occur between the common duct and duodenum; however, a colecystocolic fistula may occasionally occur. Carcinoma of the gallbladder or liver may also occasionally fistulize into the colon. Renal infections may lead to fistulas between the colon and perinephric space.

Primary peritoneal processes may also involve the colon, although the small bowel is more frequently involved. Postoperative adhesions and bands rarely obstruct the colon, but may cause some deformity or fixation of the contour. Lymphocysts and aneurysms may cause smooth impressions typical of extrinsic noninvasive mass lesions. Inflammatory processes, such as peritoneal tuberculosis or retractile mesenteritis, may occasionally involve the colon. Lymphomas may manifest with invasive or noninvasive changes of the colon.

Because of the frequency with which it occurs and its multiple manifestations, involvement of the colon by pancreatic disease deserves special mention. Most of the length of the pancreas is directly connected to the transverse colon by the transverse mesocolon. This extends from about midline to the splenic flexure, where the tail of the pancreas ends at the splenic hilum. The transverse mesocolon arises on the anterior aspect of the pancreas and travels caudad to end at the mesocolic taenia on the posterior aspect of the transverse colon.

Evidence of acute pancreatitis may sometimes be seen on a plain film of the abdomen when the distal transverse colon is narrowed, or along the splenic flexure with proximal distension of the bowel and a relative absence of bowel gas distal to this region. This appearance, or colon cutoff sign, is not pathognomonic and may be found with carcinoma or other inflammatory processes such as left perinephric abscess or colonic stricture.

On barium examination, the region of the cutoff may be found to be an area of spasm, which distends normally. More often, there is bowel wall edema and there may be rigidity, spiculation of folds and other evidence of infiltration. The inferior margin of the transverse colon, which is the site of attachment of the

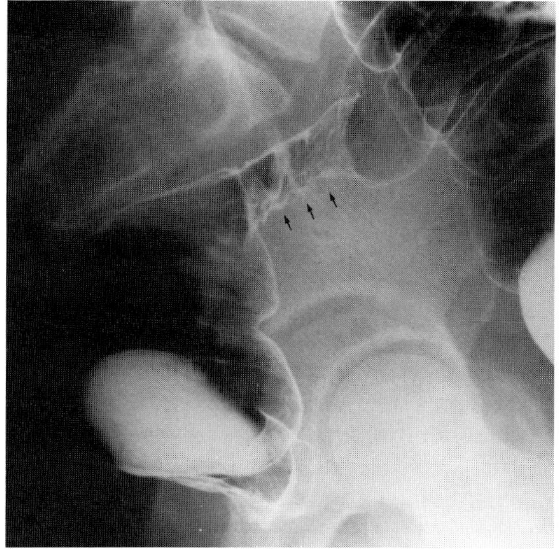
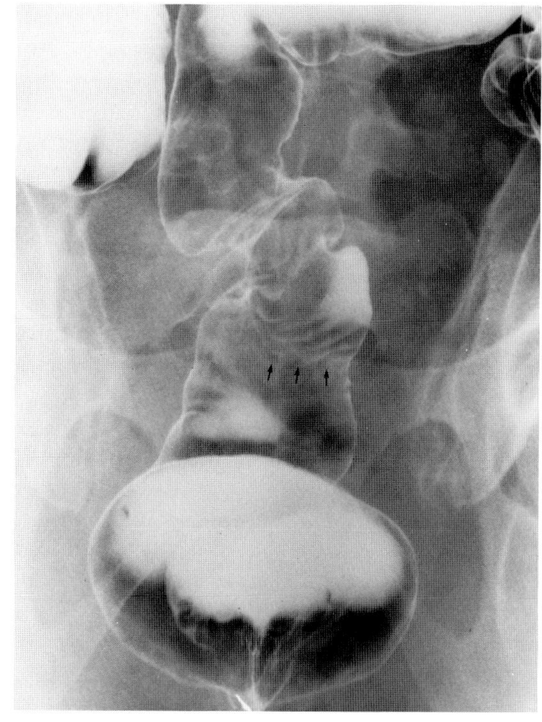

Fig. 4-45 Metastatic disease. **(A)** Lateral view of the rectum showing a narrow, straightened distal sigmoid encased by tumor. There is tethering of the folds on the anterior surface *(arrows)*. **(B)** Prone-angled view of the rectosigmoid in same patient demonstrating the en face appearance of the metastatic involvement with "striped" or crinkled mucosal surface *(arrows)*.

transverse mesocolon, is classically involved although the superior border may also be abnormal. The margin may appear straightened or spiculated. Although signs of acute pancreatitis are most often seen in the transverse colon and splenic flexure, the potent pancreatic enzymes released may also track down the mesentery or along the paracolic gutters to involve other areas of the colon, including the cecum and the ascending and descending colon. Fistula formation and perforation secondary to necrosis are unusual complications.

Development of pancreatic pseudocysts leads to another aspect of secondary involvement of the colon. Whereas changes of acute pancreatitis, including pancreatic phlegmons, abscesses, and even hemorrhagic pancreatitis are essentially inflammatory, evolution of a well-encapsulated pseudocyst will cause a smooth extrinsic impression. Pseudocysts usually arise from the body or tail of the pancreas. They vary widely in size and location within the abdomen and may extend into the pelvis to involve cecum, sigmoid or rectum, and the transverse colon. Ultrasound is the modality of choice for following the maturation of pseudocysts.

Carcinoma of the pancreas also may spread along the transverse mesocolon; focal and an asymmetric mass effect occur along the transverse colon. Areas of mass effect may be more discrete than those seen with pancreatitis. Intraperitoneal seeding, as described above, also occurs.

TRAUMA

Colonic trauma is relatively uncommon, accounting for about 5 percent of abdominal trauma. Most often, the trauma results from a motor vehicle accident, shooting, or stabbing. Blunt trauma may compress the bowel or mesentery against the spine and lead to hemorrhage or contusions that may result in ischemic changes. Penetrating trauma may result in bowel perforation and plain abdominal radiographs will then demonstrate pneumoperitoneum. Contrast studies are rarely necessary. An emergency colostomy may be required for traumatic bowel perforations. With blunt trauma, conservative treatment is usually all that is required.

Ingested foreign bodies may cause bowel obstructions or perforations. These are more likely to occur in the terminal ileum or appendix than in the colon. Rarely, foreign bodies may be identified on plain abdominal films. Foreign bodies inserted into the rectum may be a source of trauma in children, psychotics, or homosexuals. A nonspecific proctitis may result from acute or chronic irritation. Perforation may occur and may be extra- or intraperitoneal.

THE POSTSURGICAL COLON

Most colonic surgery is performed for carcinoma and diverticulitis. Inflammatory bowel disease and trauma account for most other sources of colon surgery. After segmental resections, the colon may be anastomosed, either end-to-end, end-to-side, or side-to-side, to small bowel or colon.

Right hemicolectomies for carcinoma, angiodysplasia, or ileocecal Crohn disease are repaired with ileocolotomies. Invagination of the bowel wall may frequently be identified on radiographs taken during postoperative barium enema examinations. Small, nodular filling defects may occur as a result of healing. A baseline postoperative double-contrast study, best performed 8 to 12 weeks after surgery, will distinguish these from recurrence.

Colostomies are performed as definitive surgery for low rectal carcinomas, ulcerative colitis, or exenterations for pelvic malignancies. They may also be performed as definitive or interim procedures for diverticulitis, trauma, and other lesions. If the bowel distal to the colostomy is not removed, it can be tied-off (Hartmann pouch) or left as a mucous fistula or a double-barreled colostomy. Barium enemas are performed as follow-up examinations or prior to reanat-

omosis. Depending on the anatomy, the distal limb may be examined per rectum or via the colostomy. Many catheter and enema arrangements have been devised for both single- and double-contrast colostomy enemas. If a balloon catheter is used, it must be inflated outside the patient and held against the skin. Unfortunately, none of the methods mentioned works in all cases, and colostomy enemas can be quite messy.

Ulcerative colitis and familial polyposis have traditionally been treated by proctocolectomy and ileostomy, but a trend toward the rectal-sparing ileoproctotomy plus close endoscopic surveillance, has been increasing. This procedure is usually performed with an end-to-side anastomosis. Ileoanal anastomosis, in which the rectal mucosa is stripped and the sphincters preserved, is another procedure used to treat ulcerative colitis and familial polyposis.

Immediate complications after colon surgery are primarily leaks and abscess formation. These may be evaluated by contrast enema, fistulogram or CT, depending on the individual case. Late complications may be stricture formation, recurrent tumor, or metachronous lesions.

On postoperative radiographs taken during double-contrast barium enema examinations, invagination of the bowel wall can usually be identified at colocolic anastomoses. One or more nodular filling defects may be seen adjacent to the anastomosis, caused by stitch granulomas. These defects should be identified on an initial postoperative evaluation. Over time, they regress or stay the same size. Any increase in nodularity, irregularity, or eccentricity of the anastomosis should raise the suspicion of tumor recurrence. After abdominoperineal resection, CT best evaluates pelvic recurrence (see Fig. 4-20).

CONGENITAL AND DEVELOPMENTAL ANOMALIES

Manifestations of some of the aberrations that result from anomalous rotation or abnormal mesenteric attachments in adults are discussed in this section. The reader is referred to pediatric gastrointestinal radiology texts for radiologic manifestations in childhood.

5
Radiology of the Liver

Harvey V. Steinberg
Michael E. Bernardino

ANATOMY OF THE LIVER

Gross Morphology

The liver is the largest solid organ in the human body, weighing 1 to 2 kg in the adult. Individual variations in size and configuration are both common and considerable. The adult liver lies in the right and midportions of the upper abdomen and measures approximately 10 to 12.5 cm in its anteroposterior dimension, 20 to 22.5 cm in its transverse diameter, and 15 to 17.5 cm vertically.

The liver is composed of a large right lobe, a smaller left lobe, and an anatomically distinct caudate lobe. The main lobar fissure divides the liver into right and left lobes. This fissure corresponds to a drawn line that extends from the gallbladder fossa to the inferior vena cava. The right lobe, approximately six times larger than the left, is further divided into anterior and posterior segments by the right intersegmental fissure. The right lobe has a rounded contour with rather smooth margins. Occasionally, in women more commonly than men, a tongue of liver tissue is seen to extend caudally from the right lobe of the liver to form the so-called Riedel lobe. The left lobe is divided into medial and lateral segments by the left intersegmental fissure (fissure of the ligamentum teres). The caudal and anterior portions of the left intersegmental fissure are contiguous with the falciform ligament — an extrahepatic remnant of the fetal ventral mesentery. Fibrofatty tissue within the fissure of the ligamentum teres and the falciform ligament frequently produces an echogenic cleft on ultrasound, which corresponds to an area of low attenuation on computed tomographic (CT) scans.

The caudate lobe is a posterior portion of the liver bound by the fissure of the ligamentum venosum anteriorly and the fossa of the inferior vena cava (IVC) posteriorly. Separating the caudate lobe from the more anteriorly located lateral segment of the left lobe, the fissure of the ligamentum venosum is commonly seen as a strong specular reflection in both longitudinal and transverse sonograms but is only rarely seen on CT scans. Arterial and portal venous branches from both the right and left lobe of the liver supply the caudate lobe. In addition, however, the veins from the caudate lobe empty directly into the inferior vena cava, thus accounting for relative sparing of this portion of the liver in certain diffuse parenchymal diseases (i.e., cirrhosis, Budd-Chiari syndrome).

Hepatic Vasculature

The hepatic veins comprise the efferent vascular system of the liver. Three major hepatic trunks — the right, middle, and left—drain into the IVC at the superior margin of the liver. The right hepatic vein runs through the right intersegmental fissure, and thus divides the right lobe into anterior and posterior segments. The middle hepatic vein courses through the interlobar fissure to help define the boundary between the right and left lobes of the liver. The left hepatic vein is located within the left intersegmental fissure. It serves as a landmark in separating the medial and lateral segments of the left lobe of the liver. The hepatic veins can vary in caliber between individuals and can become quite large in size with a strenuous Valsalva maneuver or right-sided heart failure.

The hepatic veins and their tributaries can, most commonly, be recognized on longitudinal ultrasound scans as tubular, oval, or round thin-walled sonolucencies in the liver parenchyma. (In less than one-third of cases, hepatic veins exhibit echogenic walls.) In contrast, thick-walled portal veins can be identified by their echogenic borders, which usually makes it possible to differentiate between hepatic and portal vein branches. Moreover, the hepatic veins can be traced back to their junction with the IVC by serially scanning in oblique planes (Fig. 5-1). Furthermore, the caliber of the portal vein increases toward the porta hepatis, whereas that of the hepatic vein increases toward the diaphragm and IVC.

The hepatic veins can be seen on CT images after a bolus of iodinated contrast material is rapidly administered. They appear as areas of increased attenuation when compared with the surrounding liver parenchyma. As with ultrasound, the hepatic veins can be seen to empty into the IVC.

Direct hepatic vein visualization requires a selective hepatic vein injection. This can be accomplished via a femoral, brachial, or transjugular approach. The main hepatic injection is performed with an end- and side-hole catheter. Injection rates of 10 to 12 ml/sec for a total of 25 to 30 ml (of 76 percent contrast) into the main hepatic vein provide optimal hepatic vein visualization. Alternatively, wedged hepatic venography can be performed, using a catheter with only an end-hole. Performed under fluoroscopic observation, lower volumes of contrast—generally 2 ml/sec for a total of 8 to 10 ml—are used with this technique. The pressure measured in wedged hepatic venography reflects portal pressure, which normally ranges between 40 and 150 mm of saline. Pressures greater than 150 mm are consistent with portal hypertension.

In normal individuals, 75 to 80 percent of the total hepatic blood flow comes from the portal vein, and the remainder comes from the hepatic artery. The larger portal venous structures course through the liver transversely and are thus best assessed when imaged in the transverse plane. The main portal vein crosses just anterior to the IVC, branching into an anterior left branch and then into a more laterally directed right branch in the porta hepatis. The left portal vein, smaller in caliber than the right, originates slightly to the right of midline and then passes anteriorly and to the left. The right portal vein divides into anterior and posterior branches, supplying the corresponding segments of the right hepatic lobe. Unlike the hepatic venous trunks, which run in the fissures separating the major hepatic segments, the portal vein branches run within the hepatic parenchyma itself.

The portal venous structures are generally well visualized in the venous phase of splenic and superior mesenteric artery (SMA) arteriography. A vasodilator, i.e., 25 to 50 mg tolazoline (Priscoline) injected directly into the SMA approximately 45 seconds before contrast injection, further enhances the portal phase. The filming sequence is always tailored to the specific clinical problem, but must include an evaluation of both the systemic arterial supply as well as the portal circulation. Thus, initial rapid filming is followed by a longer, slower sequence, and should be carried out for at least 25 seconds (Table 5-1).

Transhepatic portography or splenoportography are less commonly used to visualize the portal structures. Portography is generally reserved for those uncommon cases of unsatisfactory portal vein visualization with standard arteriography, or for therapeutic applications such as variceal emoblization.

The hepatic artery proper usually arises from the celiac axis and continues as the common hepatic artery after giving off the gastroduodenal artery, before dividing into right and left branches within the porta hepatis. Transverse images at the level of the porta hepatis show the portal vein to be posterior and the

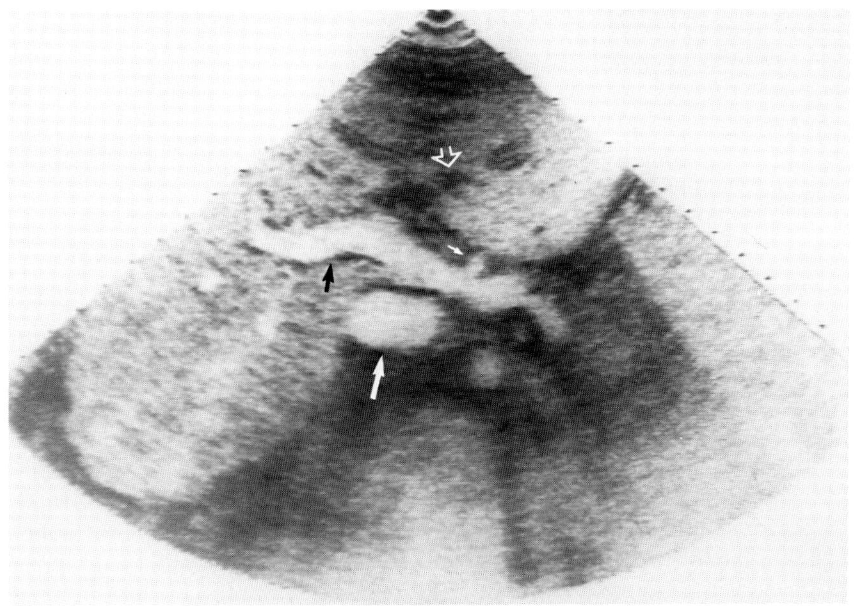

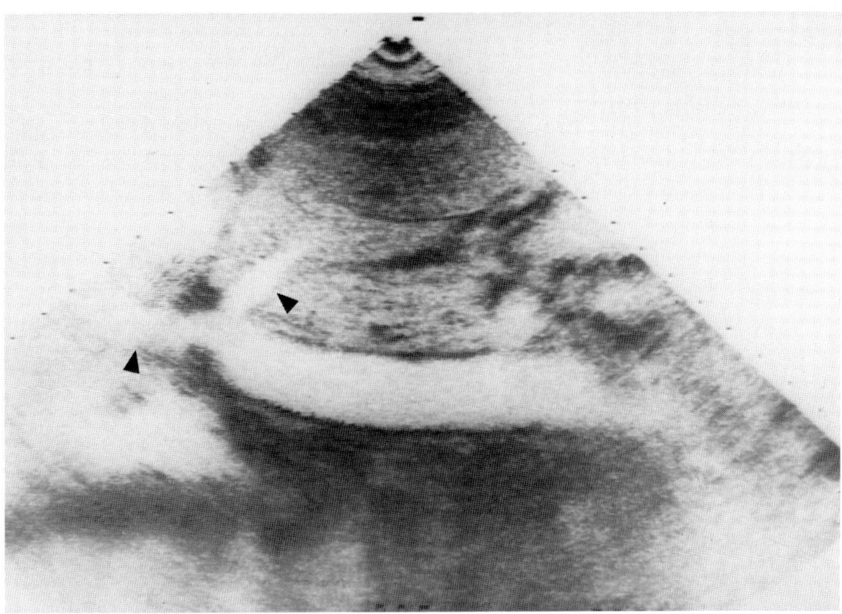

Fig. 5-1 (A) A transverse sonographic image shows the clearly identified portal vein *(black arrow)* anterior to the inferior vena cava *(long white arrow)*. The portal vein has distinct echogenic borders. A small, rounded lucency, anterior to the portal vein on this transverse image, corresponds to a portion of the hepatic artery *(short white arrow)*. The liver parenchyma itself is of homogeneous and normal echogenicity. A linear focus of echogenicity corresponds to fibrofatty tissue in a portion of the falciform ligament *(open white arrow)*. **(B)** On a longitudinal sonographic image, thin-walled hepatic veins *(black arrowheads)* are seen as they drain into the inferior vena cava.

Table 5-1 Angiography of the Liver

Site	Dose (cc)	Rate (cc/sec)
Celiac artery	50–60	6–10
Superior mesenteric artery	50–70	6–10
Common hepatic artery	40–50	6–8
Main hepatic venography	25–30	10–12
Wedged hepatic venography	8–10	2

common bile duct anterior, with the hepatic artery sandwiched between the two. Partial or complete replacement of the common, left, and right hepatic arteries is present in up to 45 percent of the population. The left hepatic artery arises from the left gastric artery in about 25 percent of individuals. Half of these variations are partial replacements. The origin of the right hepatic artery from the SMA is completely replaced in about 14 percent of the population and partially replaced in 8 percent. Other anomalies of the origins of the common, right, and left hepatic arteries occur less frequently.

Hepatic Parenchyma

The normal adult hepatic parenchyma has a homogeneous echogenicity slightly greater than that of the renal cortex and slightly less than that of the pancreas on ultrasound.

When imaged by computed tomography, the normal nonenhanced hepatic parenchyma has a slightly higher density than other upper abdominal organs (spleen, kidneys, pancreas). Normal adult liver attenuation values are somewhat variable — between 40 to 80 Hounsfield units (HU). However, the range of each individual liver is much narrower, resulting in a relatively homogeneous parenchymal pattern.

Most commonly, the hepatic parenchyma has a greater attenuation than that of blood. Thus, the portal and hepatic venous systems appear as relatively low density branching structures when compared to the surrounding parenchyma on noncontrast CT scans. Distinction can usually be made between dilated bile ducts and normal vascular structures by anatomic position and CT density. However, venous structures are best differentiated from dilated ducts by injecting the contrast material intravenously. Although contrast material increases the density of the hepatic venous structures and liver parenchyma, it causes no such effect on the biliary system. Following the intravenous administration of iodinated contrast material,

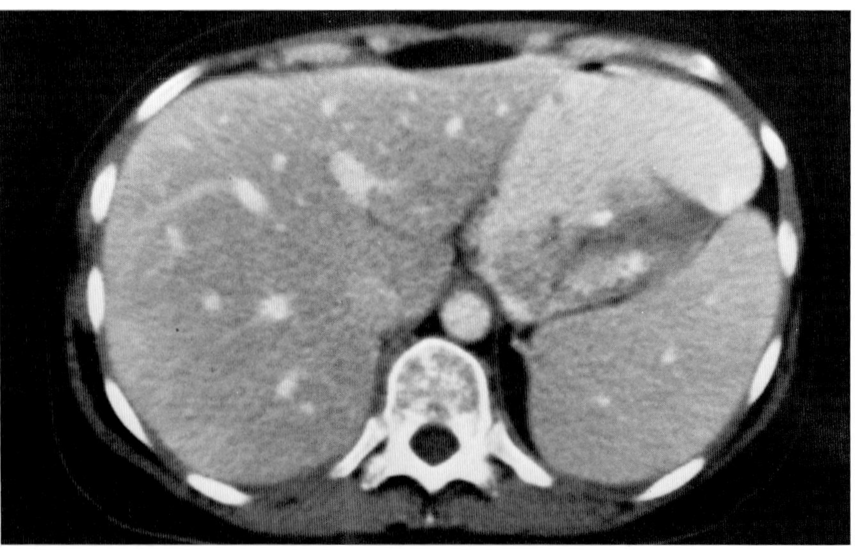

Fig. 5-2 An axial CT image through the liver after a bolus injection of iodinated contrast demonstrates enhancement of the aorta, hepatic vasculature and, to a lesser extent, the inferior vena cava and spleen.

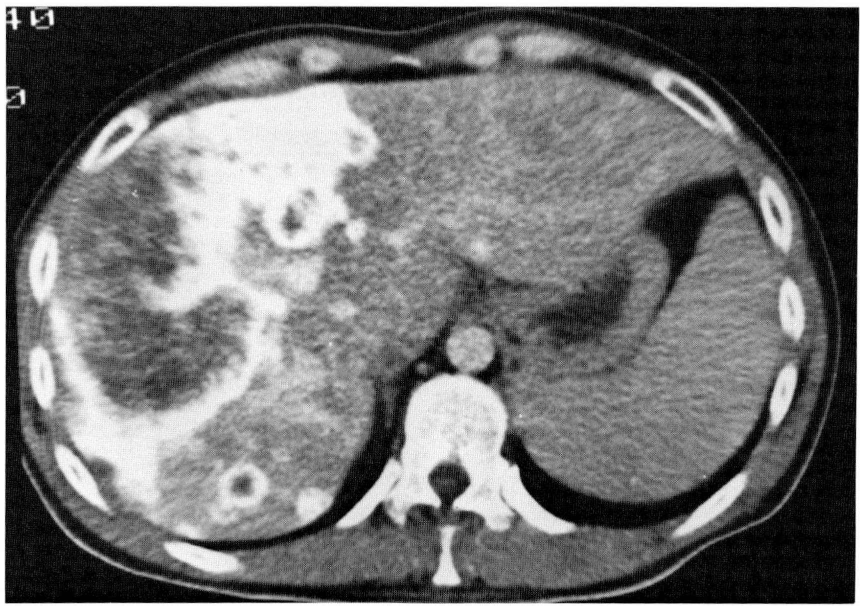

Fig. 5-3 A CTA reveals a large metastatic focus in the liver, as well as multiple smaller lesions.

the attenuation value of the normal liver parenchyma increases in a dose-related fashion, often to as high as 120 to 140 HU (Fig. 5-2). While some advocate the routine use of pre- and post-intravenous contrast scans when evaluating for focal hepatic disease, the use of high-dose intravenous iodine alone (50 to 60 g) followed by rapid CT scanning, is just as accurate, sensitive, and specific, according to recent reports in the literature.

Computed angiotomography (CTA) is a technique whereby a catheter is selectively placed in or near the hepatic artery or SMA (or their branches) and iodinated contrast material is infused through the catheter as a CT scan is being done. When third and fourth generation CT scanners are used for such scans, a somewhat dilute contrast material (30 percent) should be administered. Literature reports claim that this technique detects more focal lesions compared with routine computed tomography or selective angiography. Most of the new lesions detected, as compared with angiography, are in the left hepatic lobe and subcapsular area, classically the two most difficult hepatic regions to evaluate angiographically (Fig. 5-3).

Delayed iodine contrast scanning — i.e., scanning 4 to 8 hours after the intravenous administration of 60 g or

greater of iodinated contrast material — can also demonstrate more focal intrahepatic masses. In addition, this technique has been shown to greater quantify the extent of such masses, compared with routine CT imaging. Delayed iodine contrast scanning utilizes the fact that normal hepatic tissue secretes 1 to 2 percent of the contrast material, whereas abnormal tissue does not concentrate iodine. This makes for a greater density contrast between normal and abnormal liver tissue with a lower attenuation coefficient.

The iodolipids (i.e., EOE-13), called hepatosplenic specific agents because they opacify the reticuloendothelial space, have fallen into disfavor, owing to their toxicity and nonspecificity.

NEOPLASMS

Overlap may exist between the appearance of benign, primary malignant, and metastatic neoplasms, as well as infections. However, by (1) combining the information available from multiple diagnostic imaging procedures, (2) detecting other possible associated abnormalities, and (3) correlating the imaging modalities with the clinical history and physical examination, a correct diagnosis can usually be made. Where uncertainties still exist and/or pathologic proof is required, needle biopsy is indicated for a definitive diagnosis.

Cavernous Hemangiomas

Cavernous hemangiomas are the most common benign tumors of the liver, occurring in up to 7 percent of the general population. Approximately 75 to 85 percent of hemangiomas occur in females and although all ages are affected, the diagnosis is rarely made before adulthood. Most hemangiomas are located in the posterior aspect of the right lobe of the liver and are subcapsular. The majority are single and less than 5 cm in diameter, although multiple hemangiomas and large lesions are not infrequently seen. Histologically, cavernous hemangiomas are composed of multiple, endothelial-lined cystic blood-filled spaces separated by fibrous septa. Occasionally, calcification may be found within them.

Most cavernous hemangiomas are asymptomatic and found incidentally. Those that are symptomatic are usually "giant hemangiomas" that may present with abdominal discomfort, an abdominal mass, or both. More rarely, spontaneous rupture and hemorrhage may occur.

Angiographically, their appearance is characteristic. The arteries supplying the liver are normal in size and demonstrate normal peripheral tapering. Multiple, small vascular spaces are opacified in the late arterial phase and, unlike other vascular tumors, they remain opacified during and well into the venous phase (Fig. 5-4). The vascular spaces often demonstrate a ringed or C-shape secondary to central fibrosis of the tumor, or central thrombosis or hemorrhage. Arteriovenous shunting, classically considered a hallmark of malignancy, although not common, has been reported in cavernous hemangiomas. However, enlarged, irregular neovascular feeding vessels should not be present.

The known histologic and angiographic appearance of hemangiomas make it possible to use other less invasive imaging modalities for diagnosis and, in almost all cases, obviate the need for further investigation.

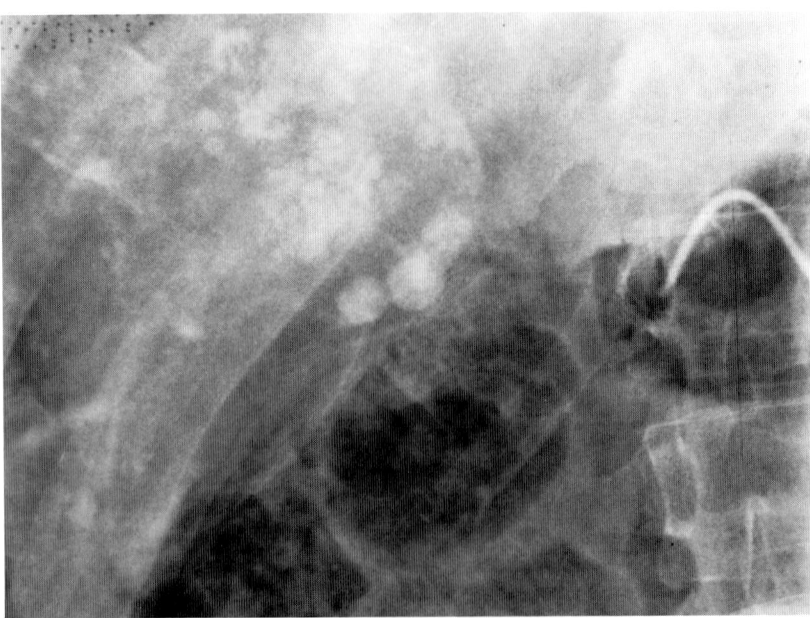

Fig. 5-4 A celiac arteriogram reveals multiple vascular lesions opacifying in the late arterial phase and remaining opacified well into the venous phase, classic for hemangiomatosis.

Prior to the intravenous injection of contrast material, hemangiomas usually appear as hypodense well-circumscribed homogeneous lesions on CT. After the administration of contrast material, a cavernous hemangioma will show sequential enhancement. The periphery will initially enhance, in contrast to the low attenuation value of the central portion of the lesion. With time, a centripetally advancing border of enhancement ensues and the central area of low density becomes progressively smaller (Fig. 5-5).

Thus, a dynamic CT scan after the administration of a bolus of iodinated contrast material (i.e., 75 to 100 ml of 60 percent) with images every 15 seconds for 1 minute, then every minute for several minutes, should be diagnostic in almost all cases of hemangiomas.

Technetium-99m red-blood cell scanning will similarly demonstrate hemangiomas as focal areas of increased activity, when delayed 1- to 2-hour blood pool images are obtained. This appearance has been shown to be both specific and sensitive.

Magnetic resonance imaging (MRI), although still relatively new, seems to hold much promise in accurately diagnosing hemangiomas. Initial work suggests that scans implementing spin-echo sequences utilizing a T_2-weighted image (i.e., TE 60 to 100, TR 2000), reveal that hemangiomas demonstrate an extremely high intensity signal (Fig. 5-6A).

On ultrasound, hemangiomas are more echogenic than the surrounding liver parenchyma (Fig. 5-6B). This increased echogenicity is related to the interface caused by the walls of the cavernous venous sinuses and the blood within these vessels. A central linear septum is frequently identified, giving the lesion a lobulated appearance. A slightly more irregular pattern develops as the hemangioma undergoes degeneration and fibrous replacement. The aforementioned findings on ultrasound may suggest hemangioma, but they are nonspecific. Further investigation and correlation with CT, nuclear medicine, and MRI, as previously outlined, is suggested.

Hepatic Adenoma

Hepatic adenomas are uncommon, usually solitary benign tumors that occur more commonly in women, especially those who have been taking oral contraceptives. However, they are also seen in men receiving hormonal therapy. Liver cell adenomas can regress or completely disappear after the birth control pills are withdrawn or hormonal therapy is discontinued. The benign well-encapsulated neoplasms, composed entirely of hepatocytes (bile ducts and Kupffer cells are not present), are prone to hemorrhage and should, therefore, be resected if they have bled.

Angiographic and radionuclide features of hepatic adenomas permit a definitive diagnosis to be made in most patients. Sulfur colloid scans demonstrate a photopenic space-occupying lesion. Angiographically, adenomas may range from hypovascular to hypervascular. Typical appearances include (1) a hypovascular lesion with displacement and draping of the hepatic arteries around the tumor, (2) a hypervascular lesion with tortuous vessels coursing through the lesion. Feeding vessels may enter from the periphery or center of the tumor. Neovascularity may be present but "pooling" and arteriovenous (AV) shunting should not be present.

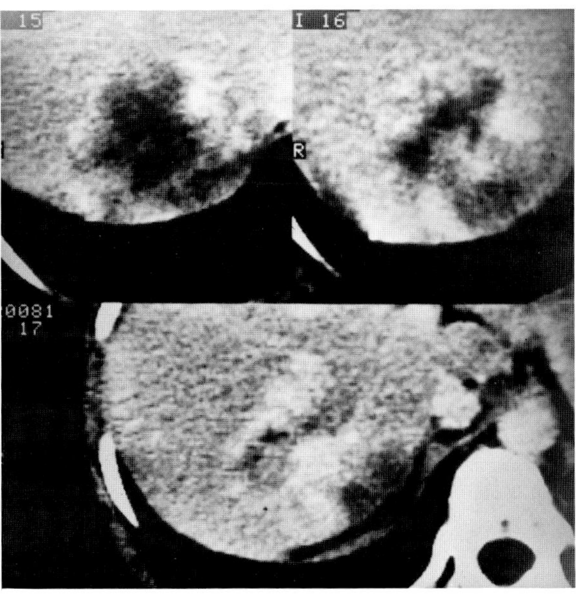

Fig. 5-5 Dynamic CT images after a bolus injection of intravenous contrast material at 15 seconds, 1 minute, and 3 minutes demonstrate a progressive centripetally advancing border of enhancement characteristic of a hemangioma.

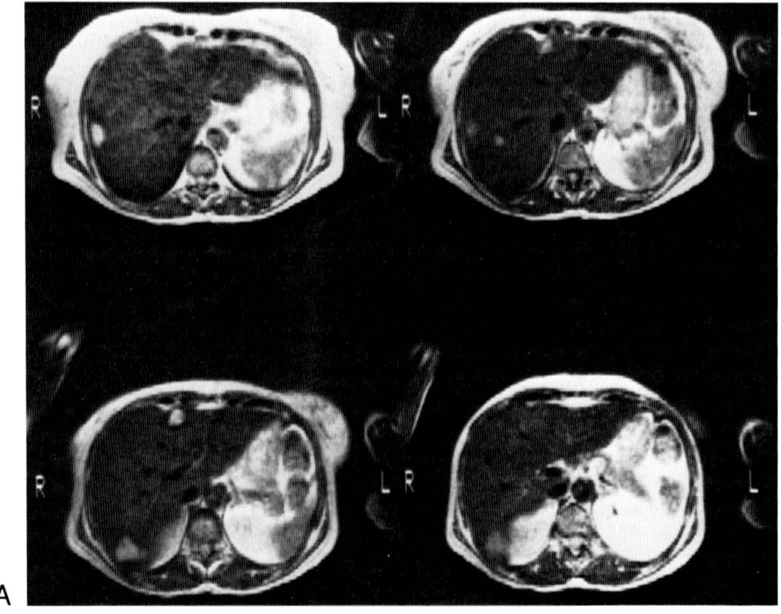

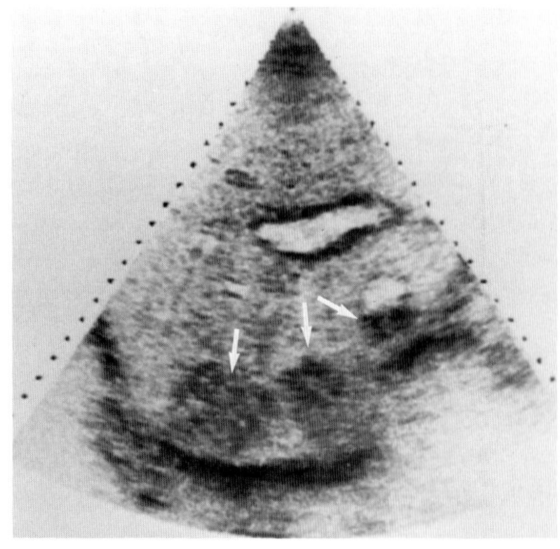

Fig. 5-6 (A) This MRI demonstrates multiple hemangiomas. Interestingly, CT demonstrated two hemangiomas, ultrasound demonstrated three hemangiomas, and the MRI, using a TE 60 msec, TR 2000 msec, demonstrates five hemangiomas, recognizable by their extremely high-intensity signal. **(B)** Ultrasonography demonstrates multiple echogenic foci consistent with, but not diagnostic of, hemangiomas *(white arrows)*.

Computed tomography and ultrasonography can detect hepatic adenomas (Fig. 5-7). However, findings using these methods are variable and nonspecific. Ultrasonography may demonstrate hepatic adenomas as solid masses of increased or decreased echogenicity. They may appear slightly less dense or isodense with the surrounding liver parenchyma on precontrast CT scans. Following intravenous contrast infusion, the appearance of adenomas may or may not be enhanced. A CT examination, showing a well-defined, nearly isodense mass with a central area of relative increased density on precontrast scans, is almost certainly a liver cell adenoma. This appearance is probably caused by an excess of lipid-laden hepatocytes comprising the capsule of the lesion, which uniformly and transiently enhances, except for the central area of hemorrhage.

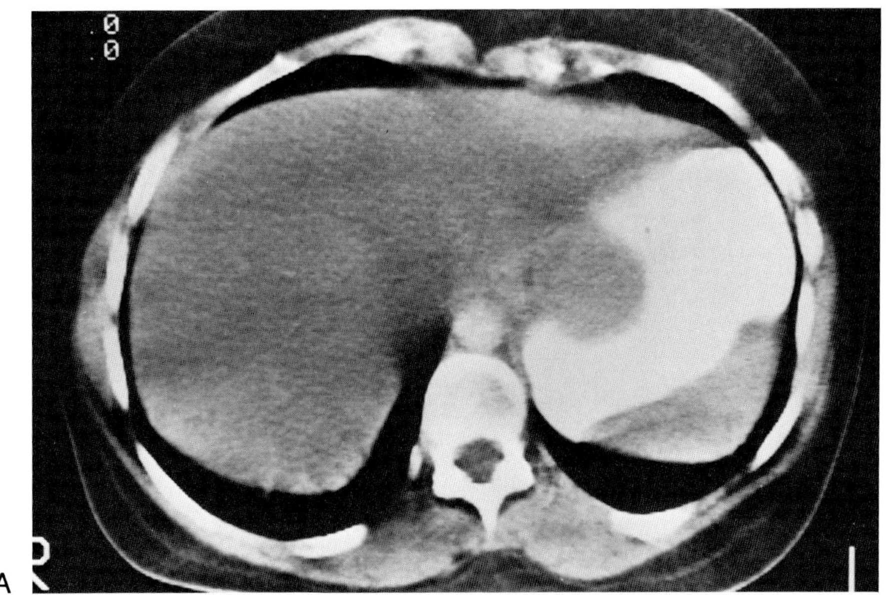

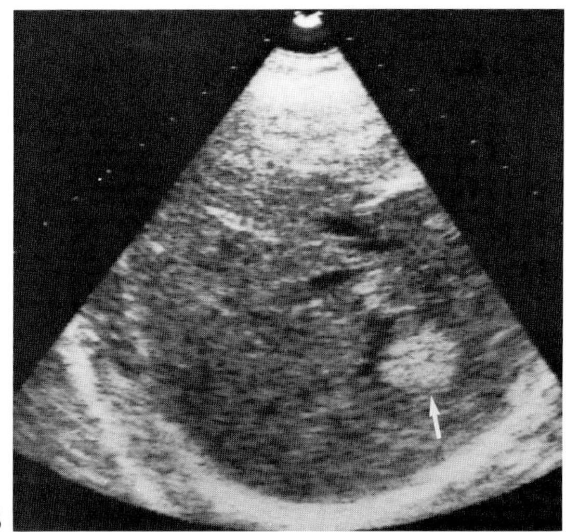

Fig. 5-7 (A) CT demonstrates a soft tissue mass smoothly indenting the lesser curvature of the stomach. The diagnosis suggested was leiomyoma of the stomach. However, no clear demarcation between this soft tissue mass and the liver is identified. Thus, a mass arising from the liver could not be excluded. At surgery, this mass was found to represent an adenoma of the liver. **(B)** Ultrasonography of a different patient reveals an echogenic focus in the liver *(white arrow)*. A CT (not shown) revealed minimal enhancement of this lesion, making the diagnosis of hemangioma unlikely. The diagnosis of a hepatic adenoma was made by percutaneous needle biopsy.

Focal Nodular Hyperplasia

Focal nodular hyperplasia (FNH) is a rare, benign liver lesion composed of hepatocytes, Kupffer cells, and bile ducts. The presence of the latter two elements helps to differentiate FNH from hepatic adenomas. The vast majority are asymptomatic, with hemorrhage a rare complication. Lesions may be multiple in approximately 13 to 20 percent of cases. The female to male ratio is 4:1; no definite association with oral contraceptives has been shown. Tumors are usually subcapsular in location or may be pedunculated.

Due to the presence of hepatocytes and Kupffer cells, most radionuclide scintigrams are reported as normal, although the uptake of radiocolloid is variable, ranging from cold to hot.

Classically, on angiography FNH appears as a well-defined, circumscribed, hypervascular lesion with tortuous neovascularity. Feeding vessels may appear to arise in the center of the lesion and radiate to the periphery; a central stellate scar may be seen. Rarely has AV-shunting been seen. However, a lack of encasement may help to distinguish FNH from hepatoma, which may present a similar angiographic appearance. By correlating the radionuclide study and angiography, FNH can usually be diagnosed. Biopsy may be needed, especially when the nuclide scan shows a photopenic focus or the angiogram is not typical for FNH.

Sonography and CT can detect FNH but, as in cases of hepatic adenomas, the findings are nonspecific. Hypoechoic, hyperechoic, and a mixed-echo pattern have been reported with ultrasound in FNH. CT shows FNH lesions as hypodense or isodense on noncontrast enhanced scans, with a variable change in attenuation after the intravenous administration of contrast. However, if a moderately sized, nearly isodense mass enhances transiently and diffusely except for a central stellate scar, the diagnosis of FNH should be strongly considered (Fig. 5-8).

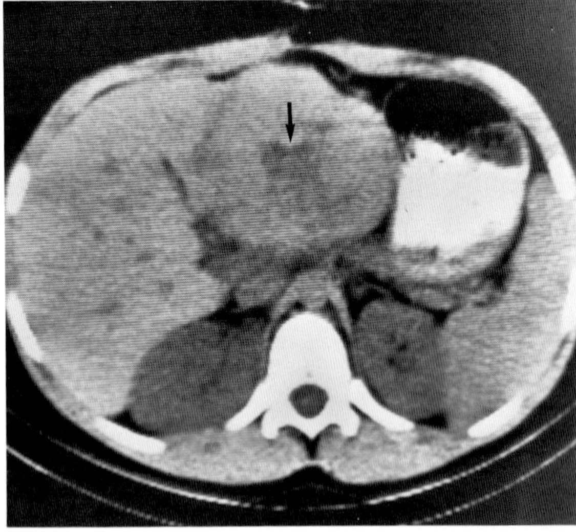

Fig. 5-8 A noncontrast enhanced CT scan through the liver reveals a large mass occupying and expanding the contour of the left lobe. In addition, a central stellate scar is appreciated *(black arrow)*. This mass represents focal nodular hyperplasia (proven by percutaneous needle biopsy).

Cysts

Hepatic cysts occur in congenital and acquired forms, congenital lesions being more frequent. Congenital cysts develop secondary to an excess of intrahepatic ductules that fail to involute. Acquired cysts are usually the result of previous inflammatory disease or trauma. Hepatic cysts are rather common; they are present in 2 to 7 percent of the population at autopsy. These cysts may vary in size from several millimeters to several centimeters. They may occur singly, in small numbers, or as innumerable multifocal cysts in polycystic liver disease. They appear as sharply delineated, round or oval-shaped lesions. On CT scans, hepatic cysts are well-circumscribed, homogeneous areas of near-water density (0 ± 15 HU), which do not enhance with intravenous contrast. Occasionally, cysts can hemorrhage, become infected, or contain debris within them, resulting in increased attenuation, fluid-fluid levels, or both. Some cysts may have slightly irregular walls or septations (Fig. 5-9).

On ultrasound, hepatic cysts reveal characteristics similar to those found in any other region of the body. Specifically, they are well-circumscribed, anechoic, and possess sharply defined posterior walls with enhanced through-sound transmission. The most common cystic lesions in the liver, which occasionally can mimic benign hepatic cysts, include old hematomas (usually not as well-defined), abscesses (usually poorly defined, with thicker, irregular walls, and containing debris), and cystic metastases. Aspiration is recommended in those rare cases in which some degree of uncertainty exists.

Hepatocellular Carcinoma (Hepatoma)

Hepatomas represent the most common primary malignant tumors seen in the liver. They represent over 80 percent of all primary hepatic malignancies. Hepatomas may present as solitary lesions (approximately 50 percent of the time), multifocal tumors (approximately 20 percent of the time), or diffuse lesions (approximately 30 percent of the time). There is an increased incidence of hepatocellular carcinoma in patients afflicted with cirrhosis, hepatitis, hemochromatosis, and syphilis. In addition, a higher incidence of hepatocellular carcinoma is seen in both

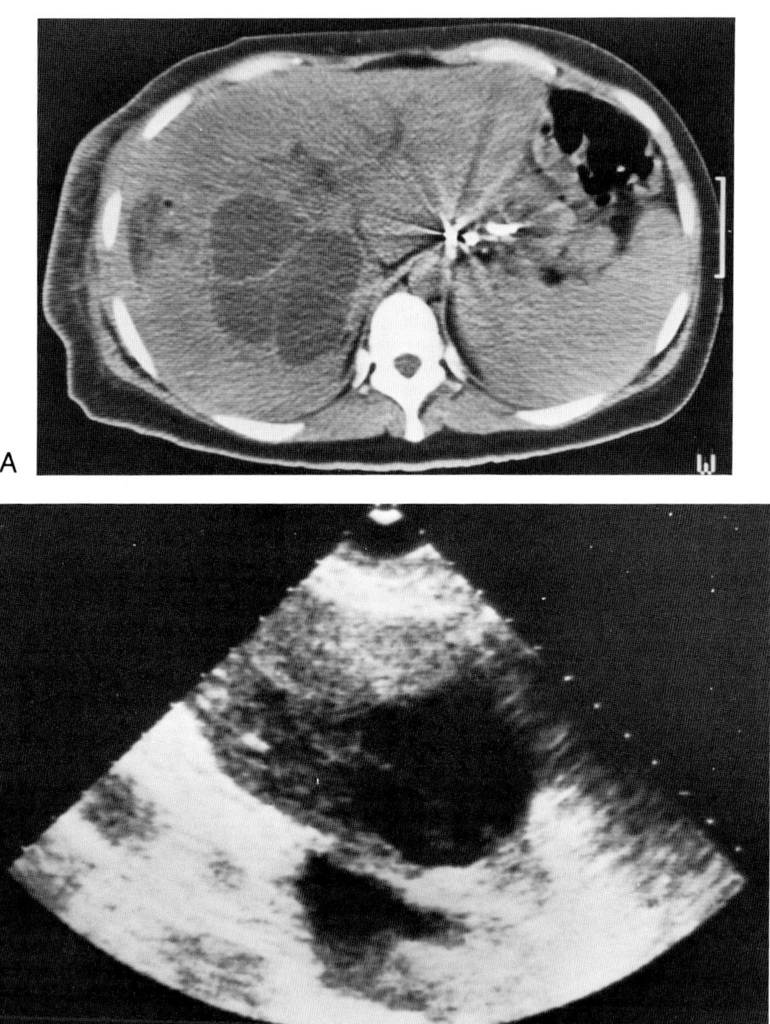

Fig. 5-9 (A) A multilocular low density lesion is noted in the right lobe of the liver. Metallic surgical clips are noted from previous partial gastrectomy. Incidentally, an area of low density, resulting from previous surgery, is noted along the lateral margin of the liver. **(B)** Ultrasound reveals this lesion to be fluid-filled with good through transmission. However, septations are noted within it, making it impossible to fully exclude a malignant process. Percutaneous needle biopsy confirmed this to be a septated benign hepatic cyst.

the Chinese and the black African populations. Elevated alpha-fetoprotein levels are usually present.

The detection of hepatomas may be difficult in patients with diseased livers (i.e., cirrhosis). In such instances, the normal homogeneous liver architecture has frequently undergone a metamorphosis, resulting in areas of lobulation and changes in density, possibly secondary to fibrosis, fatty degeneration, and/or regenerating nodules. Thus, not only can it be difficult to appreciate subtle density changes secondary to malignant tumor involvement, but when subtle differences are appreciated, benign and malignant processes cannot always be differentiated. In these cases, percutaneous biopsy is recommended.

The CT appearance of hepatocellular carcinoma is varied (Fig. 5-10). Most frequently, hepatomas produce single or multiple hepatic mass lesions less than 2.5 cm in diameter. On precontrast CT scans they appear as areas of low attenuation with respect to normal liver parenchyma (approximately 30 to 50 HU). Occasionally, hepatomas may be isodense with the surrounding hepatic parenchyma, and may be detected solely by a change in hepatic contour. Approximately 25 percent of hepatomas exhibit calcification. After the administration of intravenous contrast material, the CT appearance of hepatocellular carcinoma is variable. However, in most instances, the infusion of iodinated contrast material results in a slight increase in the density differences between normal liver and hepatomas, thus resulting in higher detectability and better definition of the tumor.

When evaluating a hepatoma, it is important to determine whether the portal vein or the hepatic veins are involved. Involvement of the IVC via extension from the hepatic veins is also possible. Both before and after the intravenous administration of contrast agent, thrombus within the portal vein or IVC appears as an area of relative decreased attenuation, compared with blood in the aorta. The diameter of the thrombosed vein may appear to be enlarged. Following an intravenous bolus of contrast, the walls of the vein may be transiently enhanced. Additionally, there may be areas of decreased attenuation in the entire lobe or in segments supplied by a branch of the portal vein and invaded by the hepatoma secondary to decreased perfusion of the affected area. A similar patchy enhancement has been described in cases of Budd-Chiari syndrome involving the lobe or segment drained by the involved hepatic vein.

On ultrasonography, the appearance of hepatomas may be quite variable (Fig. 5-11). Echogenic masses, diffuse distortions of the hepatic parenchyma—i.e., irregular tortuous vessels—and, less commonly, hypoechoic masses are included in the spectrum of appearances.

Angiographically, most hepatomas are very vascular; a dilated hepatic arterial supply, bizarre and irregular tumor neovascularity, and contrast accumulation in irregular vascular lakes are observed. Anaplastic lesions in the diffuse infiltrative form of hepatoma may be hypovascular. AV shunting is highly suggestive of hepatoma. Invasion of the portal vein, hepatic vein, or IVC may be appreciated. Although MRI is still in its early stages, it appears to show much promise, not only in detecting focal liver lesions but, more importantly, in evaluating the vasculature for tumor thrombus.

Recently, a distinct entity known as fibrolamellar hepatocellular carcinoma has been recognized. This variant form of hepatocellular carcinoma (HCC) is (1) found to affect mostly the adolescent and young adult population, (2) not associated with epidemiologic risk factors, and (3) associated with normal alpha-fetoprotein levels. Furthermore, fibrolamellar HCC is associated with a significantly better prognosis.

These tumors are usually large and well-defined. Small central calcifications may be seen, and satellite lesions are not infrequently present. Microscopically, eosinophilic hepatocyte-like cells, with an abundant fibrous stroma, are typically seen.

Fibrolamellar HCCs are echogenic ultrasonographically, cold on sulfur colloid scintigraphy, and nearly always hypervascular angiographically. Using CT, a hypodense mass that enhances after intravenous contrast administration is typically seen. Compartmentalization secondary to fibrous septa may be demonstrated by CT, angiography, or both techniques.

Cholangiocarcinoma

Cholangiocarcinomas are slow-growing tumors, most commonly located in the common bile duct between the cystic duct and the ampulla of Vater. They may involve the porta hepatis, common hepatic duct, and intrahepatic ducts. Painless jaundice is the most common presenting symptom. Despite being quite small when first detected, the tumor commonly has invaded adjacent vessels or viscera by the time it is first diagnosed. Although curative surgical intervention is

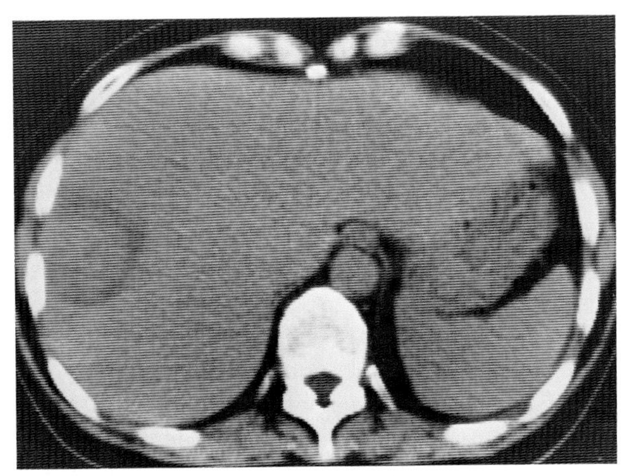

A

Fig. 5-10 (A) The CT appearance of hepatomas is variable. A single focal lesion in the liver shows significant enhancement after the administration of intravenous contrast material. **(B)** Multiple areas of low attenuation in the left lobe of the liver represent multifocal hepatomas. **(C)** A hepatoma involving the greater portion of the right lobe of the liver is seen. Speckled areas of gas are noted within the mass, corresponding to tumor necrosis.

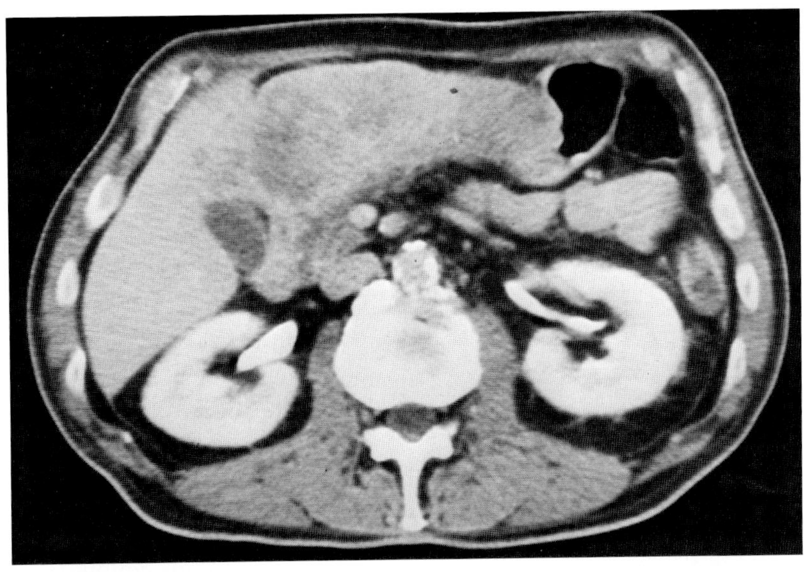

B

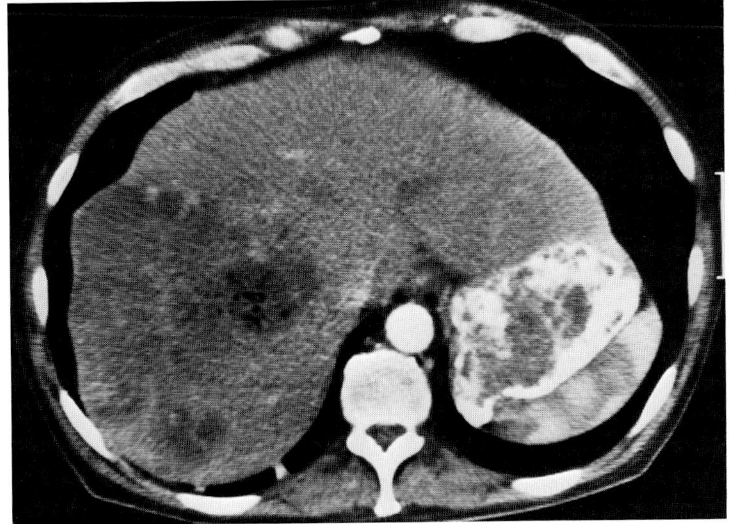

C

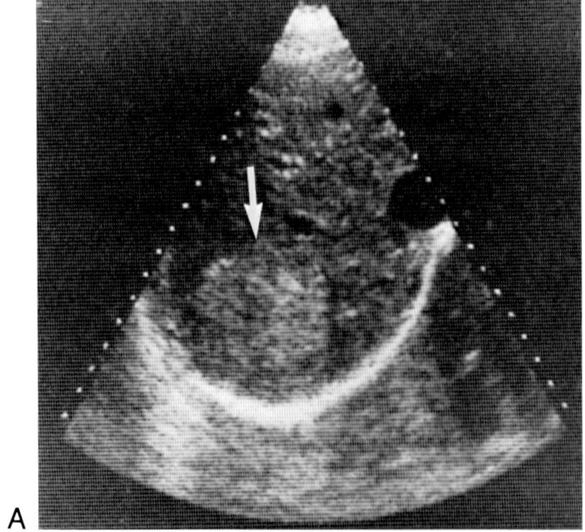

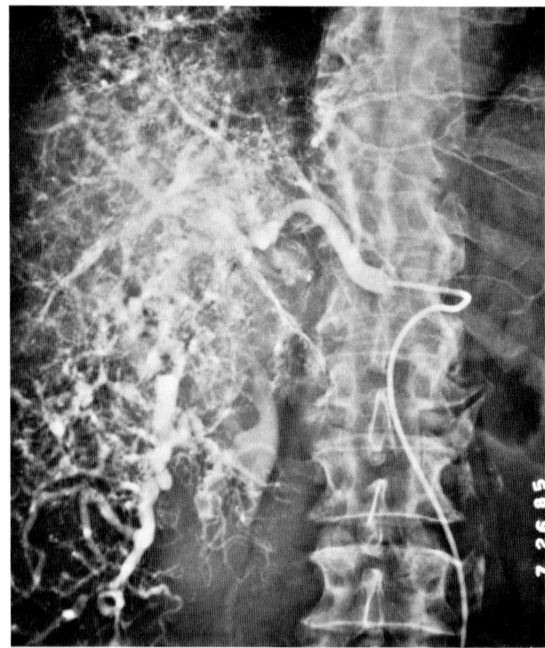

Fig. 5-11 (A) This large, relatively hyperechoic liver mass is a biopsy-proved hepatoma *(white arrow)*. **(B)** The angiogram of a different patient reveals marked hypervascularity and neovascularity in this surgically proved hepatoma. AV shunting is also evident.

rarely possible, adequate biliary drainage results in prolonged survival. CT, ultrasound, angiography, and percutaneous transhepatic cholangiograms are the radiologic imaging modalities used to evaluate cholangiocarcinoma. Focal or generalized biliary obstruction is the hallmark finding. The level of obstruction can be determined by following the dilated biliary system to the point at which it becomes obliterated.

The primary angiographic finding in cholangiocarcinoma is arterial infiltration resulting in a serrated or serpiginous appearance. Cholangiocarcinomas are more readily appreciated on CT than on ultrasound, with the density of the tumor being variable; it is usually hypodense, with some degree of enhancement following contrast administration. However, the tumor may not be appreciated because of its small size or infiltrative nature.

Hepatoblastoma

Most primary pediatric hepatic tumors, the most common of which are hepatoblastoma (34 percent) and hepatoma (26 percent), are malignant. Hepatoblastomas usually present as palpable masses associated with anorexia and weight loss. The right hepatic lobe is involved more often than the left, but both lobes are affected in 30 to 45 percent of cases. The CT, ultrasound, and angiographic findings of hepatoblastoma are indistinguishable from those of hepatocellular carcinoma, which have been previously described (Fig. 5-12).

Angiosarcoma

Angiosarcoma, a rare malignancy of the liver, has been linked epidemiologically, in 40 percent of cases, with exposure to several substances such as vinyl chloride, thorotrast, arsenicals, and radium. Thorotrast has been linked with an increased incidence of sarcomas, hepatomas, cholangiocarcinomas, and endotheliomas. Development of these tumors is related to the concentration of radioactive thorium in the reticuloendothelial element of the liver.

On CT, angiosarcomas appear as solitary or multiple hypodense lesions that are dramatically enhanced by the intravenous administration of iodinated contrast material. The arteriographic findings include normal sized hepatic arteries, peripheral tumor staining and puddling that lasts long beyond the arterial phase, and a central area of hypovascularity.

Lymphoma

This tumor only rarely arises in the liver as a primary malignancy, but it is found as a secondary site of involvement in 60 percent of patients with Hodgkin disease and in 50 percent of those with non-Hodgkin lymphoma. Diffuse infiltration is more frequent in Hodgkin disease, whereas diffuse and nodular hepatic involvement are present with equal frequency in non-Hodgkin lymphoma (Fig. 5-13).

CT and ultrasound have relatively low detection rates in lymphomatous involvement of the liver. This is secondary to the fact that infiltrative foci are commonly only several millimeters in diameter. When positive, CT usually demonstrates solid hypodense masses. Appreciation of diffuse hepatic involvement is less common. Ultrasound, when positive, most commonly reveals hypoechoic lesions (43 percent). Diffuse changes in hepatic architecture (35 percent), echogenic lesions (13 percent), and target lesions (9 percent) are less commonly seen. The echogenic and target lesions seem to be associated with non-Hodgkin lymphoma.

Hepatomegaly alone should not be interpreted as evidence of lymphomatous involvement of the liver, as lymphoma is histologically absent in 43 percent of patients with non-Hodgkin lymphoma and hepatomegaly. By the same token, its normal size does not necessarily indicate that the liver is free of disease.

Metastatic Disease

Primary tumors of the gastrointestinal tract are the most common malignancies that metastasize to the liver (Fig. 5-14). Primary breast and genitourinary carcinomas also frequently metastasize to the liver.

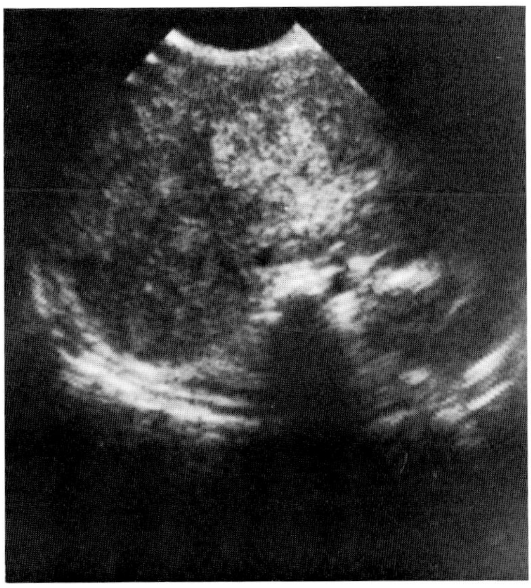

A

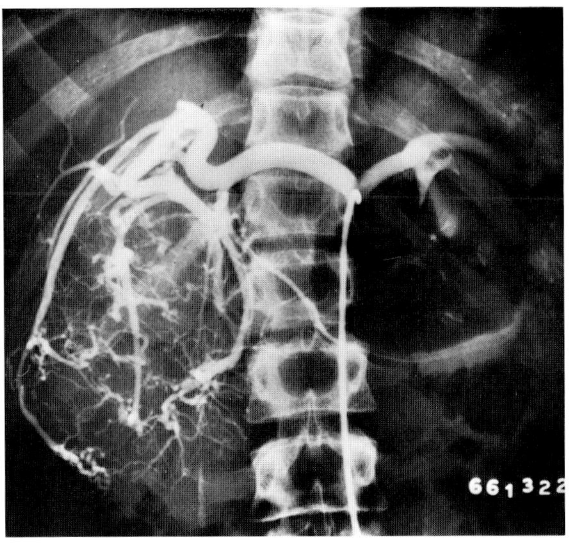

B

Fig. 5-12 (A) This transverse realtime ultrasonographic image of the liver in a child reveals a hyperechoic mass. This represents a biopsy-proved hepatoblastoma. **(B)** Angiogram of a different patient reveals a large mass in the liver causing displacement, distortion, and encasement of hepatic artery branches in this surgically proved hepatoblastoma. Significant neovascularity is also demonstrated.

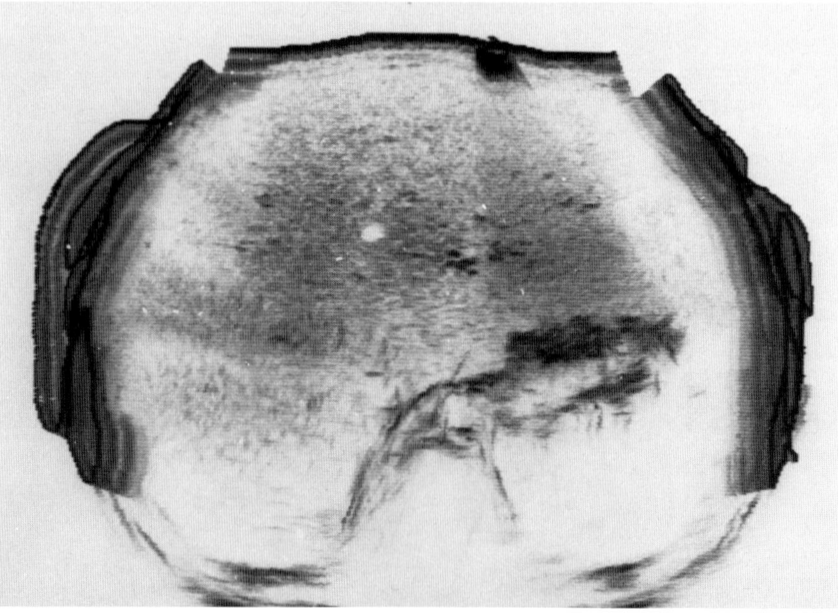

Fig. 5-13 This static transverse ultrasonographic image of the upper abdomen reveals hepatomegaly and diffuse alteration of the normal hepatic architecture. These findings are secondary to lymphomatous involvement of the liver.

Taken as a group, metastases are the most common source of malignant tumors of the liver.

Noncontrast CT scans usually demonstrate metastases as single or multiple mass lesions of the liver, exhibiting lower density than the surrounding normal hepatic parenchyma. Most metastatic lesions appear as relatively well-marginated, solid masses. However, some may be poorly circumscribed, may have areas of decreased attenuation (secondary to necrosis, hemorrhage, or both), or may appear cystlike with densities similar to water. Metastatic mucinous ovarian or colonic carcinoma, melanoma, carcinoid, leiomyosarcoma, and lung tumors are responsible for most cystic or necrotic liver metastases. Peritoneal implants juxtaposed to the liver are seen most commonly in metastatic ovarian carcinoma, breast carcinoma, and pseudomyxoma peritonei. Liver metastases with punctate or amorphous calcification in the areas of decreased density are occasionally seen, most likely secondary to mucin-producing metastatic colon carcinoma. However, metastatic deposits from ovar-

ian, pancreatic islet cell, stomach, kidney, breast, melanoma, and neuroblastoma may also be partially calcified. In fact, any tumor that undergoes necrosis may calcify.

Contrast-enhanced CT of the liver in metastatic disease most commonly demonstrates lesions as centrally hypodense with a peripheral rim of enhancement. Other lesions may become uniformly hyperdense or may show no enhancement at all (Fig. 5-15).

Ultrasonographically, metastatic liver disease may present with a myriad of appearances. Lesions may be highly echogenic, hypoechoic, or of mixed echogenicity. No correlation can be made between the histologic makeup of the lesion and ultrasonographic findings.

From an angiographic point of view, hepatic metastases fall into three groups — hypervascular (i.e., hypernephroma, endocrine carcinoma, carcinoid, leio-

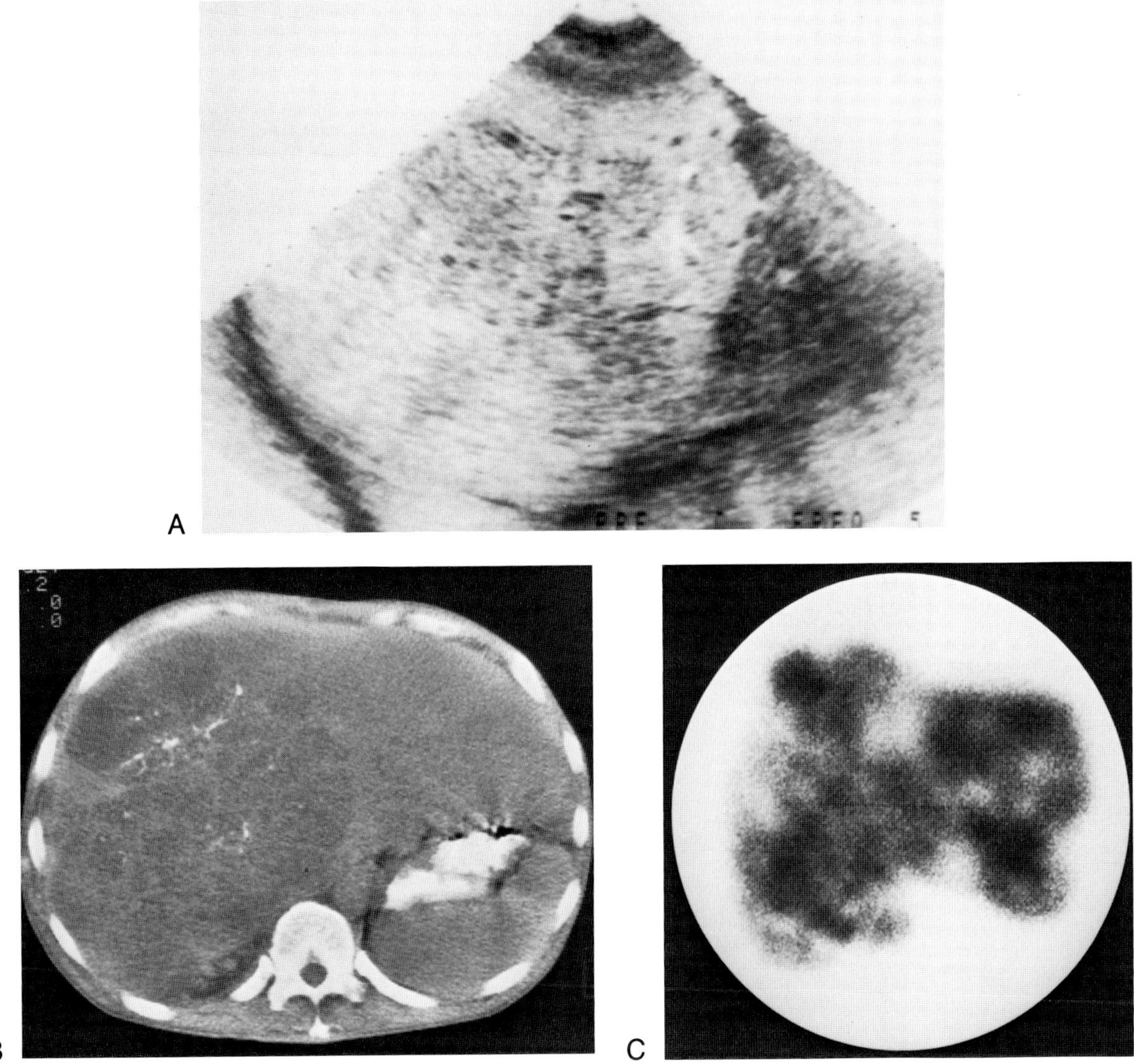

Fig. 5-14 Diffuse metastatic involvement of the liver secondary to a primary colonic carcinoma demonstrated by **(A)** ultrasound, **(B)** CT, and **(C)** ^{99m}Tc sulfur colloid liver scan. Note the punctate calcifications seen on the CT scan.

myosarcoma, choriocarcinoma); hypovascular (i.e., breast, most gastrointestinal tumors, lung, and pancreas); and those having essentially the same vascularity as the normal parenchyma.

Technetium-99m sulfur colloid may be used to evaluate metastatic disease. Its overall sensitivity and specificity is approximately 85 percent. False-negative re-sults are frequent in patients with a liver of normal size or with metastatic lesions less than 2 cm. When detected, metastatic lesions most commonly appear as photopenic defects. Occasionally, metastatic disease results in a nonspecific, diffuse or patchy colloid distribution, making it difficult to distinguish from other parenchymal diseases of the liver (i.e., cirrhosis).

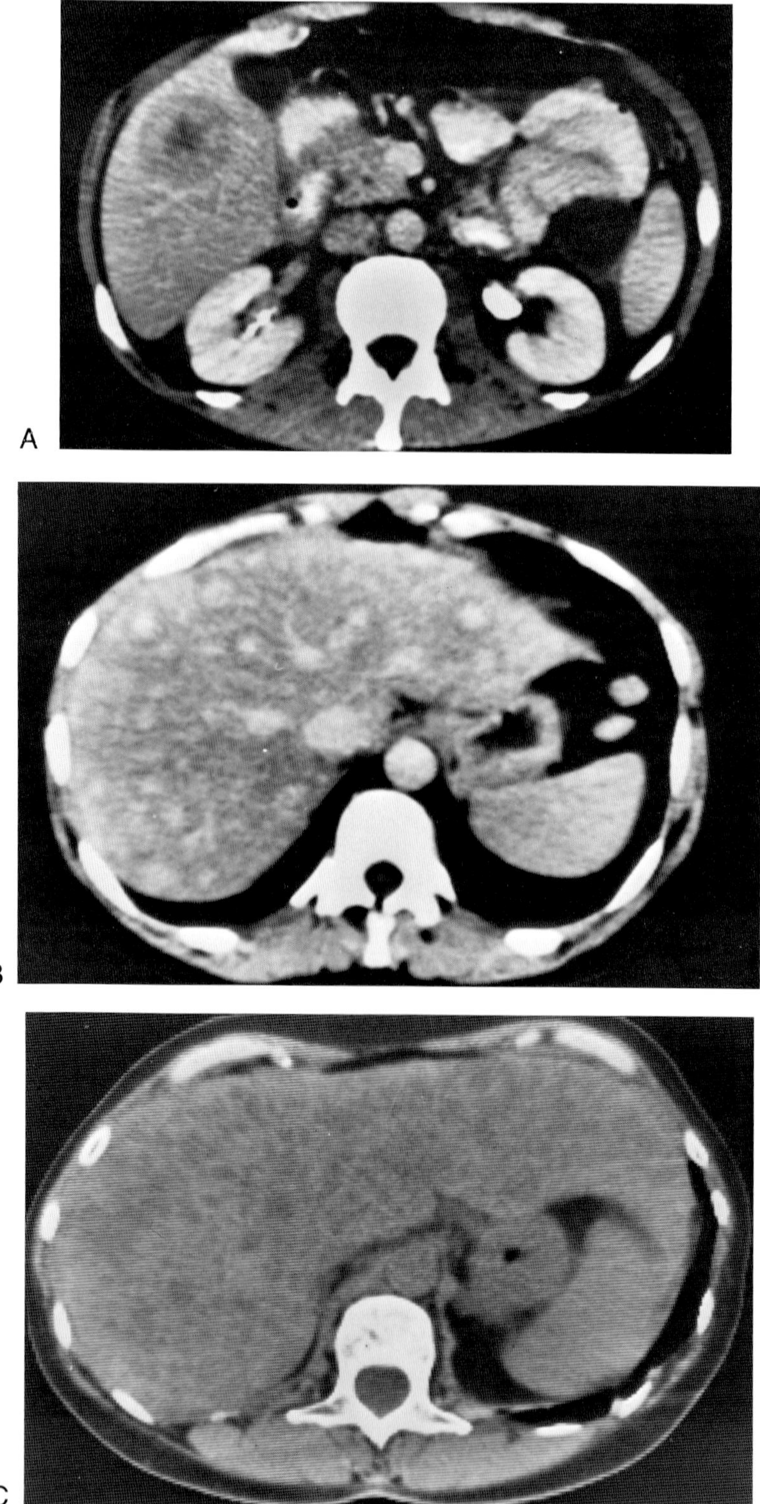

Fig. 5-15 (A) A single metastatic focus in the right lobe of the liver is seen on a contrast-enhanced CT scan. It is relatively hypodense, with a thick rim of enhancement noted peripherally. **(B)** Following a rapid bolus injection of iodinated contrast material multiple hyperdense lesions are demonstrated in this patient with metastatic carcinoid. **(C)** The liver is diffusely infiltrated by numerous small, hypodense lesions in this patient with metastatic breast carcinoma.

INFILTRATING DISEASES

Fatty Infiltration

Fatty infiltration of the liver is the result of excessive deposition of triglycerides in the liver. Although indicative of significant hepatic abnormality, it is reversible. A variety of diseases can cause fatty infiltration, as seen below. The most common cause of fatty infiltration is alcoholic cirrhosis.

DISEASES CAUSING FATTY INFILTRATION OF THE LIVER

Alcoholic cirrhosis

Chemotherapy

Cushing disease (or iatrogenic corticosteroidism)

Cystic fibrosis

Diabetes mellitus

Glycogen storage disease

Hepatitis

Hypertriglyceridemia

Intravenous hyperalimentation

Jejunoileal bypass surgery

Kwashiorkor disease

A-beta-lipoproteinemia

Malnourishment

Obesity

Radiation hepatitis

Reye syndrome

Toxic ingestion (i.e., carbon tetrachloride)

Using CT, the density of the spleen serves as a basis for comparison in evaluating the liver for fatty infiltration. Normally, the liver is approximately 8 HU greater than the spleen. It has been determined experimentally that for each milligram of triglyceride deposited in a gram of liver, hepatic attenuation decreases by 1.6 HU. Thus, it is possible not only to determine fatty infiltration, but to quantify it.

In many patients, fat deposition in the liver is uniform and diffuse. The portal veins in a diffusely fatty liver appear as high density structures surrounded by a background of low density, caused by the hepatic fat. These differences are further accentuated after IV contrast enhancement (Fig. 5-16A).

In some patients fatty infiltration occurs in a more focal or a less uniform manner. Although any of the causes listed here may result in focal fatty change, alcoholism and cirrhosis are the more common offenders. Occasionally, such areas of focal fatty infiltration can produce a CT appearance that resembles neoplasia. The observation that normal portal vessels traverse the area in question, with no evidence of mass effect or encasement, usually permits conclusive distinction between fatty infiltration and tumorous mass (Fig. 5-16B). However, a percutaneous needle biopsy may be required to provide definitive proof in some cases.

The sonographic appearance of a liver with fatty infiltration is characteristic. The overall echo pattern of the liver is increased, sound transmission is markedly diminished, and vascular structures in the liver are poorly visualized (Fig. 5-16C). The same findings may be apparent in a liver infiltrated by fibrosis.

Routine liver-spleen scintigraphy and MRI are most often normal in patients with fatty infiltration.[133]Xe ventilation scans of the liver, on the other hand, reveal an increase in uptake and retention of the radionuclide in the presence of fatty infiltration. This phenomenon is secondary to the fact that xenon gas is highly fat-soluble.

Cirrhosis

Cirrhosis results from a variety of etiologies, the most common of which, in the United States, is chronic alcoholism. On a worldwide basis, schistosomiasis is the most prevalent cause. The basic pathologic process of cirrhosis involves the extensive deposition of collagen, replacing hepatocytes and distorting the normal hepatic lobular architecture. In early cirrhosis, the liver may sometimes be enlarged, smooth, and uniformly replaced with fat. A small liver, with a nodular contour resulting from focal atrophy, fibrosis, and/or regenerating nodules, is commonly seen in more advanced forms of cirrhosis. In addition, the increased incidence of hepatocellular carcinoma in patients with cirrhosis has been well documented and cannot be overemphasized (Fig. 5-16). Hepatomas are particularly likely to occur in patients with hepatitis B surface antigen-positive cirrhosis (Fig. 5-17). Frequently, ascites, splenomegaly and dilated collateral veins (varices) may be noted (Figs. 5-18 and 5-19). The Cruveilhier-Baumgarten syndrome is characterized by splenomegaly, distended paraumbilical vein (caput-medusa), and esophageal varices. This syndrome, a reflection of portal hypertension, is commonly seen in cirrhotics.

The most significant portosystemic collateral veins in patients with cirrhosis and portal hypertension develop from the left gastric (coronary) and short gastric veins via the esophageal veins to the azygous system. These collaterals are responsible for bleeding esophageal varices, the major cause of death in patients with portal hypertension.

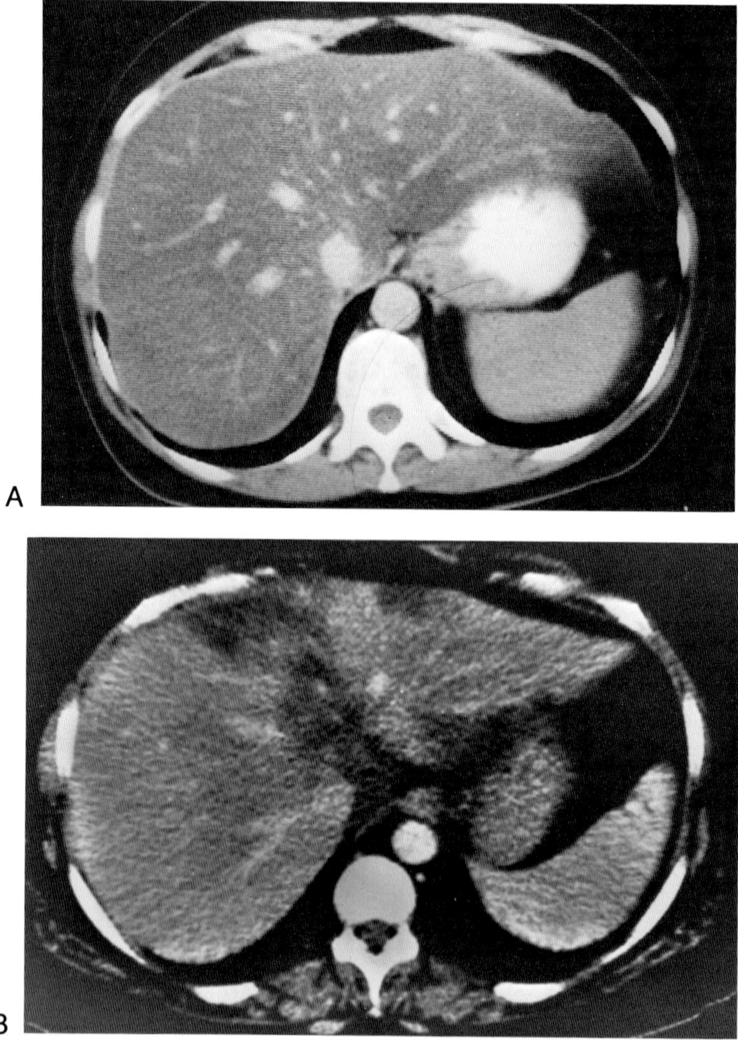

Fig. 5-16 (A) Fatty infiltration. A contrast-enhanced CT scan reveals the liver to be less dense than the spleen. Note the accentuation in contrast between the hepatic vessels and liver parenchyma. **(B)** A focal area of decreased attenuation is seen. Note the lack of mass effect, suggesting the biopsy-proved diagnosis of focal fatty infiltration in this Cushingoid patient. *(Figure continues.)*

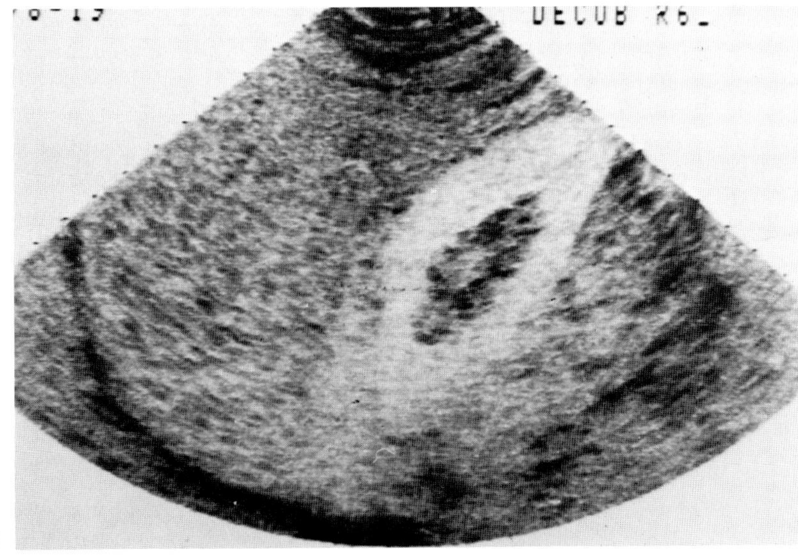

Fig. 5-16 *(Continued)* **(C)** A marked increase in echogenicity of the liver is noted by ultrasound. Note the accentuated difference in echogenicity between the liver and renal cortex.

The veins in the hilum of the spleen communicate with retroperitoneal veins and these, in turn, communicate with the anterior abdominal wall, inferior phrenic, and renal veins. This network of vessels comprises a now well-known pathway — the spontaneous splenorenal shunt. Recanalization of the paraumbilical veins results in the connection between the left portal vein and the umbilicus, and thence to the systemic veins of the anterior abdominal wall. In addition, the inferior mesenteric vein has communica-

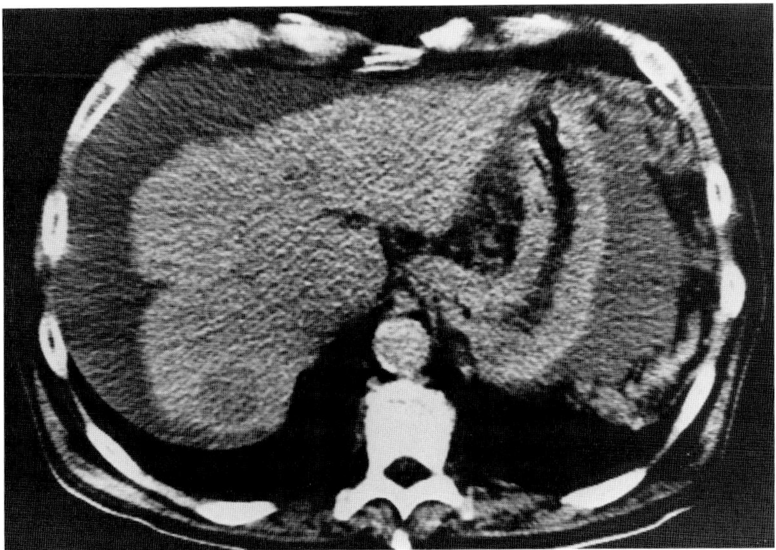

Fig. 5-17 The liver is small and has a nodular contour. Ascitic fluid is seen. Within this cirrhotic liver is an area of decreased attenuation in the posterior segment of the right lobe, representing a hepatoma.

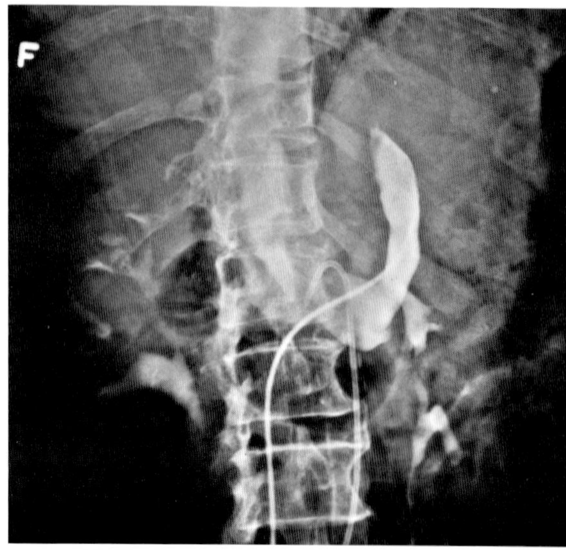

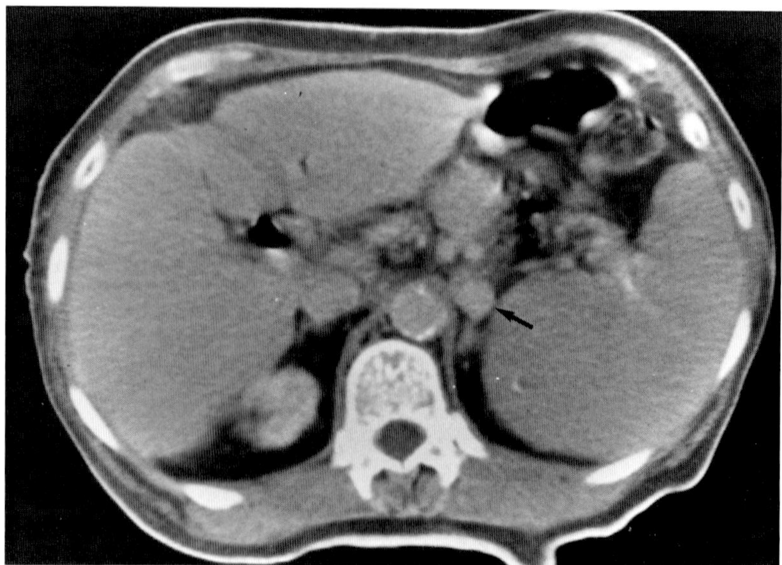

Fig. 5-18 (A) A venous injection demonstrates a splenorenal shunt. **(B)** This same shunt can be appreciated on CT *(black arrow)*. It is identified as a small, tubular soft tissue density extending from the splenic hilus, which, on more caudad images, extended to and joined the left renal vein (not shown). Incidentally noted is air in the biliary tree secondary to a choledochojejunostomy.

tions through the superior hemorrhoidal veins to the inferior hemorrhoidal and the internal iliac veins. Moreover, there are numerous, small portal tributaries along the bowel wall and in the mesentery, which connect with small veins that drain into the IVC. These collateral veins, rarely demonstrated radiographically, produce a characteristic discoloration of the peritoneum in patients with portal hypertension, and account for most of the blood loss during dissection of the IVC and portal vein in a portocaval shunt operation. Rarely, the colonic veins may communicate with the inferior mesenteric vein via the marginal vein, accounting for the colonic varices in patients with portal hypertension.

The radiologist may study varices by using angiography, ultrasound, CT, or MRI. These collaterals appear as tortuous, serpiginous vessels on angiography, ultrasound, and MRI, and as enhancing lobulated masses or rounded tubular soft-tissue densities on CT.

In cirrhosis, the right lobe of the liver may shrink dramatically; thus, the gallbladder will rotate posteriorly, extensively assuming a lateral position. The medial segment of the left lobe of the liver may either remain unchanged in size or shrink somewhat. The lateral segment of the left lobe of the liver, however, will often show a bulging appearance and gross hypertrophy. Hypertrophy of the caudate lobe is common in cirrhosis. With hypertrophy of the caudate lobe and shrinkage of the right lobe, the ratio between the transverse width of the caudate lobe and the right lobe has become the most reliable indicator in differentiating normal from cirrhotic livers when using CT or ultrasound to image the abdomen. The mean value of the ratio for normal liver volumes is 0.37 ± 0.16 with a mean volume for cirrhotic livers of 0.83 ± 0.20. This formula has been shown to be highly sensitive, specific, and accurate in differentiating cirrhotic from noncirrhotic livers.

Angiography in patients with cirrhosis reveals diffuse stretching of hepatic arterial branches. A so-called corkscrew pattern of hepatic artery branches is commonly observed secondary to progressive scarring and fibrosis of the liver. With increased fibrosis, there is increased resistance to portal blood flow and resultant portal hypertension. In severe cirrhosis, portal blood flow is reversed. As resistance to portal flow increases, its contribution to total hepatic flow decreases with compensatory dilatation of the hepatic artery. The hepatic parenchyma stains inhomogeneously.

Regeneration of the hepatic parenchyma is an integral part of the cirrhotic process. Large regenerating nodules can develop and must be differentiated from hepatomas. Regenerating nodules appear as focal masses. Stretched arterial branches are seen to penetrate their centers. The supplying arteries may have fewer side branches than the surrounding parenchyma. The parenchymal phase is homogeneous, and an enlarged portal branch is often found to extend through the nodule. Diffuse hypervascularity can occur, but without the wild neovascularity seen in most hepatomas. Arteriovenous shunting is rare. Regenerating nodules are most often isodense with the normal liver parenchyma on CT, although there is some variability. On sonography, they appear as areas of focal enlargement and decreased echogenicity.

As mentioned earlier, fatty infiltration of the liver may be seen in association with cirrhosis, resulting in areas of decreased attenuation on CT. Ultrasonographically, the cirrhotic liver reveals a coarse echo texture caused by fatty infiltration, fibrosis, or both.

Hemochromatosis

Extensive total body iron storage, resulting from either a primary process (idiopathic hemochromatosis) or as a secondary disorder (secondary hemochromatosis) can be seen. The most common cause of secondary hemochromatosis is multiple blood transfusions. It is frequently seen in patients with blood dyscrasias or with chronic bleeding.

Increased iron deposition in patients with idiopathic hemochromatosis is caused by a defect in the intestinal mucosa. Patients usually present with cirrhosis, diabetes mellitus, and hyperpigmentation (so-called bronze diabetes). Primary or secondary hemochromatosis can readily be diagnosed from noncontrast enhanced CT scans by an overall increase in the density of the hepatic parenchyma (Fig. 5-20A). Scanning at energies of 120 kVp, the average CT density of the liver in patients with hemochromatosis ranges between 75 to 132 HU. As a result, the intrahepatic vessels stand out as low density tubular structures, compared with the hyperdense liver background. With CT, it is possible to quantitate the amount of iron deposited in the liver using a method called dual energy scanning.

Magnetic resonance imaging is helpful in the diagnosis of hemochromatosis. Iron decreases both T_1 and T_2 relaxation times, the latter having the predominant effect. This manifests as a decrease in signal intensity. Thus, the liver appears darker than usual (Fig. 5-20B).

Not surprisingly, hemochromatosis causes the liver to be of increased echogenicity when studied ultrasonographically. It should be noted that patients with hemochromatosis may also show increased iron deposition in the spleen, pancreas, lymph nodes, pituitary, heart, adrenals, bowel wall, parathyroid, and thyroid glands.

Glycogen Storage Disease

Glycogen storage disease is a genetic disorder of carbohydrate metabolism subdivided into six categories on the basis of a specific enzyme defect. All enzymatic defects result in faulty glycogenolysis with subsequent excessive storage of glycogen. In types I, II, and VI, the liver is a site of excessive glycogen storage deposition. Adenomas as well as hepatomas are seen with increased frequency in patients with glycogen storage disease.

With excessive glycogen deposition, the CT attenuation value of the liver is commonly greater than nor-

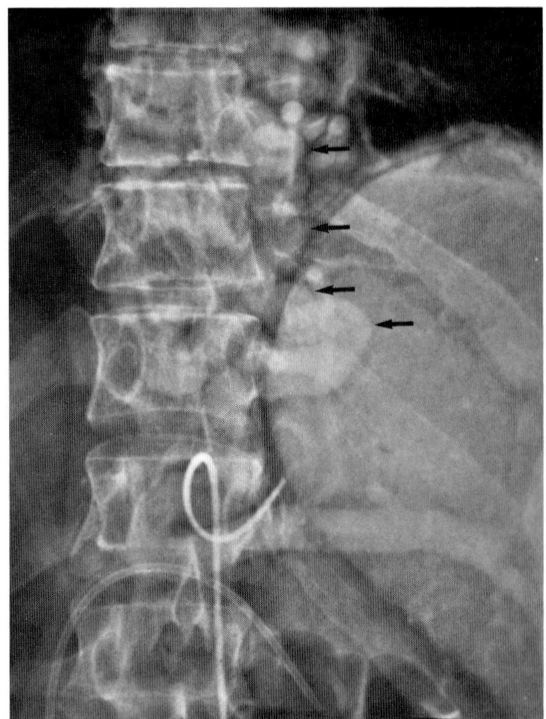

A

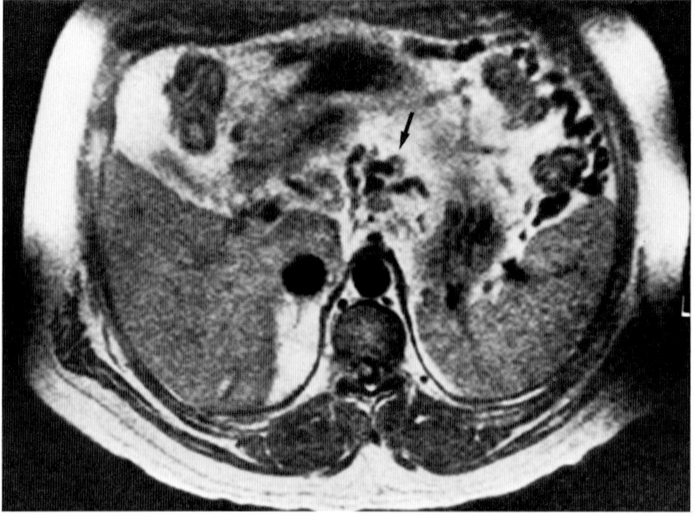

B

Fig. 5-19 Coronary and esophageal varices *(black arrows)* are demonstrated by **(A)** angiography, **(B)** MRI, and **(C)** CT. Recanalization of an umbilical vein *(white arrows)* is demonstrated by **(D)** CT and **(E)** MRI.

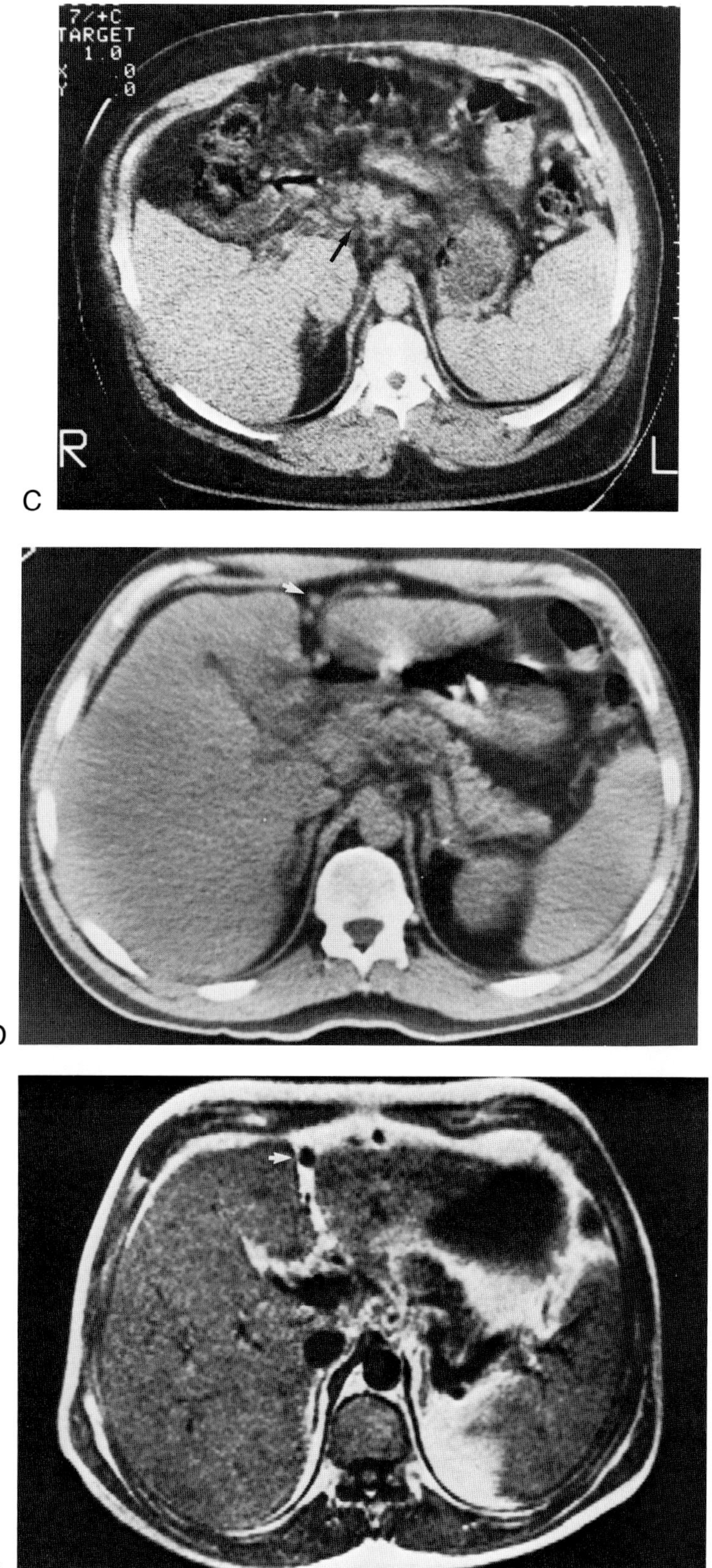

Fig. 5-19 *(Continued)*

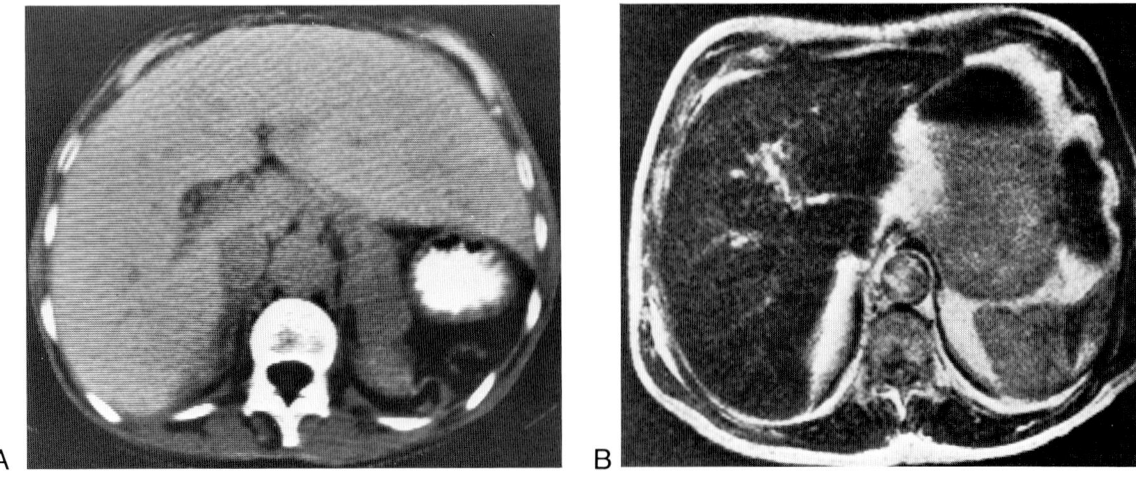

Fig. 5-20 (A) Hemochromatosis. A noncontrast CT scan of the abdomen reveals an enlarged liver of increased density. This patient has known sickle cell anemia and has had recurrent transfusions. Also note the lack of a spleen. The patient has undergone autosplenectomy secondary to recurrent infarctions of the spleen. **(B)** An MRI image of a different patient with hemochromatosis reveals the liver to be of decreased signal intensity.

mal. CT densities ranging between 55 and 90 HU on conventional CT scans are common. Longstanding glycogen storage disease may result in a decreased liver attenuation value secondary to fatty infiltration. The ultrasonic echogenicity of the liver in a patient with glycogen storage disease tends to be increased. Adenomas and hepatomas tend to appear relatively hypoechoic. Additional abnormalities that may be

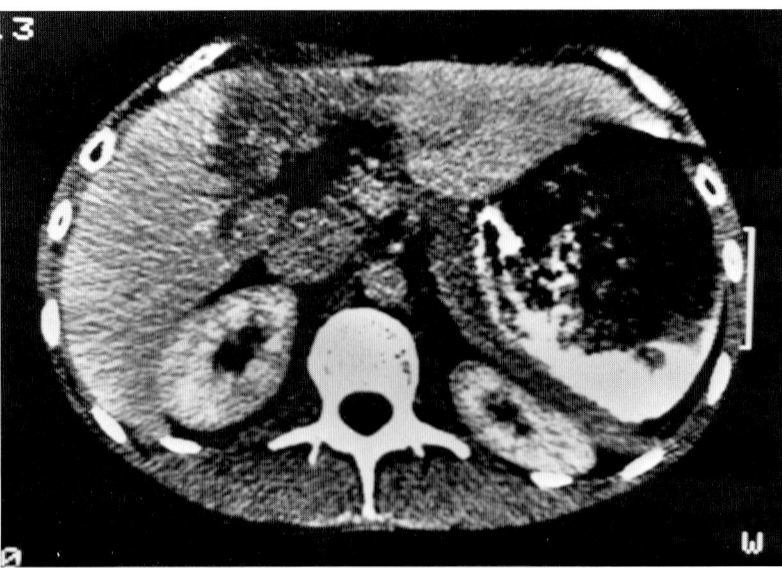

Fig. 5-21 Radiation injury. A sharply demarcated area of decreased attenuation is noted in the liver. This patient was treated 2 months earlier with radiation therapy for lymphomatous involvement of nodes in the porta hepatis.

identified in these patients include enlarged kidneys with increased cortical density (type I), renal calculi (type I), and splenomegaly (types I, III and VI).

Hepatitis

Clearly, hepatitis is not a diagnosis usually made by radiologic imaging. Interestingly, though, the ultrasonographic findings seen in hepatitis have been shown to correlate well with clinical and pathologic data. Sonographically, the echogenicity of the liver is decreased in acute hepatitis because liver cells are congested and the echogenicity of portal vein walls may be relatively accentuated. Hepatomegaly and thickening of the gallbladder wall are ancillary findings that, in acute hepatitis, may be appreciated on ultrasound or CT. In chronic hepatitis, the parenchymal echo pattern is coarsened by the presence of periportal fibrosis and chronic inflammation. It should be noted that the findings in both acute and chronic hepatitis are not specific and may be seen in a multitude of infiltrative diseases of the liver. In addition, as previously mentioned, fatty infiltration may be a secondary result of hepatitis.

Radiation Injury

Hepatocellular damage induced by radiation therapy is characterized histologically, in the acute phase, by panlobar congestion, hemorrhagic foci, decreased numbers of hepatocytes, variable amounts of fatty change, lipid-laden macrophages, and marked venous occlusion. In patients studied within several months after radiation to the liver, CT typically reveals a low density region with a sharp, straight border, corresponding to the radiation port (Fig. 5-21). If the liver is scanned 3 to 18 months later, usually total or at least partial resolution is apparent.

As would be expected, in acute radiation damage to the liver, sharply demarcated areas of decreased echogenicity are appreciated on ultrasonography.

INFLAMMATORY MASSES

Abscesses

Abscesses comprise the majority of inflammatory masses found in the liver. They occur most often in the posterior segment of the right lobe of the liver and are usually solitary. Patients with liver abscesses usually present with fever and abdominal pain. Elevated liver function tests and hepatomegaly are observed. Approximately 20 to 30 percent of pyogenic abscesses contain gas, whereas amoebic abscesses do not contain gas, unless secondarily infected (Fig. 5-22A). Despite the variable appearance of an abscess on CT or ultrasound, the patient's clinical history usually leads one to the correct diagnosis.

On CT, a liver abscess usually appears as a sharply defined area with a density usually greater than that of a hepatic cyst but lower than that of normal liver parenchyma. Overlap, however, between the appearance of abscesses and cysts and abscesses and hepatic neoplasms does exist. Hepatic abscesses have a thick capsule and somewhat irregular inner margins. The actual density of an abscess depends on the evolution of the inflammatory process itself (Fig. 5-22B).

After the intravenous administration of contrast material, the wall of an abscess cavity may enhance, becoming more dense than the liver. This rim sign is not specific for abscesses, as it may be seen in primary or metastatic tumors. The central, inner portion of the abscess — the cavity — should not enhance because it is avascular. Uniform enhancement of a liver lesion should thus lead one away from the diagnosis of abscess and toward neoplasm.

Early sonographic findings of liver abscesses may be manifested as focal or diffuse areas of increased or decreased parenchymal echoes. With time, a well-defined cavity, demonstrating irregular, thick inner walls and varying degrees of echogenicity may develop. Microabscesses may appear as target lesions, with sonolucent peripheries and echogenic centers. Abscesses with a high protein or lipid content and/or gas will result in areas of increased echogenicity.

Both gallium 67 (^{67}Ga) and indium 111 (^{111}In) oxine-labeled autologous leukocytes have been successfully used to detect hepatic abscesses. The scan patterns with ^{67}Ga of pyogenic abscesses and hepatomas are similar. Gallium does not concentrate in amoebic abscesses, although its circumferential concentration can frequently be seen at the periphery of an amoebic abscess. Work with ^{111}In is still not complete, but

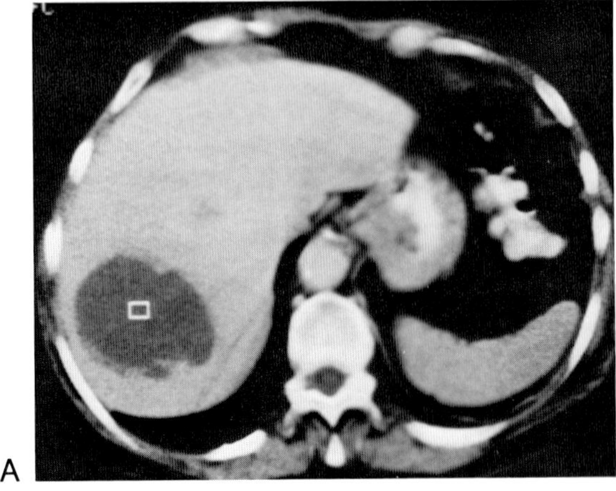 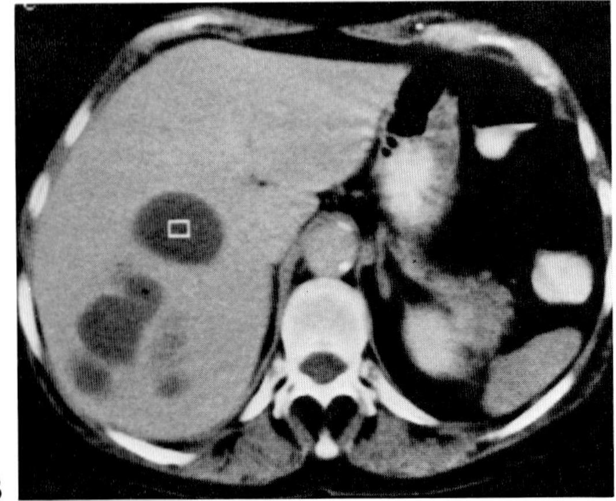

Fig. 5-22 (A) Hepatic abscess. A single focus of decreased attenuation is noted in the posterior segment of the right lobe of the liver. This amoebic abscess was drained percutaneously. **(B)** Multiple areas of decreased attenuation are noted in the right lobe of the liver. Within one of these lesions, a small amount of gas is seen. These pyogenic abscesses were treated surgically because they were multiple.

there appears to be great promise in its ability to detect acute and subacute focal sepsis.

Percutaneous drainage of hepatic abscesses has now become the treatment of choice, in conjunction with appropriate antibiotic therapy. For guidance, most radiologists favor CT.

Hydatid Disease

In humans, the liver is the organ most frequently involved in hydatid disease. The offending parasites are *Echinococcus granulosis,* which is endemic in sheep-raising areas of Europe, Asia, Africa, Australia, New Zealand, and the Mediterranean; and *Echinococcus alveolaris,* found in Central Europe, Russia, Japan and the United States. Abdominal pain, fever, and hepatomegaly, with or without jaundice, are clinical signs and symptoms seen in echinococcal involvement of the liver. The CT and ultrasonographic findings in cysts of *E. granulosis* and *E. alveolaris* are distinctly different.

E. granulosis tends to produce cysts that are well delineated and usually multilocular, although they may be unilocular. The surrounding wall of the cyst is frequently partially or completely calcified. Distinct internal daughter cysts, appearing as miniature cysts within larger cysts, are virtually pathognomonic of *E. granulosis.*

E. alveolaris produces infiltrative lesions without sharp margins. True cystic structures are rare, and calcification is amorphous or nodular, not ringlike. Its appearance may closely resemble infiltrating diseases and, thus, is more difficult to definitively diagnose by imaging alone.

Gharbi (1981) has described five classifications of hydatid cysts with respect to their evolutionary stage. A cystic intrahepatic collection with localized wall thickening is most commonly observed. A fluid collection with a floating membrane, fluid collections with septa, a collection with a heterogeneous echo pattern and, rarely, a collection with highly reflective thick walls and a cone-shaped acoustic shadow are less frequently observed.

Surgical evacuation of an echinococcal cyst is the procedure of choice. In the past, percutaneous aspiration and/or drainage of hydatid cysts have been discouraged. The fear of inducing anaphylactic shock and spreading daughter cysts to the peritoneum has deterred radiologists from draining these collections. However, successful percutaneous drainage of a hepatic echinococcal cyst has recently been described by Mueller et al (1984) in a poor surgical candidate.

TRAUMA

Injury to the liver is second only to the spleen in incidence of intraperitoneal trauma. Penetrating injuries generally have a relatively low mortality (approximately 5 percent), whereas mortality from blunt trauma to the liver ranges between 15 and 45 percent.

Lacerations of the hepatic parenchyma and capsule represent the most frequent type of injury. Other injuries include intrahepatic hematoma and frank hepatic fracture. Complications include bile pseudocyst (biloma), various fistulas, pseudoaneurysm, intraperitoneal hemorrhage, and hepatic necrosis.

Conventional plain-film radiography may give valuable information in patients with hepatic injuries. Right, lower rib fractures and fractures of the transverse processes of lumbar vertebrae are often associated with hepatic injury. Intraparenchymal and subcapsular hematomas may present with hepatomegaly and resultant displacement of the right hemidiaphragm, the hepatic flexure of the colon, or the stomach, depending on the location of the hematoma. Excessive intraperitoneal bleeding will obliterate the peritoneal recesses normally found in the abdomen and pelvis. Loss of the hepatic angle and flank stripe may be noted. The hepatorenal space (Morrison pouch) is the most common recess for blood to accumulate in liver trauma.

Evaluation of abdominal trauma by plain-film radiography is obviously somewhat limited. Radionuclide scintigraphy is simple to perform, inexpensive, and quite accurate. Disadvantages of radionuclide evaluation include its organ specificity (not allowing for evaluation of damage outside the liver and spleen) and lack of anatomic resolution. Subcapsular hematomas are manifest as a flattening of the organ contour. Damaged parenchyma and hematomas appear as photopenic defects in the organ.

Angiography is rarely used to evaluate acute hepatic trauma because it is a complex, time-consuming procedure that yields only limited, and often indirect, information. Even when angiography does detect parenchymal injury, the quantification of intraperitoneal hemorrhage and other organ damage is still lacking. Angiography is the most direct means of detecting pseudoaneurysms, arteriovenous fistulas, and arteriobiliary fistulas; hence, it may be helpful when performed electively in the subacute time frame.

Ultrasonography is not the procedure of choice in acute abdominal trauma because it is often difficult to scan the patient adequately and completely. Hepatic trauma may manifest itself sonographically as linear or echogenic foci in the parenchyma, an irregular hepatic contour, free intraperitoneal fluid (blood or bile), or fluid in or around the liver. Blood may have a variety of appearances, depending on its physical state (clotted or not) and the age of the hematoma.

Computed tomography is the procedure of choice for evaluating hepatic as well as other abdominal trauma. Intravenous and oral contrast materials are administered routinely.

Subcapsular hematomas typically appear as crescentic or lenticular shaped nonenhancing low density fluid collections located just beneath the liver capsule. They occur most often along the anterolateral surface and are frequently located under fractured ribs. The density of a fresh hematoma (70 to 80 HU) may actually be greater than that of a noncontrast-enhanced liver, but should be less than a normal contrast-enhanced liver. Over a period of days to weeks, the breakdown of blood products and the influx of fluid cause the hematoma to decrease in attenuation. As the clot continues to retract and lyse, a density as low as 20 to 25 HU may result. Since blood extravasated into the peritoneal cavity is quickly lysed, it will appear to have a relatively low density (Fig. 5-23).

Intraparenchymal hematomas, usually oval or irregular in shape, commonly have a heterogeneous density. Blood in the hepatic parenchyma remains clotted for variable periods of time and may appear as an area of higher attenuation, although an area of decreased attenuation is more common. Hepatic lacerations appear as irregular linear defects or, less commonly, may have a stellate configuration.

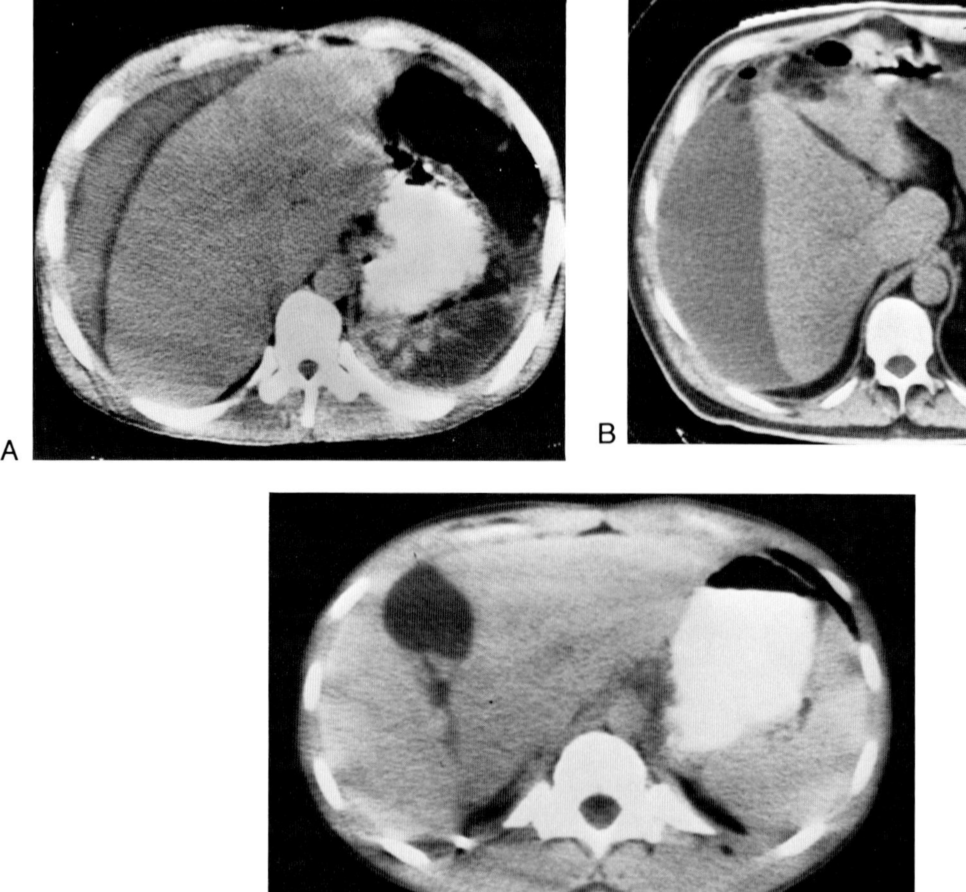

Fig. 5-23 (A) An acute subcapsular hematoma of the liver is seen. Note the crescentic shape of the collection and its high density (secondary to fresh blood). **(B)** A larger, more chronic subcapsular hematoma is shown. This lenticular-shaped collection is of relatively low attenuation (approximately 20 HU). **(C)** This patient received a gunshot wound to the abdomen several weeks earlier. CT at this time reveals a liver laceration with a fluid collection in the anterior segment of the right lobe of the liver. This biloma was percutaneously drained.

Injury to the biliary system may result in the formation of collections of bile (bilomas or bile pseudocysts). They appear as oval or rounded masses of decreased attenuation (Fig. 5-23C). Radionuclide HIDA scans may help to localize the site of, and document bile leakage.

An important advantage of CT in evaluating trauma is its ability not only to evaluate abdominal and pelvic organs but also to identify and quantify free intraperitoneal hemorrhage. These determinations are often crucial in deciding whether or not surgical intervention is warranted.

VASCULAR ABNORMALITIES

Portal Vein Thrombosis

Portal vein thrombosis may be secondary to neoplasm, cirrhosis, trauma, or infection. Chronic portal vein thrombosis results in peripheral portal hypertension, splenomegaly, and varices.

On ultrasonography, clot in the portal vein appears as an area of fixed echogenicity in the lumen of the vessel. If a Doppler examination is performed, no signal is detected because there is no blood flow. The associated varices and splenomegaly can also be depicted sonographically.

CT demonstrates a clot in the portal vein as a filling defect of decreased attenuation. After the contrast material is administered intravenously, the thrombus does not enhance, although a peripheral ring of enhancement is frequently observed. Incomplete or branched portal vein occlusion manifests itself as a segment of the liver with a relative or transient decrease in hepatic enhancement (Fig. 5-24A).

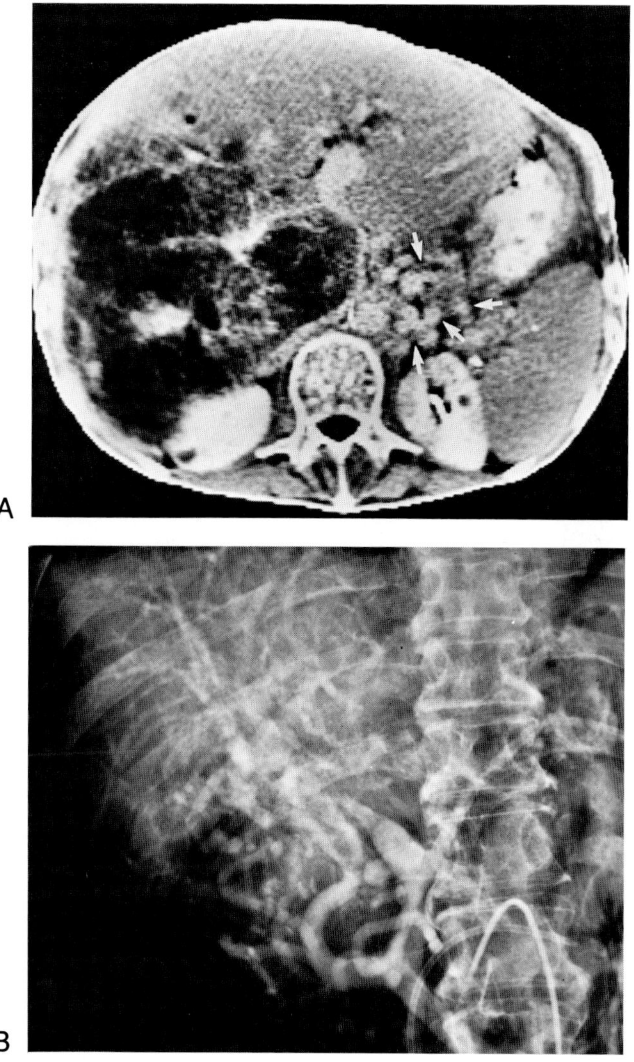

Fig. 5-24 (A) CT scan reveals marked tumor involvement of the right lobe of the liver. The left portal vein is visualized with a marked increase in attenuation of the left lobe of the liver after intravenous contrast material was administered. The right portal vein is never visualized, and there is only minimal enhancement of the right lobe of the liver. A marked number of collateral vessels (varices) are seen *(white arrows)*. These findings are secondary to tumor invasion, and subsequent occlusion of the right portal vein. Incidentally noted are bilateral small renal cysts. **(B)** The venous phase of a superior mesenteric angiogram in a different patient reveals many tortuous, wormlike collateral vessels extending along the path of the portal vein, although no portal vein is seen. These findings are diagnostic of cavernous transformation of the portal vein.

Angiography clearly demonstrates portal vein thrombosis. Complete (nonvisualization of the portal vein) or partial occlusion (a filling defect in the portal vein) with associated collateral channels may be visualized (Fig. 5-24B). Although still in its early stages, MRI shows great potential in evaluating portal flow and in detecting thrombus.

Hepatic Vein Occlusion (Budd-Chiari Syndrome)

Hepatic vein occlusion (Budd-Chiari syndrome) is a common cause of portal hypertension. The diagnosis is difficult to establish clinically, as a result it is often not diagnosed until autopsy. Most hepatic vein thromboses are idiopathic (primary). Secondary forms of hepatic vein occlusion include hypercoaguable states (secondary to polycythemia vara, sickle cell anemia, and the ingestion of birth control pills), invasion by tumor (hepatoma, hypernephroma), and trauma. The patient usually presents with hepatosplenomegaly and ascites. The patient may be asymptomatic or complain of abdominal pain. Once the Budd-Chiari syndrome is suspected, its definitive diagnosis depends on demonstrating occluded hepatic veins or the upper inferior vena cava. The inferior vena cavagram may demonstrate occlusion of the IVC at the renal or hepatic level. Direct hepatic vein injection demonstrates the so-called spider web appearance, pathognomonic for Budd-Chiari syndrome (Fig. 5-25A). This

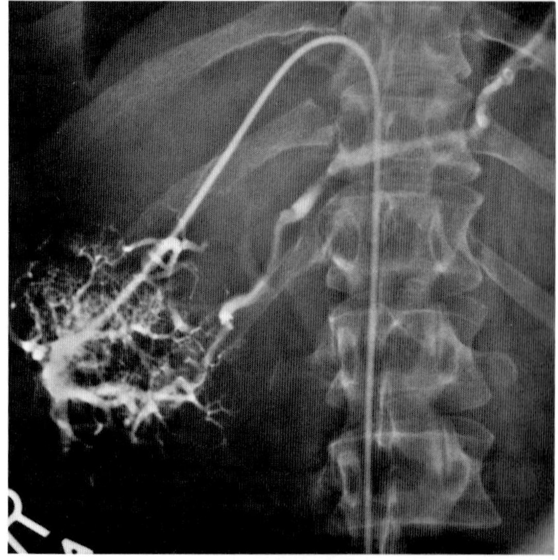

A

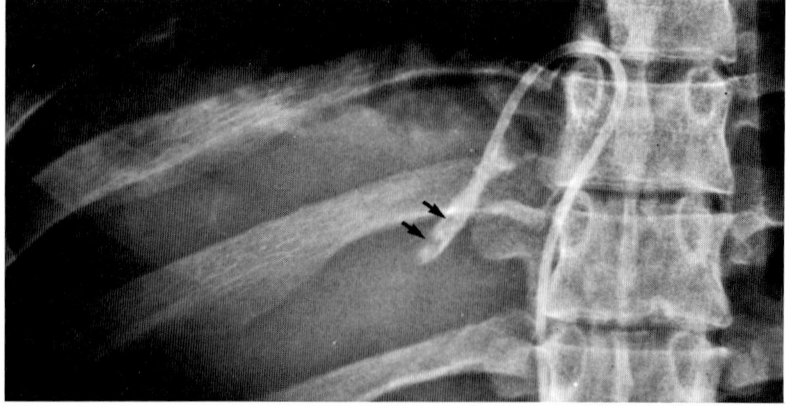

B

Fig. 5-25 (A) Direct hepatic vein injection demonstrates the so-called spider web pathognomonic for Budd-Chiari syndrome. **(B)** A selective hepatic vein injection reveals filling defects *(black arrows)* that correspond to clots.

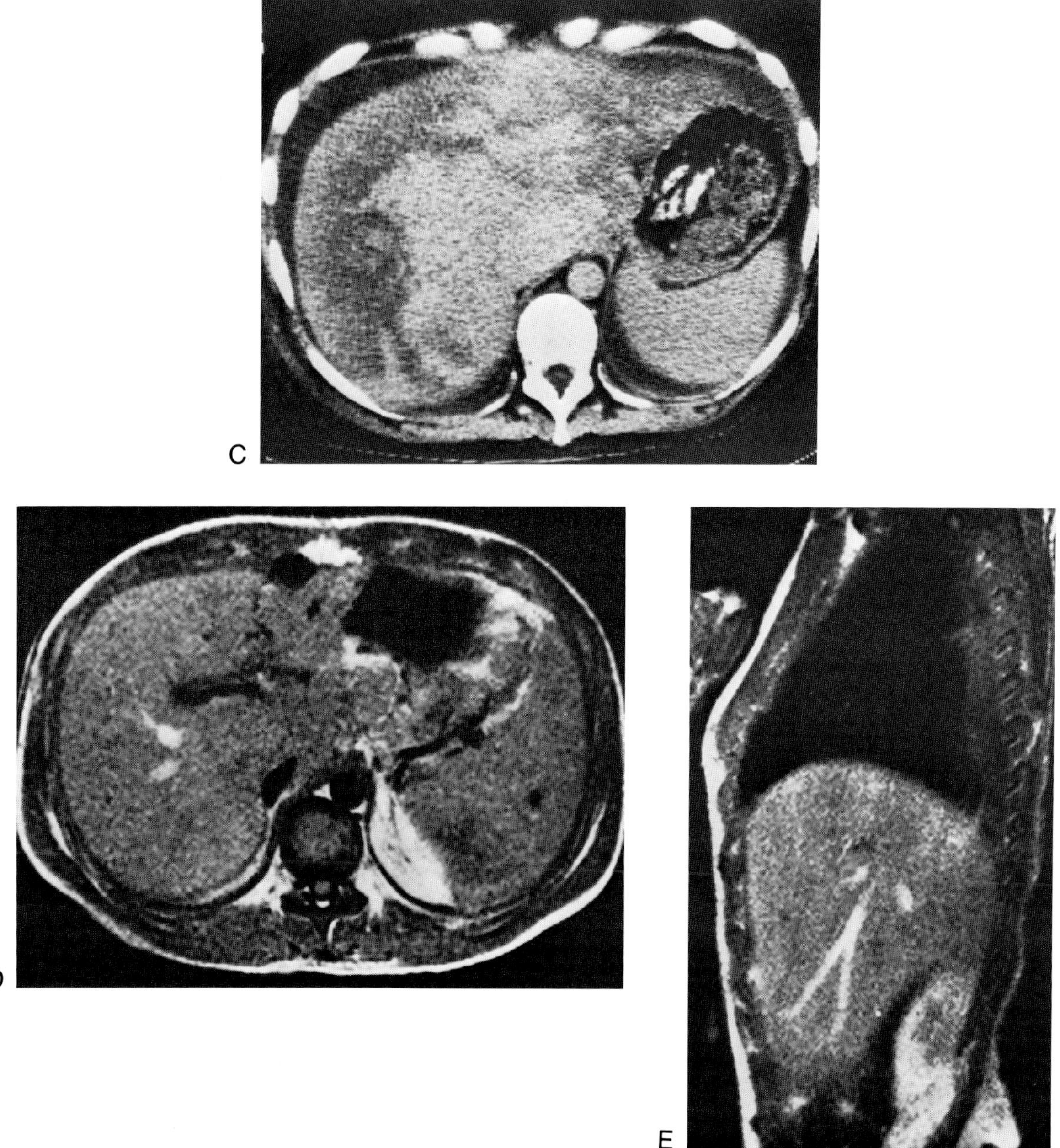

Fig. 5-25 *(Continued)* **(C)** CT scan of the upper abdomen reveals a nonhomogenously enhancing liver. Ascites is incidentally noted. **(D)** An axial MRI image reveals narrowing of the inferior vena cava. **(E)** On this sagittal MRI image, areas of high intensity are noted in the hepatic veins. These areas of increased signal intensity represent thrombus in the hepatic veins.

appearance is secondary to the many collateral channels that develop between hepatic venules and systemic veins. Selective hepatic vein injections may actually demonstrate intraluminal thrombus (Fig. 5-25B). On celiac or hepatic angiography the hepatic arteries appear stretched and bowed. In patients with longstanding disease, the hepatic arteries may dilate, and arterial-portal shunting may be demonstrated. The arterial phase is dense and prolonged.

Following the intravenous injection of contrast material, CT demonstrates a liver that poorly enhances centrally. Later scans reveal a liver with a patchy area of increased attenuation radiating in a fanlike pattern from the retrohepatic inferior vena cava (Fig. 5-25C). As in angiography, these high-density areas persist for a prolonged period of time. The caudate lobe, owing to its unique drainage (via the infrahepatic vena cava), is usually not involved in the Budd-Chiari syndrome. It exhibits a normal pattern of contrast enhancement and commonly hypertrophies in this condition.

A focal area of increased uptake, corresponding to the caudate lobe, is seen on radionuclide scans in patients with Budd-Chiari syndrome. Other causes for focal "hot spots" in the liver include superior or inferior vena cava obstruction, focal nodular hyperplasia, cirrhosis and, less commonly, hepatic tumors.

Hepatic sonography in the Budd-Chiari syndrome results in an inability to visualize normal hepatic veins. Dilatation, stenosis, thick-wall echoes, and thrombosis of hepatic veins may be seen. Abnormal intrahepatic vascular structures, which do not connect with the hepatic or portal venous systems, may also be demonstrated.

Thrombus appears as an area of increased signal intensity on MRI. Differentiation between thrombus (secondary to tumor or clot) and slow flow may be difficult at times. However, MRI offers great promise as refinements in magnetic resonance imaging tech-

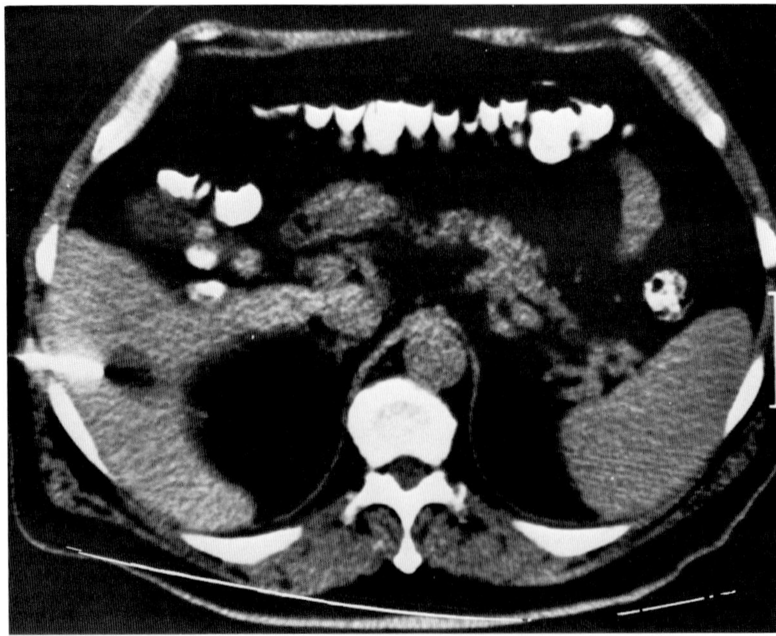

Fig. 5-26 A CT-directed percutaneous biopsy of a single low density lesion in the liver was performed using an 18-gauge CHIBA needle. Note the artifact distal to the needle is normally seen only when the x-ray beam passes through the most distal tip of the needle. Metastatic adenocarcinoma was diagnosed in this patient who has a history of colonic carcinoma.

niques continue and at the same time increase our understanding of the modality itself (Fig. 5-25).

Limited experience with percutaneous transluminal angioplasty (PTA) of hepatic veins in patients with Budd-Chiari syndrome has been somewhat successful. To properly evaluate the role and efficacy of PTA in Budd-Chiari syndrome, further experience is needed.

HEPATIC BIOPSIES AND ABSCESS DRAINAGES

Using CT or ultrasonographic guidance, percutaneous hepatic biopsies and abscess drainage have become commonplace over recent years. Small-to-medium bore needles (18 to 22 gauge) are used to evaluate focal masses for cytologic diagnosis (i.e., metastatic disease). Larger needles, up to 14-gauge in size, are used to obtain tissue when a specific histologic diagnosis is needed (i.e., cirrhosis, hepatitis). The accuracy of these biopsies is between 83 and 94 percent; the complication rate is very low (Fig. 5-26).

Catheters varying in size from 7 to 14 French are used to drain hepatic abscesses percutaneously. The size of the catheter used depends on the viscosity of the material drained. In experienced hands, the success rate is high and the complication rate low.

SUGGESTED READING

Bernardino ME, Sones PJ Jr: Hepatic Radiography. Macmillan, New York, 1984

Gharbi HA, Hassive W, Brawner MW, Depuch K: Ultrasound examination of the hydatid liver. Radiology 139:459, 1981

Lee KT, Sagel SS, Stanley J: Computed Body Tomography. Raven Press, New York, 1983

Moss AA, Gamsu G, Genant HK: Computed Tomography of the Body. WB Saunders, Philadelphia, 1983

Mueller PR, VonSonnenberg E, Ferrucci JJ: Percutaneous drainage of 250 abdominal abscesses and fluid collections. Radiology 151:337, 1984

Reuter SR, Redman HC: Gastrointestinal Angiography. 2nd Ed. WB Saunders, Philadelphia, 1977

Sardi, DA, Sample WF: Diagnostic Ultrasound. GK Hall Medical Publishers, Boston, 1980

6

Radiology of the Biliary System

Susan M. Williams
Roger K. Harned

The past two decades have ushered in a new era of biliary imaging. Rapidly advancing technology has facilitated more accurate diagnosis and has altered the traditional approaches to biliary disease. For example, sonography has replaced oral cholecystography for the diagnosis of cholelithiasis, cholescintigraphy and sonography have replaced intravenous cholangiography for the diagnosis of acute cholecystitis, and the interventional radiologist rather than the surgeon is often the first to treat biliary obstruction. This chapter is intended to provide a concise review of biliary radiology today. Following a discussion of pertinent anatomy, the more common disease entities involving the gallbladder and bile ducts are reviewed. Reference is made to imaging modalities that are most useful in each condition; one section is devoted to imaging the jaundiced patient.

Because hospitals will differ in available technology and expertise, the suggested imaging sequences are not intended to be absolute. The large amount of new, rapidly developing technology precludes a detailed description of each technique. We have tried to present an overview of what is now available, and we refer the interested reader to the suggested readings at the end of the chapter.

BILIARY ANATOMY

The liver is divided into right and left lobes on the basis of biliary drainage and portal venous anatomy (Fig. 6-1). On the external liver surface, the lobes are not clearly demarcated. However, the division plane can be approximated by a line projected between the gallbladder fossa and the inferior vena cava. Internally, the biliary ducts and blood vessels of the right and left lobes do not intercommunicate. The division is of practical importance as it identifies a potential plane for surgical resection. The left lobe is divided into medial and lateral segments by the fissure of the ligamentum teres. The medial segment of the left lobe was previously referred to by anatomists as the quadrate lobe. The right lobe is divided into posterior and anterior segments. The biliary duct to the posterior segment generally arises more proximally and superiorly from the right hepatic duct, although anatomic variations in this area are common. Each hepatic segment is further subdivided into superior and inferior subsegments. The biliary drainage of the caudate lobe is variable and may be related to the left or right duct system. Occasionally, small aberrant ducts drain into the gallbladder or cystic duct and may be a cause of persistent bile leak after cholecystectomy.

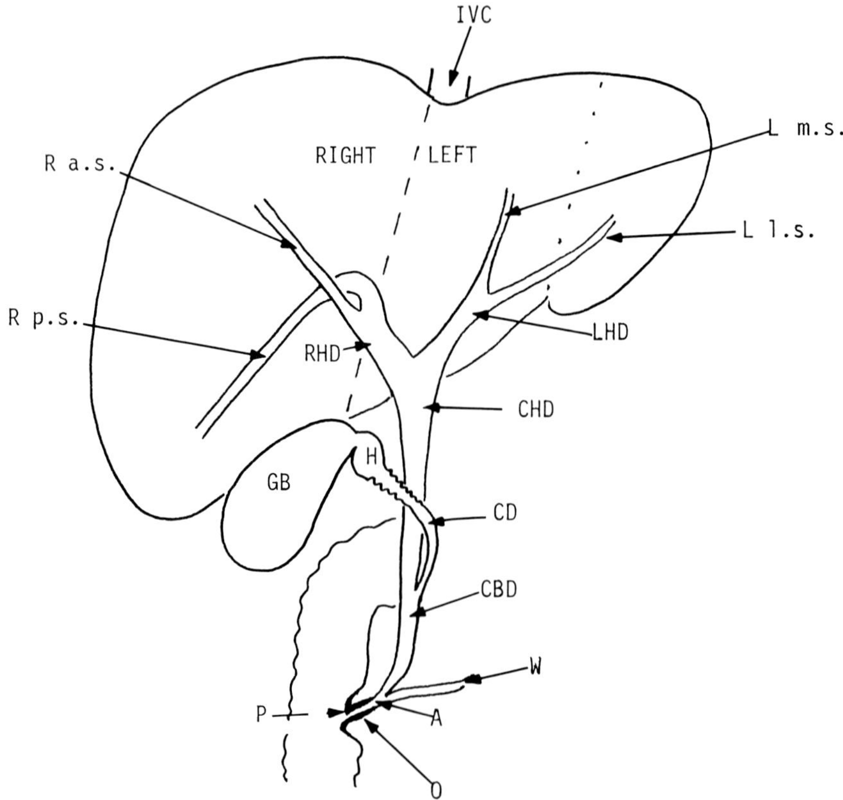

Fig. 6-1 Biliary anatomy. Inferior vena cava *(IVC)*. Right lobe of liver: anterior segment *(R a.s.)*, posterior segment *(R p.s.)*. Left lobe of liver: medial segment *(L m.s.)*, lateral segment *(L l.s.)*. Left hepatic duct *(LHD)*. Right hepatic duct *(RHD)*. Common hepatic duct *(CHD)*. Duct of Wirsung *(W)*. Ampulla of Vater *(A)*. Sphincter of Oddi *(O)*. Papilla of Vater *(P)*. Gallbladder *(G)*. Hartman pouch *(H)*.

Common Hepatic Duct

The right and left hepatic ducts join at the hilus of the liver to form the common hepatic duct (CHD). The CHD courses from the porta in the adventitia of the hepatoduodenal ligament anterior to the portal vein. Although elastic fibers in the duct wall allow distensibility, the CHD has no intrinsic muscular activity. It is joined by the cystic duct to form the common bile duct (CBD).

Common Bile Duct

The common duct passes posteromedially to the duodenal bulb and continues in a groove on the poste-rior surface of the pancreas. It opens into the medial aspect of the second portion of the duodenum at the papilla of Vater. The inferior choledochal sphincter, 5 to 10 mm in length, controls bile emptying and prevents reflux of duodenal contents into the biliary system. Elastic fibers and sparse oblique muscle fibers in the wall of the CBD allow some contractile activity. In most adults, the main pancreatic duct joins the distal CBD to form a short common channel, the ampulla of Vater. Entirely separate orifices for the CBD and pancreatic duct occur occasionally on the papilla. The average diameter of the normal CBD, as measured at sonography, is about 4 to 6 mm. Because of distension and magnification, it may appear larger at cholangiography.

Gallbladder

The gallbladder normally lies in close apposition to the inferior surface of the right lobe of the liver, and is enveloped in the peritoneum continuous with the liver surface. The depth of the gallbladder fossa is variable; thus, varying degrees of intrahepatic gallbladder may occur. Conversely, a loose peritoneal covering or mesentary may allow the gallbladder to migrate into the pelvis, left abdomen, or even into the lesser sac. Torsion may occur in these situations. Rarely, the gallbladder may be related to the left lobe of the liver. Double or septated gallbladders may occur, but are uncommon. Complete agenesis is rare and usually associated with other congenital anomalies. The gallbladder ranges from 7 to 10 cm in length, with a capacity of 30 to 50 ml. Its size may increase after vagotomy, in diabetes, or following cystic duct or CBD obstruction.

Anatomically, the gallbladder is divided into fundus, body, and neck. A pouch-like configuration of the neck is known as the Hartman pouch, a site where stones occasionally lodge. The mucosa of the gallbladder is composed of simple columnar epithelium with redundant fine mucosal folds that aid in its physiologic function of water resorption. The normal gallbladder wall is 2 to 3 mm thick. Contraction is mediated by cholecystokinin released from the duodenal mucosa in response to fats, peptones, and hydrogen ions.

Cystic Duct

The cystic duct is 3 to 4 cm in length. Its mucous membrane forms prominent crescenteric folds known as the spiral valves. The level at which the cystic duct enters to form the CBD is variable; the cystic duct frequently lies parallel to the CHD in a common sheath for several centimeters before it opens into the lumen. Thus, to avoid injury to the common duct, a cystic duct remnant is usually left following cholecystectomy.

CHOLELITHIASIS

Incidence and Predisposition

Cholelithiasis is common, occurring in 10 to 20 percent of the Western population. The incidence is

twice as great in females as in males and increases with age. It is more common in whites than blacks, and is especially common in certain tribes of American Indians. Obesity is correlated with an increased incidence of gallstones in both sexes. Several conditions predispose to the development of cholelithiasis. Patients with hemolytic anemia are at increased risk of developing pigment stones. Similarly, hemolysis in patients with prosthetic cardiac valves or hypersplenism may lead to cholelithiasis. Abnormal enterohepatic recirculation of bile salts in patients with severe small bowel disease, such as Crohn ileitis or extensive distal small bowel resections, leads to a gradual bile salt deficiency and subsequent gallstone formation. Cholelithiasis is also reported with an increased incidence in diabetes mellitus, cirrhosis, hy-

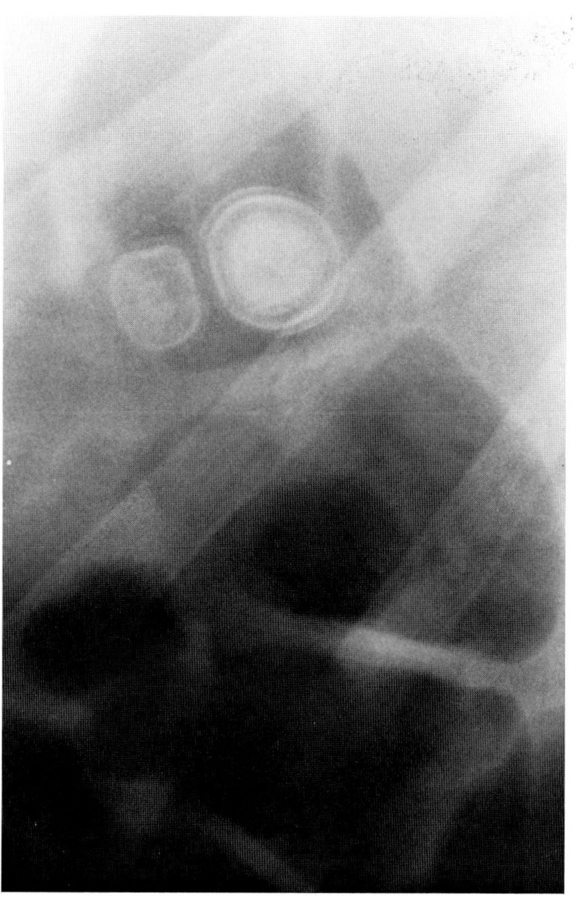

Fig. 6-2 Cholelithiasis. Only 10 to 15 percent of gallstones are visible on plain abdominal radiographs.

perparathyroidism, and postvagotomy. Estrogen therapy induces increased saturation of bile with cholesterol and may accelerate stone formation.

Radiographic Detection

Gallstones are composed of varying proportions of bilirubin, cholesterol, and calcium carbonate. Although relatively pure cholesterol or bilirubin pigment stones occur, most stones are of mixed composition. Between 10 and 15 percent of gallstones contain enough calcium to permit visualization on plain abdominal radiographs (Fig. 6-2). Cholesterol crystals shrink as the stones become dehydrated, resulting in dendritic cracks in the center of the stones. These

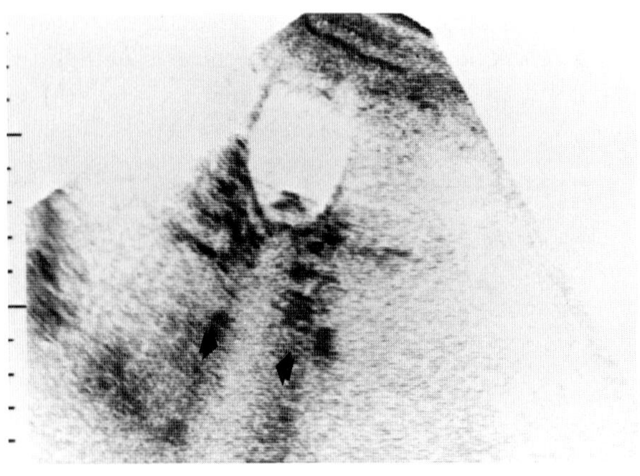

Fig. 6-4 Cholelithiasis. Echogenic foci in the gallbladder lumen projecting an acoustic shadow *(arrowheads)*.

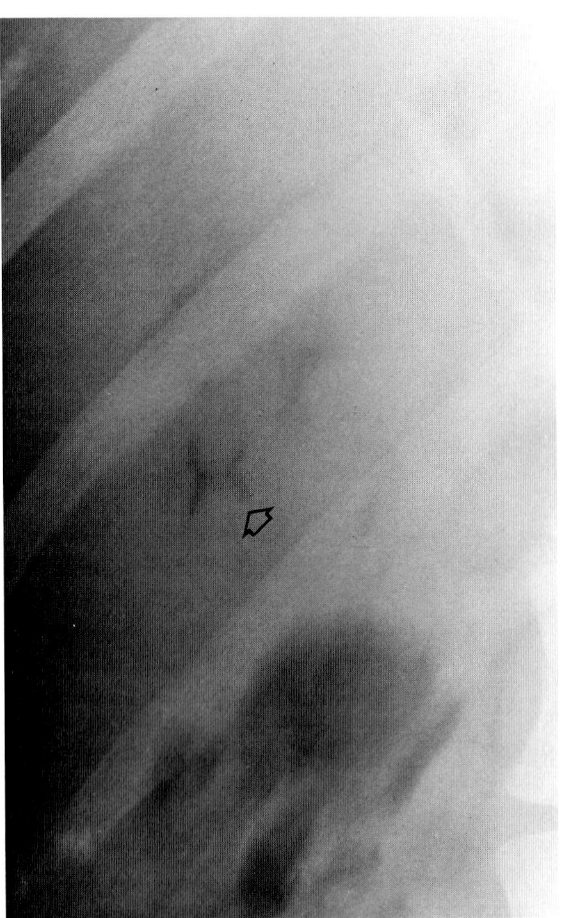

Fig. 6-3 The "Mercedes Benz" sign *(arrowhead)* permits the radiologist to diagnose cholelithiasis on the plain abdominal radiograph.

cracks accumulate nitrogen gas by diffusion. Occasionally the stellate gas pattern is prominent enough to be detected on plain abdominal radiographs. This has been referred to as the Mercedes Benz sign because of its resemblance to the automobile insignia (Fig. 6-3).

Currently, sonography is the procedure of choice for detection of cholelithiasis. The exam is easily and quickly performed on fasting patients, requires no medication or ionizing radiation, and detects calculi with an accuracy exceeding 96 percent. The diagnosis of cholelithiasis is made by demonstrating nonfixed, echogenic foci within the gallbladder lumen. The stones usually occupy a dependent position in the gallbladder and shift as the patient changes position. Acoustic shadowing is often demonstrable and depends on the technique employed (Fig. 6-4). The diameter of the sonic beam in relation to the diameter of the stone is the most important factor in demonstrating shadowing, which depends on the size and position of the stone and the frequency and focal length of the transducer. The majority of nonshadowing, movable, intraluminal opacities are small calculi. However, pus, sludge, mucin, or blood clots may occasionally have a similar appearance. Because sonography can identify the gallbladder in almost all normal fasting patients, failure to visualize it is highly correlated with disease. Nonvisualized gallbladders are usually contracted and totally filled with stones. Generally, in such cases, an echogenic focus and acoustic shadow will originate from the gallbladder fossa.

The success of ultrasound has made oral cholecystography a secondary test for the diagnosis of cholelithiasis. Although a properly performed oral cholecystogram with adequate opacification of the gallbladder is greater than 92 percent accurate in identifying calculi, the technique has certain relative limitations. (1) It requires a contrast agent with the potential for adverse reactions; (2) it is dependent on liver function and inconsistent intestinal absorption of the contrast; (3) it involves exposure to ionizing radiation; and (4) the significance of a nonvisualized gallbladder is not always certain.

Oral cholecystography is now reserved for cases in which ultrasound is equivocal or unavailable, or compelling clinical symptoms suggest gallbladder disease, even if sonography is normal. The appearance of calculi at oral cholecystography does not clearly predict stone composition; thus, it is of limited value in predicting the success of pharmacologic dissolution. Many stones have a specific gravity less than that of contrast-laden bile and, as seen on horizontal-beam radiographs (Fig. 6-5), they frequently layer out.

ACUTE CHOLECYSTITIS

Between 90 and 95 percent of the cases of acute cholecystitis are caused by acute calculus obstruction of the cystic duct. It is estimated that this complication will develop in 3 to 10 percent of patients who harbor gallstones. The obstructed gallbladder then becomes distended, edematous, congested, and ischemic. Secondary bacterial infection occurs. Clinically, the patients typically present with colicky, right upper quadrant pain, tenderness, fever, nausea, and vomiting. If the obstruction is unrelieved, the disease may progress to gangrene and perforation. If the inflammation subsides but the cystic duct remains obstructed, the gallbladder may become distended with sterile mucous. This condition is referred to as hydrops of the gallbladder.

Diagnosis of Acute Cholecystitis

^{99m}Tc-labeled iminodiacetic acid (^{99m}Tc-IDA) derivatives have recently been perfected for biliary imaging. Following intravenous injection, the nuclide is excreted by the hepatocytes into the biliary ducts. If the cystic duct is patent, radionuclide accumulates in the gallbladder. The absence of activity in the gallbladder indicates cystic duct obstruction. Because acute cholecystitis is almost associated with cystic duct obstruction, cholescintigraphy is a sensitive and specific diagnostic test (Fig. 6-6). The overall accuracy of cholescintigraphy in patients with acute symptoms approaches 98 percent. If the gallbladder is visualized within 1 hour of injection, acute cholecystitis can be confidently excluded. If no visualization is identified, delayed images up to 4 hours must be made. Occasionally, chronic cholecystitis results in a 1 to 4 hour delayed visualization. Rare false positives may occur in patients with chronic cholecystitis or in patients on long-term hyperalimentation with biliary stasis. False negatives, less than 5 percent, may occur in acalculus cholecystitis, usually in patients with delayed visualization.

Sonography is also widely utilized in the diagnosis of acute cholecystitis. However, because of the 11 percent incidence of asymptomatic cholelithiasis in the general population, the demonstration of calculi alone does not necessarily indicate that the gallbladder is the source of acute clinical symptoms. Several other sonographic signs contribute to the diagnosis of acute cholecystitis. Focal tenderness, elicited when the transducer is directly over the gallbladder, is a subjective finding that suggests acute inflammation. The gallbladder wall may thicken from edema and

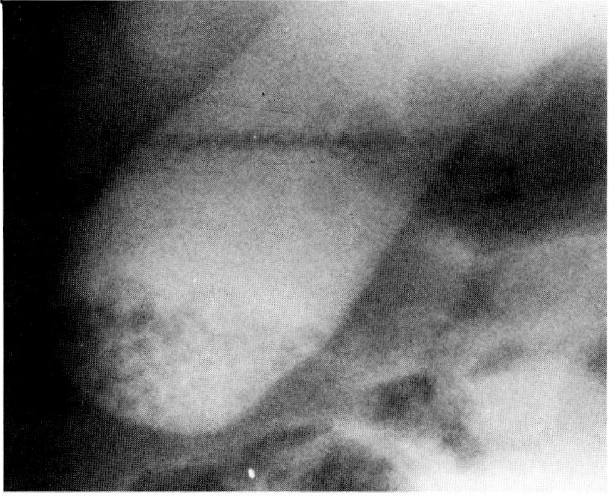

Fig. 6-5 Gallstones frequently form layers on upright spot radiographs.

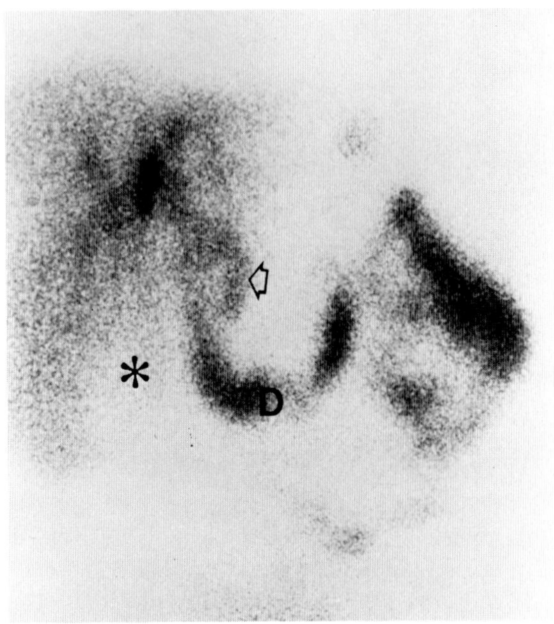

Fig. 6-6 Acute cholecystitis diagnosed by scintigraphy. Activity is present in the common bile duct *(arrow)* and duodenum *(D)*, but not in the gallbladder fossa (*).

congestion in acute cholecystitis. The anterior wall is the best site for sonographic measurement and normally is less than 2 mm in thickness; 5 mm is definitely abnormal. Caution is required in the presence of ascites, as the wall may appear erroneously thickened in this condition. Congestive heart failure, hypoproteinemia, chronic cholecystitis, carcinoma, viral hepatitis, and varices also cause the gallbladder wall to thicken and should be considered in the differential diagnosis. In nonfasting patients, a normal contracted gallbladder may also have a thickened wall. Finally, pericholecystic fluid may be demonstrable in severe cases of acute cholecystitis, aiding the sonographic diagnosis.

Intravenous cholangiography has been replaced by cholescintigraphy and ultrasound and no longer has a role in the evaluation of acute cholecystitis. Findings of acute cholecystitis, including calculi, thickened gallbladder wall, and pericholecystic fluid are demonstrable by computed tomography (CT). However, CT is not recommended as a cost-effective initial study.

Acalculus Cholecystitis

Between 5 and 10 percent of the cases of acute cholecystitis occur in the absence of calculi. The pathogenesis of this disorder is unclear, but postulated etiologic factors include ischemia, bacterial infection, and irritation by hyperconcentrated bile or refluxed pancreatic enzymes. Acute acalculus cholecystitis is most common in older patients with multisystemic disease. The clinical and radiographic diagnosis is often elusive; morbidity and mortality are high. Because edema and inflammation cause functional cystic duct obstruction in most patients, cholescintigraphy is often diagnostic. However, false-negative rates as high as 25 to 30 percent have been reported. Sonography is occasionally useful in the diagnosis, if a thickened gallbladder wall or pericholecystic fluid can be demonstrated.

Emphysematous Cholecystitis

Emphysematous cholecystitis is a variant of acute cholecystitis. Infection with gas-forming bacteria causes gas to accumulate in the lumen and wall of the gallbladder, and occasionally in the pericholecystic soft tissues. This condition is more common in males; 20 to 30 percent of the cases occur in patients with diabetes mellitus. The pathogenesis may be related to ischemia, and calculi are not always present. The infecting organisms include *Clostridia, Escherichia coli, Aerobacter aerogenes, Klebsiella,* and nonhemolytic streptococcus. The condition carries a greater risk of gangrene and perforation than does nonemphysematous cholecystitis. The diagnosis may be made on the plain abdominal radiograph when gas is visible in the gallbladder lumen, wall, or both (Fig. 6-7). Large extraluminal gas collections suggest that perforation has already occurred and pericholecystic abscess has developed. The cystic duct is usually obstructed by edema and inflammation but gas is rarely visible in the biliary ducts.

CHRONIC CHOLECYSTITIS

The histologic criteria for the diagnosis of chronic cholecystitis are not clearly defined. They include minimal to severe inflammatory infiltrate in the gallbladder wall, varying degrees of transmural thickening and fibrosis, and epithelial crypts extending intramurally (Rokitansky-Aschoff sinusus). In 90 to 95 percent of the cases, gallstones are present. Almost all patients undergoing cholecystectomy for biliary symptoms and cholelithiasis have some histologic changes of cholecystitis. However, autopsy series and operative series of incidentally removed asymptomatic gallbladders indicate some degree of inflammatory change is often present. Additionally, cholelithiasis may occasionally be present without cholecystitis and conversely, chronic acalculus cholecystitis may occur.

The preoperative diagnosis of chronic cholecystitis is based on the presence of calculi in patients with symptoms suggesting gallbladder disease. Chronic or

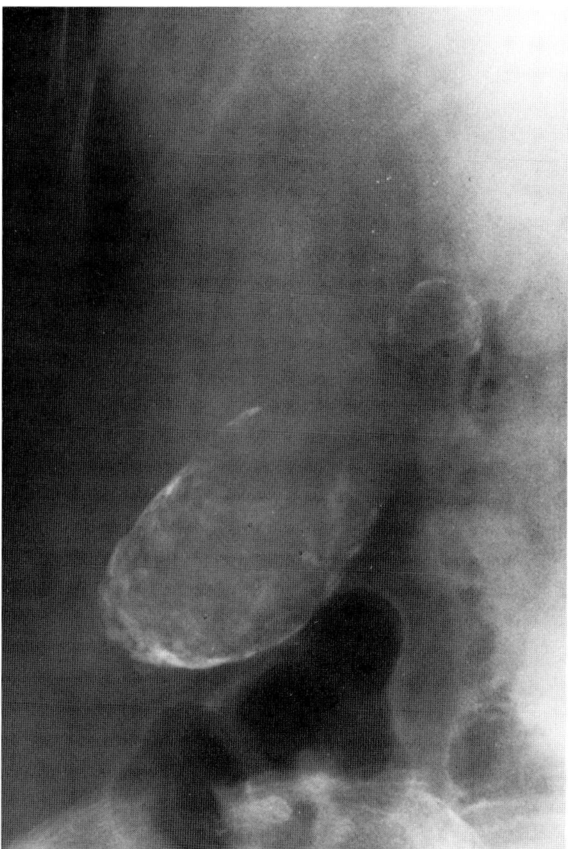

Fig. 6-8 Porcelain gallbladder. The calcified gallbladder is evident on the plain abdominal radiograph.

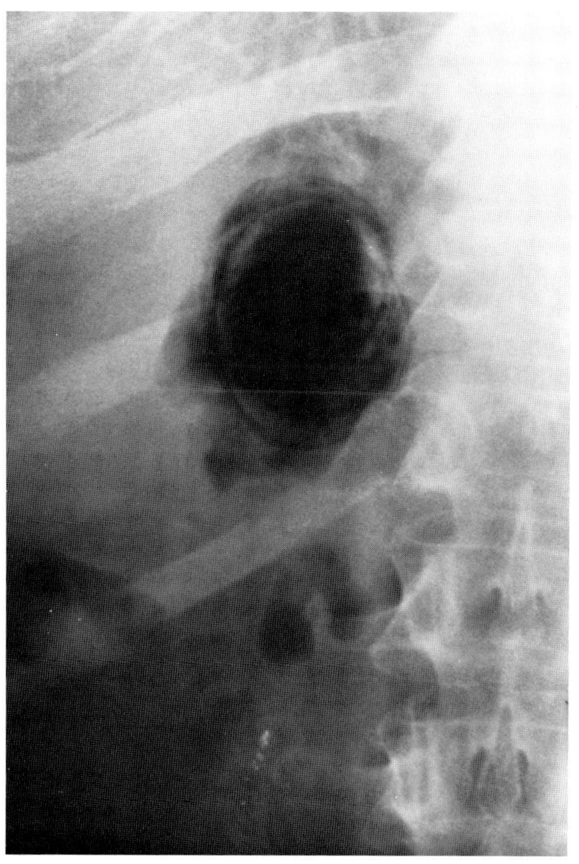

Fig. 6-7 Emphysematous cholecystitis. Gas is present in the lumen and wall of the gallbladder, as well as in the pericholecystic soft tissues.

episodic upper abdominal pain, fatty food intolerance, and flatulence are commonly associated symptoms.

If clinical symptoms suggest gallbladder disease but radiographic studies fail to demonstrate calculi or other abnormality, the problem becomes much more difficult. A variety of attempts have been made to define and diagnose such disorders as acalculus chronic cholecystitis and biliary dyskinesia. Prolonged opacification of the gallbladder after oral cholecystography has been suggested as one diagnostic sign, but it is more likely related to inadequate fat in the diet or to the enterohepatic recirculation of iopanoic acid. In either case, its significance has not been proved. Quantitation of the contractile and symptomatic response to cholecystokinin is being widely investigated as a diagnostic test. To date, no definitive study is available to prove that the response to cholecystokinin can predict gallbladder histology or identify patients that will benefit from cholecystectomy.

Porcelain Gallbladder

The inflammatory changes of chronic cholecystitis may result in calcification of the gallbladder wall. The descriptive term porcelain gallbladder is used to describe this condition. Histologically, the calcification is of two types: multiple punctate calcifications in the glandular spaces, or a diffuse band of calcification in the muscularis. Stones are usually present and the cystic duct is frequently obstructed. The diagnosis is based on the characteristic appearance of the calcified gallbladder on plain abdominal radiographs (Fig. 6-8). The patients are often asymptomatic and the

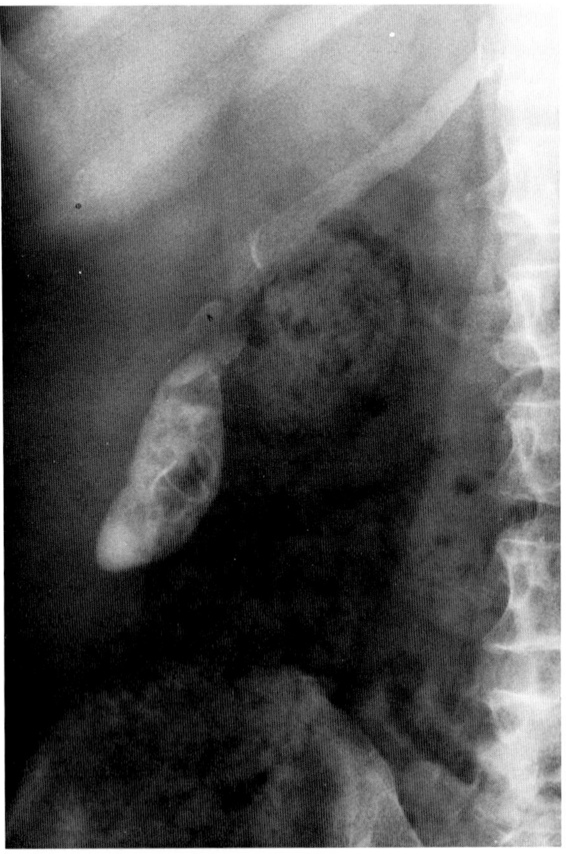

Fig. 6-9 Milk of calcium bile. This patient has received no contrast. Note the presence of several calculi.

condition is usually an incidental finding. The true incidence is difficult to determine with certainty, but extensive calcification is found in less than 1 percent of cholecystectomy specimens.

Several series have reported a high incidence (12 to 60 percent) of adenocarcinoma in porcelain gallbladder. Although the mechanism of this association is not proven, prophylactic cholecystectomy should be considered when a porcelain gallbladder is encountered.

Milk of Calcium Bile

Occasionally, in longstanding cystic duct obstruction the concentration of calcium salts in intraluminal bile becomes sufficient to opacify the gallbladder on plain radiographs. This is known as milk of calcium bile or limey bile syndrome. The radiographic appearance is similar to that of a gallbladder opacified following oral cholecystography (Fig. 6-9). Larger stones are often seen to float in the opaque bile. Although these gallbladders do manifest histologic changes of chronic cholecystitis, an increased incidence of carcinoma has not been reported.

BILIARY-ENTERIC FISTULA AND GALLSTONE ILEUS

Chronic or recurrent inflammatory episodes may cause the gallbladder to become adherent to adjacent bowel. Gallstones may then spontaneously erode into the bowel lumen. This is the most common etiology of noniatrogenic biliary-enteric fistula. Penetrating peptic ulcer, trauma, or neoplasm are less common causes. The duodenum is the most common site of erosion, but fistulization to stomach, colon, or other organs may occur. Usually the stones pass spontaneously, but a large calculus may become lodged in the pylorus or ileocecal valve, causing obstruction. Small bowel obstruction caused by a gallstone is referred to as gallstone ileus. It is an important cause of small bowel obstruction in patients over 65 and, if not diagnosed promptly, it is accompanied by high morbidity and mortality.

The classic triad of radiographic findings, as first described by Rigler is (1) dilated air- and fluid-filled loops of small bowel, (2) air in the biliary tree, and (3) ectopic gallstone in the abdomen. Biliary gas can be identified in about two-thirds of the cases. The stone itself is visible in less than half. Biliary gas should be differentiated from portal venous gas, which is usually due to intestinal ischemia. Portal gas tends to collect in the periphery of the liver, whereas biliary gas collects in the more central ducts near the porta. Because gallstone ileus is a potentially curable condition, it is important to look carefully for the radiographic clues when an elderly patient presents with small bowel obstruction.

CHOLESTEROLOSIS

Cholesterolosis is a benign condition in which triglycerides and cholesterol esters are deposited in the macrophages of the gallbladder wall, mainly within the lamina propria. The yellowish lipid deposits are visible grossly, causing the gallbladder mucosa to resemble a strawberry. Thus, the term "strawberry gallbladder" is often used to describe this condition.

Cholesterolosis is common and can be identified in 10 to 20 percent of gallbladders in surgical and autopsy series. The size and distribution of the lipid deposits varies. Most are diffuse and less than 1 mm in size. Larger, discrete, polypoid deposits, up to 1 cm in diameter, also occur. These polyps contain no glandular tissue and are not true neoplasms. They may have a short epithelial pedicle. Inflammation is not a prominent histologic feature of cholesterolosis, which has often been classified with adenomyomatosis as one of the hyperplastic cholecystoses. Actually, the two conditions are histologically distinct entities and grouping them together serves no purpose.

Radiographically, the larger polypoid cholesterol deposits appear as fixed lucencies within the opacified gallbladder lumen at oral cholecystography (Fig. 6-10). They are distinguished from calculi by their failure to move with compression and positional changes. Sonography also detects the lesions as nonmobile, nonshadowing intraluminal echos. Other associated signs, including hypercontractility and hyperconcentration, have been described but their sensitivity and specificity for cholesterolosis is questionable. If clinical symptoms occur, they are usually vague and poorly defined. Unless compelling biliary

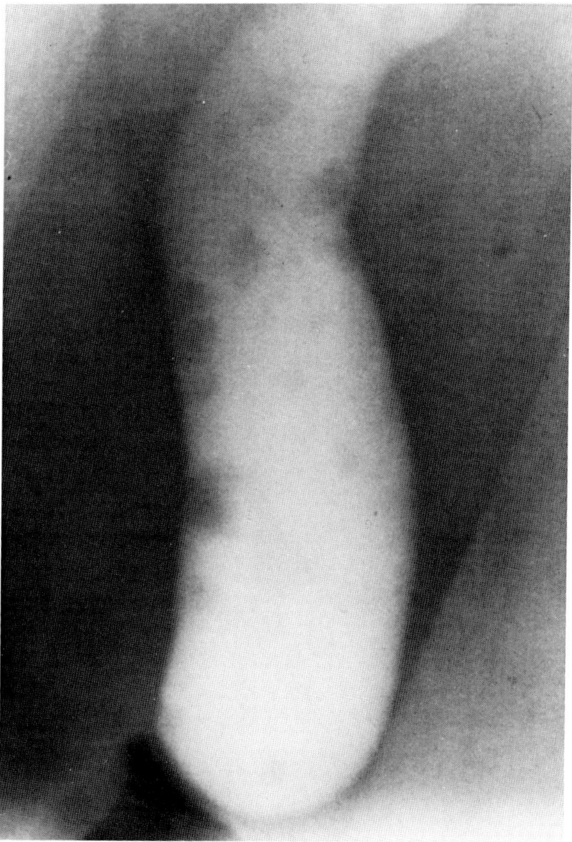

Fig. 6-10 Cholesterolosis diagnosed by oral cholecystography. The lucent polyps in the gallbladder lumen are fixed on this upright spot radiograph.

colic is present or gallstones coexist, cholecystectomy is probably not indicated.

ADENOMYOMATOSIS

Adenomyomatosis is a hyperplastic degenerative disease of the gallbladder. It is the most common of a group of conditions known as hyperplastic cholecystoses. The histopathology consists of hyperplasia of the mucosa and muscular wall. Epithelium herniates into the lamina propria and muscularis, forming small crypts or intramural diverticula (Rokitansky-Aschoff sinusus). Inflammation is not a characteristic feature. The disease may be diffuse, segmental, or localized and any portion of the gallbladder may be involved. A localized form, occurring in the fundus, is often termed adenomyoma. Unfortunately, the term adenomyoma may be confusing because it is not a true neoplasm. There is no malignant potential. The etiology of adenomyomatosis is unknown. The condition is more common in women and calculi often coexist.

Radiographic diagnosis is only possible in advanced cases. The larger Rokitansky-Aschoff sinuses may communicate with the lumen and fill with contrast at oral cholecystography. These contrast-filled sinuses resemble small beads, in the gallbladder wall, surrounding the lumen (Fig. 6-11). This characteristic appearance is best identified in the partially contracted gallbladder with compression filming. A focal narrowing of the lumen, or thick annular septum, is often associated. The diagnostic findings of localized fundal

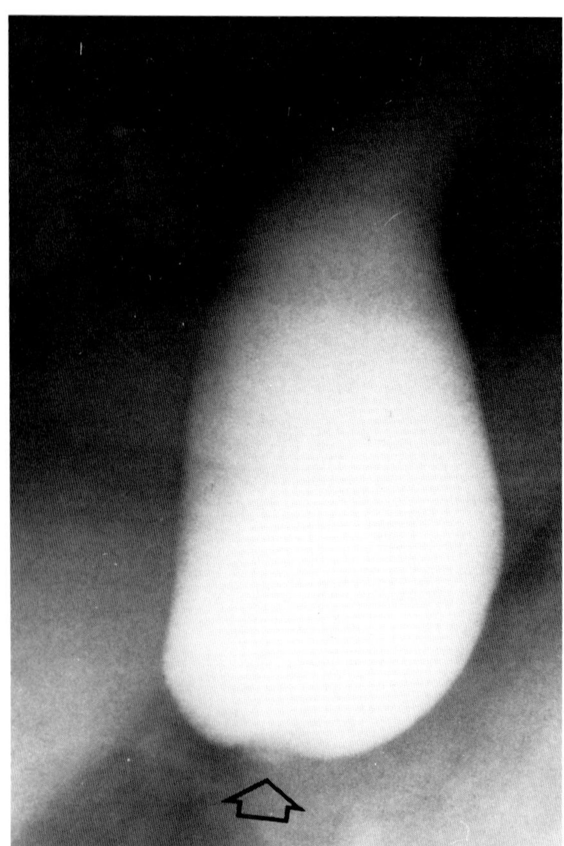

Fig. 6-12 Localized adenomyomatosis (adenomyoma) in the fundus of the gallbladder *(arrowhead)*.

adenomyomatosis may be subtle and include a small mass or focal thickening of the wall (Fig. 6-12). As in cholesterolosis, hyperconcentration and hypercontractility have been described in association with adenomyomatosis. These are nonspecific signs and are of little aid, unless the pathologic changes in the gallbladder wall are also demonstrated. Adenomyomatosis may also occasionally be diagnosed by sonography if the small, cystic, anechoic, Rokitansky-Aschoff spaces are detected. Thickening of the gallbladder wall is the most prominent sonographic finding, but is nonspecific.

Adenomyomatosis is a benign degenerative condition without specific clinical findings. Many patients are asymptomatic or have only vague complaints. Cholecystectomy is probably not warranted unless calculi or persistent symptoms of biliary colic are present.

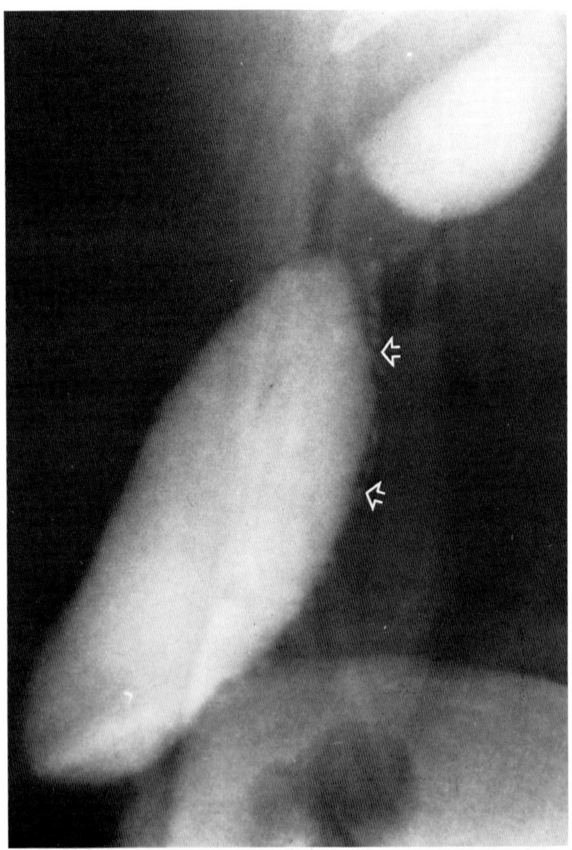

Fig. 6-11 Small contrast-filled Rokitansky-Aschoff sinuses *(arrowheads)* allow the diagnosis of adenomyomatosis. Notice a thick annular septum is also associated.

CARCINOMA OF THE GALLBLADDER

Carcinoma of the gallbladder is the fifth most common cause of death from gastrointestinal malignancy, accounting for about 3 percent of all cancer deaths. The incidence is at least three times greater in females than males, and most of the cases occur after the age of 50. In various series, 65 to 95 percent of cases are associated with cholelithiasis, although the etiologic relationship remains speculative. Unfortunately, the early stages of the disease are relatively asymptomatic. The tumor is almost always advanced by the time of detection and progresses relentlessly to death within 1 to 5 years.

Most of the lesions are well-differentiated adenocarcinoma of which greater than half are scirrhous. The remainder are papillary and mucinous forms. Unusual histologic variants include anaplastic carcinoma, squamous cell carcinoma, and adenoacanthoma. The most frequent mode of extension is by contiguous invasion, often directly into adjacent liver. Nodal spread occurs first to the pericholedochal and pancreaticoduodenal nodes and subsequently to celiac and paraaortic nodes. Biliary obstruction is common. Hematogenous metastasis and intraperitoneal seeding also occur.

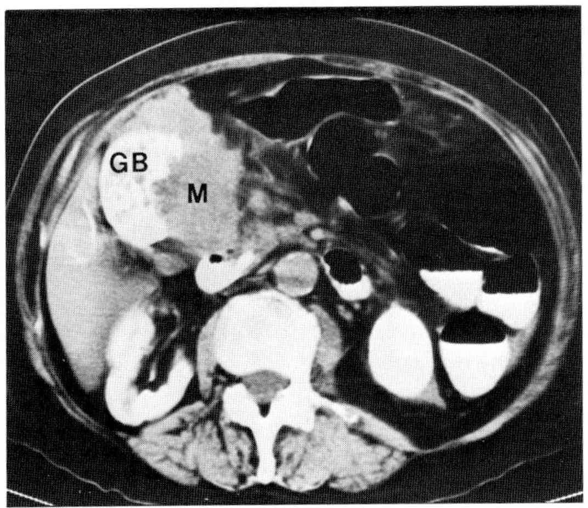

Fig. 6-13 CT demonstrates a mass *(M)* arising from the contrast-filled gallbladder *(GB)*.

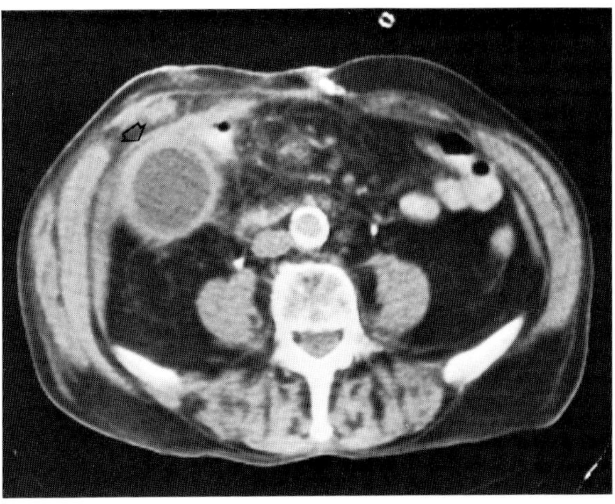

Fig. 6-14 Thickening of the gallbladder wall may also occur in cases of cholecystitis. A thin halo of fluid *(arrowhead)* around the gallbladder suggests cholecystitis in this case.

Prior to the advent of sonography and computed tomography, the diagnosis was rarely made preoperatively. Now the preoperative diagnosis is made more frequently, but diagnosis of early resectable lesions is still rare. The most frequent finding by CT and sonography is a mass in the gallbladder fossa, with extension to adjacent liver (Fig. 6-13). Other common findings include a thickened gallbladder wall, intraluminal polypoid or fungating mass, cholelithiasis, biliary obstruction, nodal involvement, and hematogenous metastases. Differentiation from advanced carcinoma of the pancreas may be difficult. Chronic cholecystitis also causes a thickened gallbladder wall, which may simulate carcinoma. It has been suggested that visualization of a thin halo of fluid around the wall indicates cholecystitis rather than carcinoma (Fig. 6-14). If an irregular intraluminal polypoid mass, greater than 1 cm, is found in the gallbladder, consideration should be given to cholecystectomy in the hope of finding a resectable carcinoma.

Primary malignancies of the gallbladder other than carcinoma are rare. Carcinoid tumors and sarcomas have been reported. Hematogenous metastatic disease, especially melanoma, may involve the gallbladder but is rarely diagnosed radiographically.

BENIGN NEOPLASMS OF THE GALLBLADDER

True benign neoplasms of the gallbladder are rare, occurring in less than 5 percent of cholecystectomy specimens. Most are papillary or nonpapillary adenomas. These may be sessile or pedunculated, solitary or multiple, and are usually smaller than 1 cm. They are identified as small, fixed, intraluminal masses at sonography or oral cholecystography (Fig. 6-15). There is no evidence to indicate malignant potential. Cholecystectomy is usually not necessary but may be considered if growth is demonstrated, or if a larger irregular polypoid mass raises the suspicion of carcinoma.

The differential diagnosis of a fixed mass in the gallbladder also includes metastasis, polypoid cholesterolosis (most common), localized adenomyomatosis, adherent gallstone, inflammatory polyp, and cyst. Ec-

topic pancreatic tissue or gastric mucosa rarely occurs in the gallbladder. Mesenchymal neoplasms are quite rare.

RADIOGRAPHY IN THE JAUNDICED PATIENT

The rapid technical advances of recent years have vastly expanded the role of radiology in the evaluation and treatment of the jaundiced patient. Although careful clinical and laboratory studies often suggest the obstructive or nonobstructive origin of jaundice, a more definitive preoperative diagnosis is usually necessary. Currently available imaging techniques allow confident diagnosis of obstructive jaundice and also define the precise level and etiology in almost all cases. In addition, a variety of radiologic and endoscopic options for palliation and treatment are available alternatives to operation in selected patients.

Intravenous Cholangiography

In past decades intravenous cholangiography (IVC) was the only method available to image the biliary ducts without surgery. Unfortunately, the usefulness of this study was limited by the toxicity of the contrast, high error rate, and frequent inadequate visualization of the bile ducts. IVC has now been largely replaced by computed tomography, sonography, percutaneous cholangiography, and endoscopic retrograde cholangiography.

Sonography in Diagnosis of Biliary Obstruction

Sonography accurately demonstrates the caliber of the intrahepatic and extrahepatic bile ducts. Because of its safety, lack of ionizing radiation, wide availability, and relative low cost, sonography is generally considered to be the initial imaging study when biliary obstruction is suspected. Intrahepatic ducts of normal caliber are not visible at sonography. However, the common hepatic duct (CHD) is almost always identifiable in the porta hepatis anterior to the portal vein.

The normal diameter of the CHD is 4 mm or less. A CHD greater than 7 mm is definitely abnormal, indi-

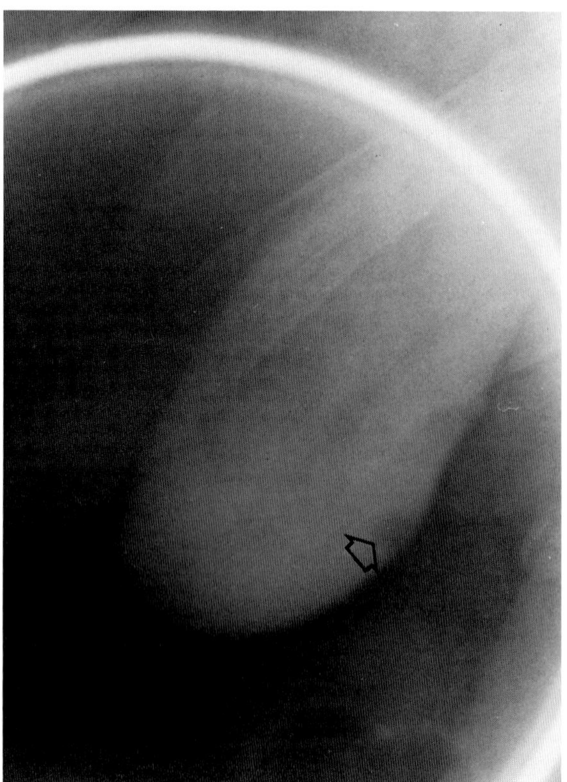

Fig. 6-15 Small adenoma of the gallbladder *(arrowhead).*

cating either present or past biliary disease. Some authors consider even a 5 to 6 mm duct to be abnormal and an indication for further study. The more distal common bile duct is less frequently visualized sonographically, as it may be obscured by adjacent gas in the duodenum or colon.

Dilated intrahepatic ducts are visible with sonography. Several signs of intrahepatic duct dilatation have been described. The "too-many-tubes" sign is created by an increased number of sonolucent channels in the liver (Fig. 6-16). The similar "parallel-channel" sign is formed by a dilated bile duct that runs anterior and parallel to a portal vein. Relative increased transmission of sound through bile, as compared to blood, results in acoustic enhancement posterior to dilated bile ducts, which may help in distinguishing them from veins.

Sonography is reported to be 83 to 97 percent accurate in diagnosing the presence of obstructive jaundice. The occasional limitation is that bile duct caliber does not always correlate exactly with the presence or absence of biliary obstruction; some patients have significant biliary obstruction in the absence of dilated ducts. Such a situation may occur when transient cholangitis is the result of a small calculus impacted at the ampulla, in some cases of sclerosing cholangitis, and in occasional cases of bile duct carcinoma. Therefore, if clinical and laboratory evidence strongly indicates biliary obstruction, further study may be warranted, even if the sonogram appears normal. Some investigators are successfully utilizing provocative tests to detect biliary obstruction in the absence of dilated ducts. Because of elastic fibers in the wall of the extrahepatic duct, rapid changes in caliber may occur with varying intraluminal pressure. Following the administration of a fatty meal or cholecystokinin to stimulate bile flow, the normal, unobstructed extrahepatic duct decreases or does not change in caliber. An increase in caliber, as bile flow is stimulated, suggests some degree of distal obstruction.

To further complicate the diagnosis of biliary obstruction, there are patients without evident biliary obstruction, who have definitely dilated biliary ducts. This situation is most likely to occur in older individuals who have had previous cholecystectomy or prior biliary tract disease. Cholecystectomy is not always followed by bile duct dilatation. But, if inflammation, age, or chronic distension have destroyed the elasticity of the bile duct wall, it may never return to normal caliber after an episode of transient biliary obstruction. The clinical problem in some of these patients is the difficulty of excluding a functional stenosis at the papilla of Vater. Bile duct manometry may prove to be of value in this situation to help select patients who might benefit from sphincterotomy.

Computed Tomography in the Diagnosis of Biliary Obstruction

Computed tomography (CT) can determine the caliber of intrahepatic and extrahepatic ducts with an accuracy comparable to that of sonography. In addition, in several recent series CT was more often useful than sonography in precisely defining the site and etiology of biliary obstruction. Intravenous contrast enhancement is necessary to accurately assess the biliary tract by CT. As with sonography, intrahepatic ducts of normal caliber are rarely visible, but dilated ducts are seen clearly against the contrast-enhanced liver as water density tubular structures converging in the porta. The normal or dilated extrahepatic duct is visible in most patients and can be followed on serial, thin consecutive sections along its course to the ampulla. Scanning, initially without the use of oral and intravenous contrast materials, increases the accuracy of diagnosis of common duct calculi (Fig. 6-17). Subsequent, dynamic scanning techniques following an

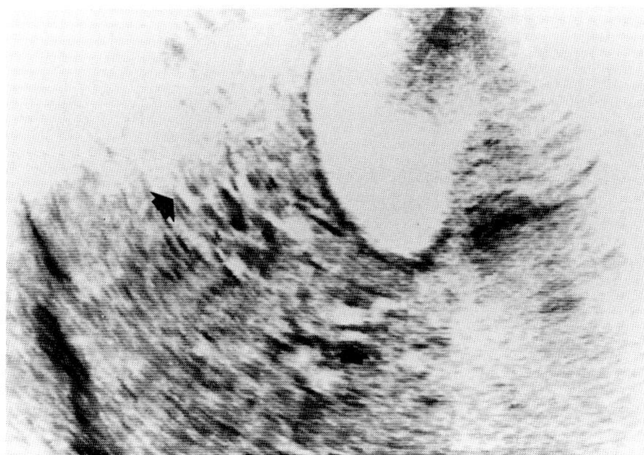

Fig. 6-16 "Too many tubes" *(arrowheads)* in the liver indicate intrahepatic bile duct dilatation at sonography.

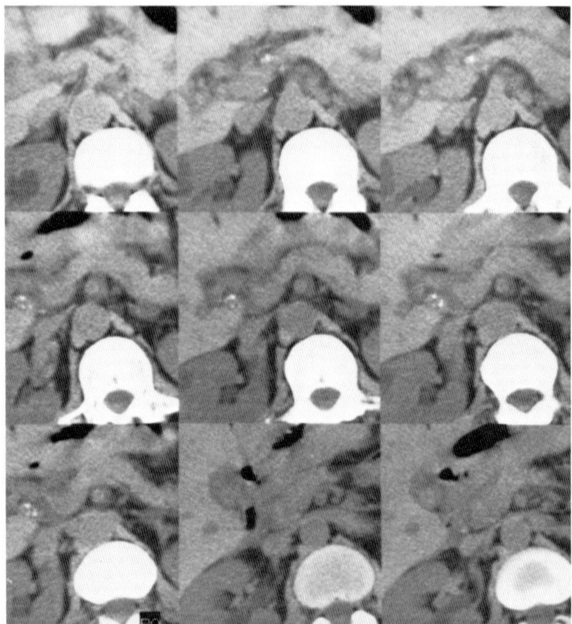

Fig. 6-17 A collage of serial CT scans taken at 4-mm intervals reveals several calculi in the common duct. Note that the absence of contrast materials facilitates this diagnosis.

intravenous contrast bolus are helpful to evaluate the area of porta hepatis and pancreatic head. Because of the cost, the necessity for intravenous contrast, and frequent scheduling delays, most centers still prefer to use sonography for the initial screening study in suspected biliary obstruction. CT is then reserved for selected cases in which sonography is equivocal, or does not provide sufficient specific evidence concerning the site and etiology of biliary obstruction.

Percutaneous Transhepatic Cholangiography

Direct cholangiography offers precise visualization of biliary anatomy as well as a variety of options for therapeutic intervention. The role of PTC has greatly expanded since the development of the fine, 22-gauge, flexible Chiba or "skinny" needle. The small caliber needle has reduced post-procedure complications. If proper technique is employed, percutaneous transhepatic cholangiography (PTC) is a safe, accurate, reliable, and widely available study. However, several precautions are necessary prior to the proce-

dure. Blood clotting studies should be obtained and any disorder corrected preoperatively, if necessary. To decrease the possibility of septic complications, preoperative intravenous antibiotic coverage is recommended. Because many patients experience pain during the procedure, mild sedation is usually necessary.

Although a detailed description of the technique is beyond the scope of this chapter, several technical points are worth emphasizing. Contrast is heavier than bile and the two liquids are not immediately miscible. Contrast flows by gravity to the most dependant portions of the biliary system. Therefore, when the patient is supine, the ducts of the right lobe fill preferentially. In the presence of biliary obstruc-

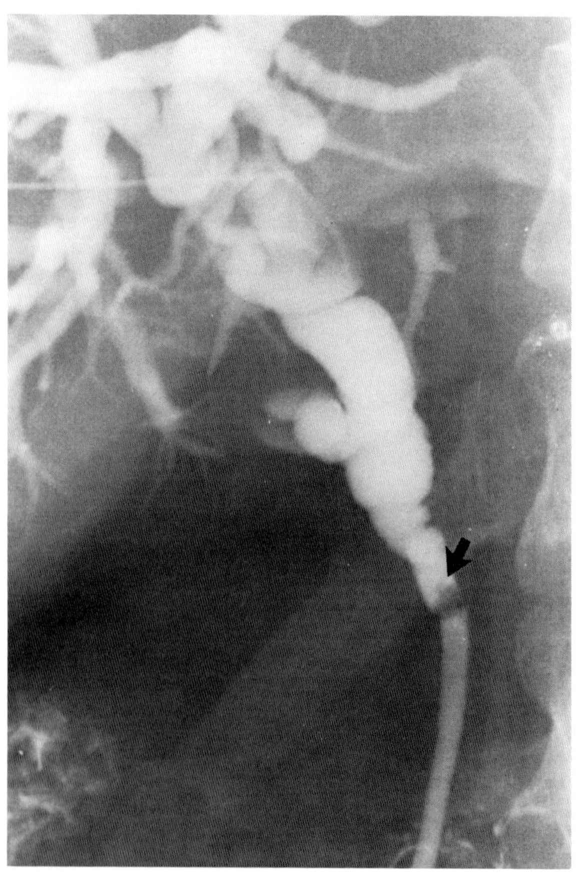

Fig. 6-18 PTC allows detailed visualization of biliary anatomy. A small calculus *(arrow)* is causing partial biliary obstruction.

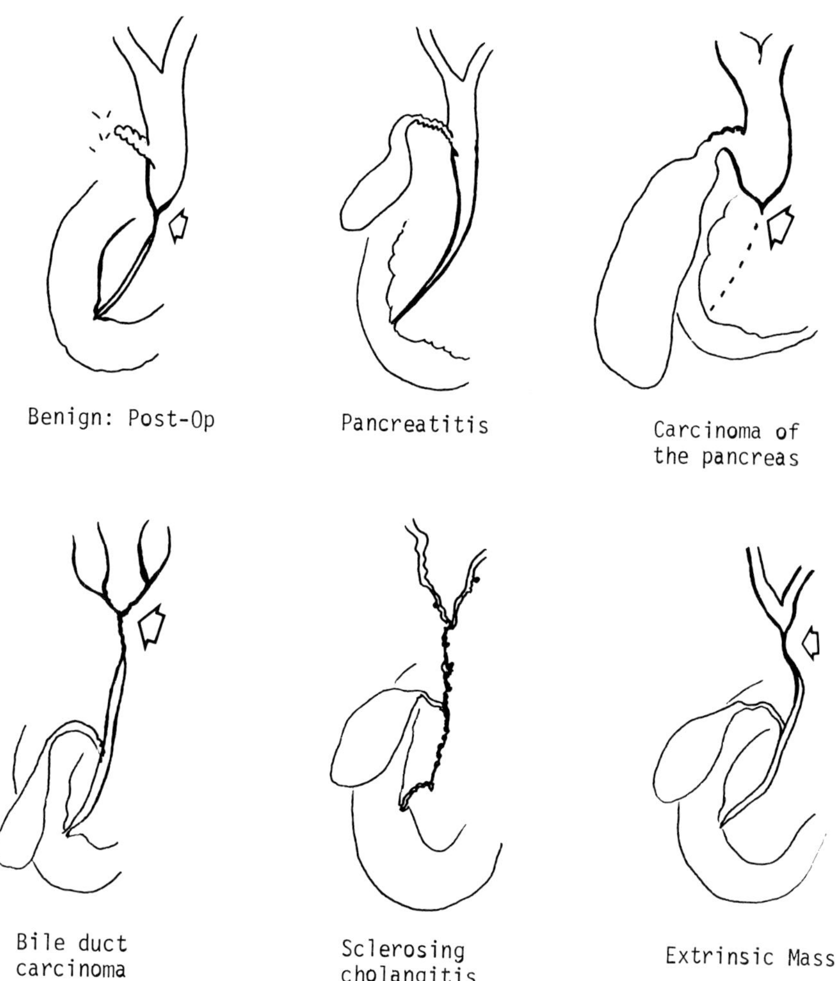

Fig. 6-19 Differential diagnosis of common biliary strictures.

tion, it is usually necessary to tilt the table partially erect to allow the contrast to flow by gravity to the site of distal obstruction. Utilizing gravity avoids error in estimating the site of obstruction and avoids overdistension of the biliary system, which may result in sepsis. Careful spot filming in several projections is essential. Percutaneous transhepatic cholangiography accurately identifies choledocholithiasis (Fig. 6-18). The cholangiographic appearance of benign and malignant strictures is often sufficiently characteristic to suggest the specific diagnosis (Fig. 6-19). Fine-needle aspiration biopsy or cytology expedites the histologic diagnosis.

Transhepatic Interventional Procedures

The transhepatic route offers a variety of therapeutic options as well as an accurate diagnosis. External biliary decompression via a percutaneous catheter is occasionally useful. In cases of septic cholangitis, decompression allows the patient's condition to stabilize preoperatively. Because of high operative morbidity and mortality in patients with massive hyperbilirubinemia (greater than 20 mg/dl), it has been postulated that preoperative biliary decompression may be advisable. Although some investigators have observed a decrease in operative complications after biliary decompression, this has not been uniformly confirmed. The possibility of additional complications from the decompression procedure itself may outweigh the value of lowered serum bilirubin. Severe complications include sepsis, hemorrhage, and bile leakage.

Decompression catheters can often be passed beyond sites of malignant biliary obstruction, thus allowing more physiologic internal biliary decompression (Fig. 6-20). Reestablishing biliary flow may aid palliation of terminal cancer patients by improving appetite and nutrition, and eliminating pruritic jaundice. Internal biliary drainage is particularly useful in patients with slowly growing neoplasms, who may survive several years. The catheters may also be used effectively as conduits for radioactive nuclides to deliver local radiation therapy to the tumor mass (brachytherapy). Unfortunately, problems do occur; the catheters may be-

come occluded or dislodged and must be exchanged. The protruding catheter hub at the skin may cause discomfort and be a source of psychological stress to some patients, as a constant reminder of their disease.

Another decompression alternative is a totally internalized stint. Long-term patency of these stints may be a problem since convenient reaccess to replace the catheter is lost. Some can be retrieved and replaced endoscopically, if necessary. The option of a totally internal stint is utilized most often in patients with a short life expectancy, or in patients who would not care for an external catheter.

The percutaneous route is currently under investigation for dilatation of strictures, biliary manometry, and stone removal.

Endoscopic Retrograde Cholangiography

Side viewing endoscopes allow an experienced endoscopist to cannulate the pancreatic and biliary ducts. In most centers the cannulation is done by a gastroenterologist in cooperation with a radiologist who insures careful fluoroscopic monitoring and optimal spot filming for diagnosis. The bile duct can be cannulated successfully in more than 90 percent of cases. The success rate and complication rate is similar to PTC. The choice of procedure for direct cholangiography depends on the clinical situation and the availability of a skilled endoscopist. Endoscopic retrograde cholangiography (ERC) has an additional advantage in that the pancreatic duct can be visualized. Ancillary options include therapeutic endoscopic sphincterotomy for choledocholithiasis or ampullary stenosis, balloon dilatation of strictures, and placement of internal biliary stints. Biopsy forceps can be passed through the endoscope for mucosal biopsy, and fluid can be obtained for cytology.

Further sections will discuss the use of the above procedures in individual disease entities and discuss in more detail the interpretation of diagnostic cholangiograms.

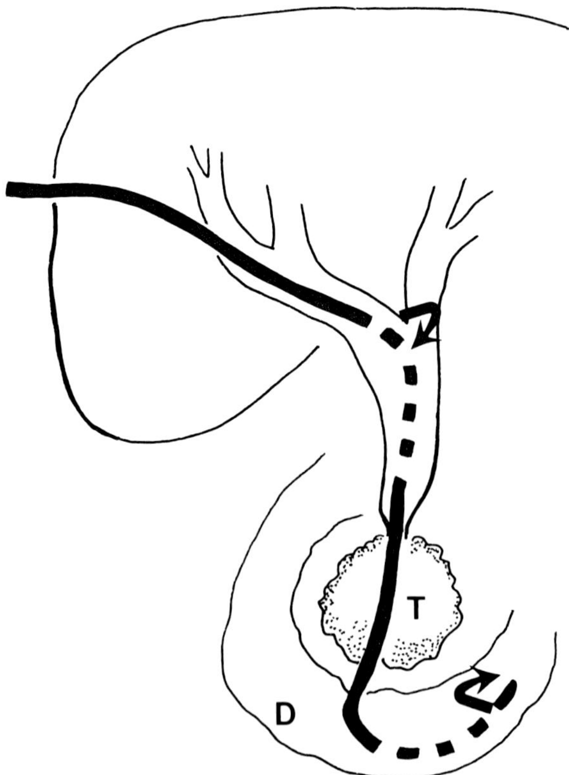

Fig. 6-20 Diagram illustrating internal biliary decompression. Sideholes *(arrows)* above and below the tumor mass *(T)* allow bile to flow into the duodenum *(D)*.

CHOLEDOCHOLITHIASIS

Calculi can form primarily within the biliary ducts, usually in conditions in which biliary stasis and infec-

and improving the yield of common duct exploration (Fig. 6-21). All patients undergoing cholecystectomy should have operative cholangiography. Accuracy demands meticulous technique and close cooperation between the surgeon and radiologist.

Postoperative T-tube cholangiography should detect any residual calculi left at the time of operation. Most of these calculi can be successfully removed percutaneously, via the T-tube tract, after the tract has matured 4 to 5 weeks postoperatively. This widely utilized technique was developed by Burhenne and utilizes basket extraction with a steerable catheter system.

Choledocholithiasis, which presents at a time remote from cholecystectomy, may be more difficult to diagnose and manage. The classic clinical symptoms of biliary colic and jaundice occur in 75 to 80 percent of the cases. Complications may be severe and include septic cholangitis, hepatic abscess, liver damage progressing to cirrhosis, and acute pancreatitis. Sonography is less successful in detecting calculi in the common duct than in the gallbladder. Most authors report accuracy in the range of 15 to 25 percent (Fig. 6-22). High resolution computed tomography is more useful because most calculi are of mixed composition and contain enough calcium to be visible. With 5-mm sections through the duct, accuracies up to 90 percent are reported.

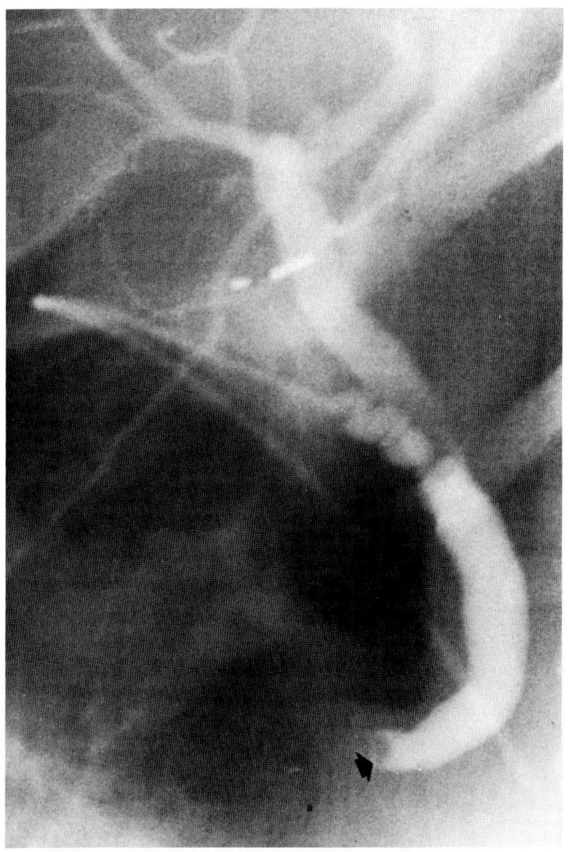

Fig. 6-21 A small calculus impacted at the ampulla *(arrow)* was discovered by operative cholangiography.

tion are present. However, the majority of common bile duct calculi originate in the gallbladder and migrate to the common duct, where they may be overlooked at the time of cholecystectomy. Approximately 10 to 15 percent of patients undergoing cholecystectomy for cholelithiasis also have concomitant choledocholithiasis. Since surgeons cannot reliably detect CBD calculi by palpation at the time of cholecystectomy, the common duct is frequently opened and explored, if calculi are suspected on clinical grounds. However, a negative common duct exploration unnecessarily increases the morbidity of the operation, necessitates T-tube placement, and prolongs hospitalization. Even following duct exploration, the incidence of residual stones is about 5 to 10 percent. Carefully performed, operative cholangiography can detect choledocholithiasis with 80 to 99 percent accuracy, thereby decreasing the frequency

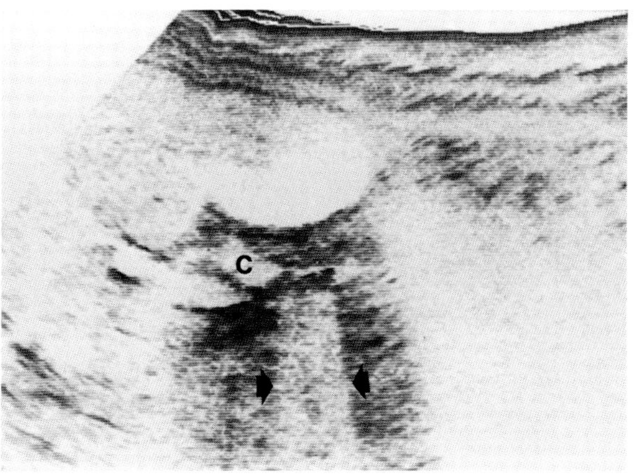

Fig. 6-22 Several calculi within the CBD *(C)* are evident at sonography. The acoustic shadow *(arrowheads)* confirms the diagnosis. (Case courtesy of Dr. Joseph C. Anderson.)

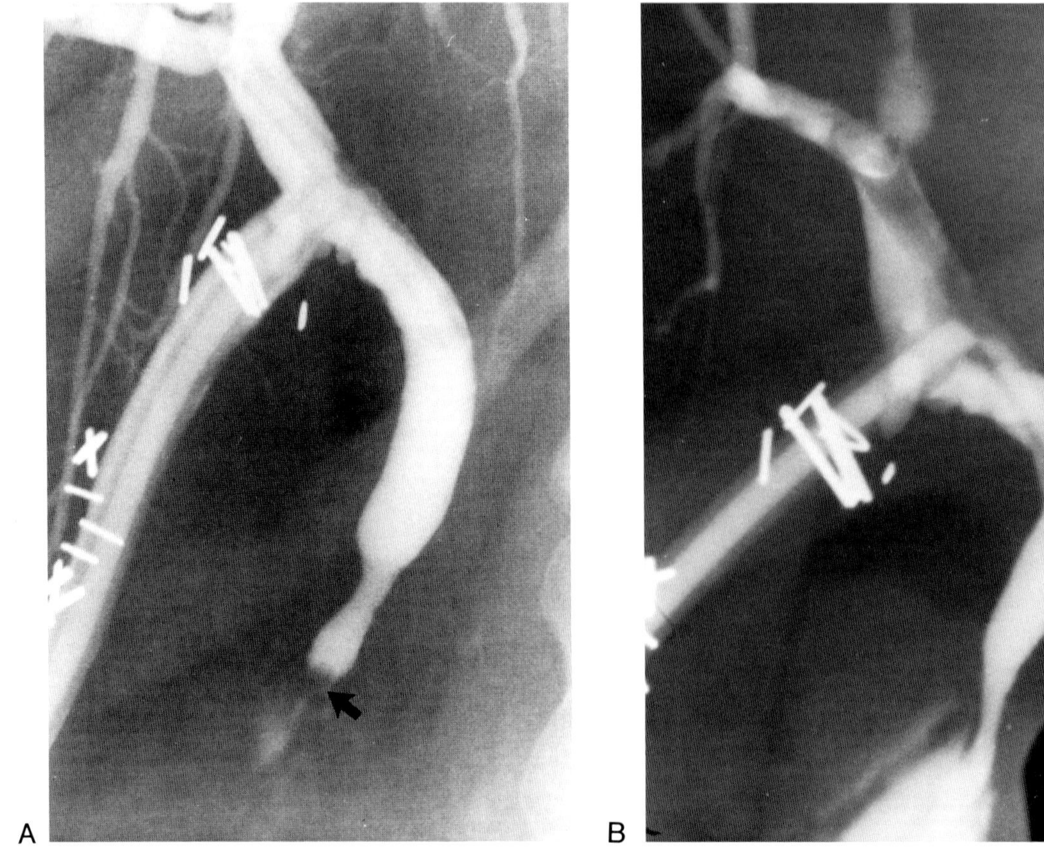

Fig. 6-23 (A) Pseudocalculus appearance caused by the inferior choledochal sphincter *(arrow)*.
(B) Spot radiograph after glucagon administration demonstrates relaxation of the sphincter.

Direct cholangiography (PTC or ERC) is the most sensitive and specific means of radiographic diagnosis. Rarely is a papillary intraluminal neoplasm or blood clot mistaken for a calculus. Also, care must be taken to avoid the false positive interpretation of intraluminal calculi caused by poor admixture of contrast and viscous bile. The inferior choledochal sphincter, when contracted, may give a "pseudocalculus" appearance (Fig. 6-23). Careful fluoroscopic observation and spot filming the duct should eliminate any confusion.

Endoscopic sphincterotomy combined with basket or balloon extraction currently offers an alternative to reoperation in patients with common duct calculi. This method is especially useful in patients who would be at an increased operative risk because of age, previous operations, or debilatated medical condition.

A skilled endoscopist can usually remove stones, less than 2 to 3 cm in size, with a low complication rate compared to operative removal. Although long-term follow-up is not yet available, the results to date do not indicate a significant problem with restenosis at the papillotomy site. New techniques to aid the management of choledocholithiasis are currently under investigation. These include infusion of the cholesterol solvent, monooctanoin, into the biliary ducts to dissolve calculi and percutaneous manipulation or irrigation of stones into the duodenum.

MIRIZZI SYNDROME

Mirizzi syndrome is an unusual cause of partial common bile duct obstruction. The syndrome consists of an impacted stone in a cystic duct that lies close and parallel to the common bile duct. The mass of the stone itself as well as its surrounding inflammatory reaction causes partial obstruction of the common bile duct. Cholangitis may occur and progress to biliary cirrhosis. The cholangiographic appearance is that of a smooth extrinsic impression on the common hepatic duct. The differential diagnosis includes enlarged portal lymph nodes or metastatic neoplasm.

PYOGENIC CHOLANGITIS

Pyogenic cholangitis or acute ascending cholangitis results from bacterial infection of obstructed biliary ducts. Choledocholithiasis is most commonly the cause, although malignant obstruction may rarely be responsible. *Escherichia coli* is frequently the infecting organism. The classic clinical presentation is chills, fever, pain, and jaundice. Sonography demonstrates the dilated ducts, but direct cholangiography is generally necessary to confirm the site and etiology of the obstruction. Percutaneous biliary decompression may be useful as initial therapy to relieve the obstruction and sepsis. Another alternative is endoscopic sphincterotomy and stone removal, if a skilled endoscopist is available.

ORIENTAL CHOLANGIOHEPATITIS

A unique form of recurrent pyogenic cholangitis occurs in Orientals and Asian immigrants. The clinical syndrome consists of recurrent attacks of chills and fever, right upper quadrant pain, jaundice, nausea, and vomiting. Young adults are most commonly affected. The usual course is one of exacerbations and remissions leading to progressive biliary destruction and cirrhosis. Liver abscess and septic shock may complicate the syndrome. The intrahepatic and extrahepatic ducts become focally and irregularly dilated owing to multiple strictured segments; distal obstruction, however, is not present. Soft intra- and extrahepatic pigment calculi and debris are present within the ducts. The disease seems to have a predilection to involve the left ductal system most severely.

Although the etiology of oriental cholangiohepatitis is not known, it is most likely caused by a combination of factors. Coliform bacteria more commonly infect the bile of patients on low protein diets, and it has been postulated that these bacteria deconjugate bilirubin and predispose to pigment calculi. Parasitic infestation, usually *Clonorchis sinensis* commonly coexists and may contribute to the pathology.

The diagnosis can frequently be suggested by sonography and computed tomography. Both modalities image the dilated ducts filled with stones, debris, and sludge. PTC and ERC are useful to delineate the anatomic details but they must be performed carefully, administering antibiotic prophylaxis to avoid exacerbation of sepsis. Long-term medical therapy is ineffective. Endoscopic sphincterotomy and stone removal, operative segmental resections, sphincteroplasty, and biliary enteric anastomoses may be of some palliative benefit. Percutaneous stricture dilatation and stone removal may also be useful in selected cases.

Primary Sclerosing Cholangitis

Primary sclerosing cholangitis is a chronic disease characterized by fibrosis and inflammation of the extrahepatic biliary ducts. Usually, the intrahepatic ducts are also involved. This is an uncommon condition, but recently is being diagnosed with increasing frequency, probably because of improved cholangiographic techniques. The etiology of primary sclerosing cholangitis is unknown. Several etiologic theories have been postulated, including abnormal hepatic copper metabolism and abnormal cellular immunity. Secondary cholangitis from postsurgical stricture or choledocholithiasis should not be diagnosed as primary sclerosing cholangitis. Sclerosing cholangitis is more common in males and is usually diagnosed in the fourth and fifth decades of life. The obliterative biliary fibrosis progresses ultimately to cirrhosis and death from liver failure. No treatment has been shown to alter the course of the disease. However, selected patients may be candidates for liver transplantation. Although primary sclerosing cholangitis may occur as an isolated entity, 50 to 70 percent of the cases are associated with inflammatory bowel disease, most commonly chronic ulcerative colitis. The temporal relationship of the two entities is variable. Sclerosing cholangitis may appear before or after the onset of symptomatic bowel disease and may even occur years after colectomy.

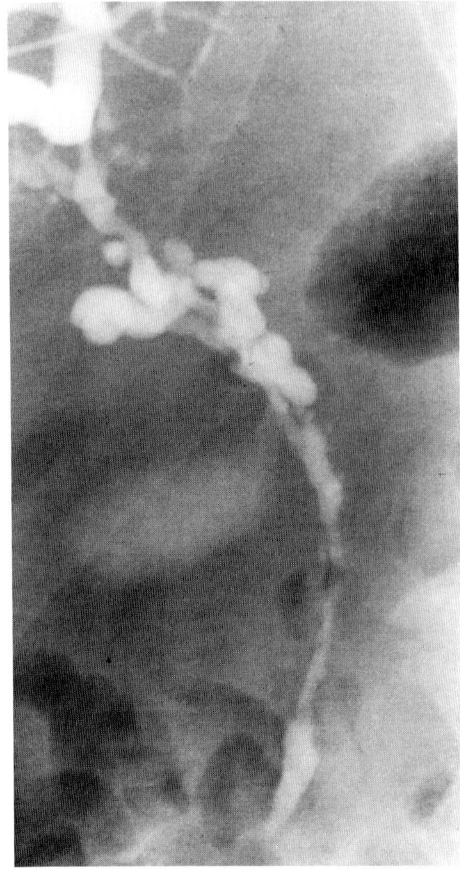

A

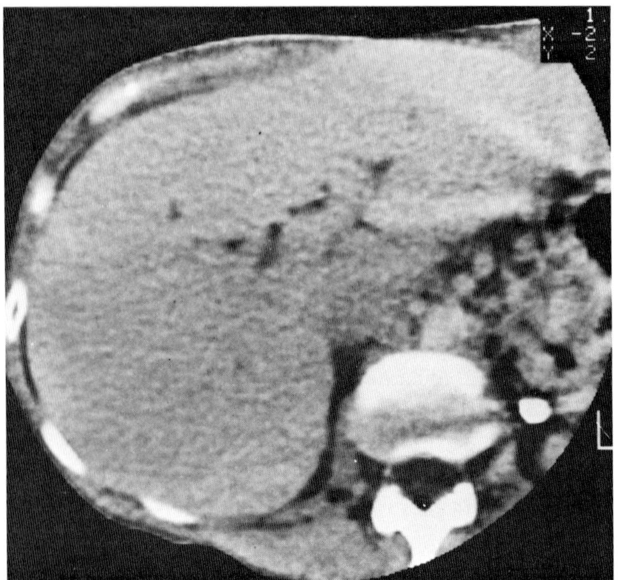

B

Fig. 6-24 (A) Typical beaded appearance of the bile ducts in sclerosing cholangitis. **(B)** CT scan reveals areas of focal dilatation in the intrahepatic ducts.

The diagnosis is based on characteristic clinical, biochemical, and radiographic features. The clinical onset is often insidious with symptoms of fatigue, pruritis, and jaundice. Serum alkaline phosphatase is elevated, usually twice normal. Either ERC or PTC may demonstrate the radiographic features, but because the intrahepatic ducts are often not uniformly dilated, ERC may more easily visualize the ducts. The biliary ducts are markedly irregular; multiple short strictures and intermittent areas of mild dilation are apparent. The appearance has been likened to a "string of beads." Small diverticulum-like outpouchings are common (Fig. 6-24).

The differential diagnosis includes primary biliary cirrhosis (PBC) and diffuse cholangiocarcinoma. Clinical findings in PBC patients are often similar to those of sclerosing cholangitis. However, because the extrahepatic ducts are not involved, PBC can be differentiated radiographically. In PBC the intrahepatic ducts are attenuated and irregular, but the common hepatic and the common bile duct are normal. The diffuse scirrhous form of cholangiocarcinoma is more difficult to differentiate because it can closely simulate the radiographic appearance of sclerosing cholangitis. To further complicate the problem, the entities may coexist. There is also some evidence to suggest that chronic sclerosing cholangitis may lead to the development of carcinoma. If biopsy is negative for malignancy, only long follow-up or autopsy completely excludes carcinoma.

MALIGNANT NEOPLASMS OF THE BILE DUCTS

Primary Bile Duct Carcinoma

Primary bile duct carcinoma or cholangiocarcinoma is less common than carcinoma of the gallbladder, the autopsy incidence of which is less than 0.5 percent. The histology is most often well-differentiated adenocarcinoma. About 10 percent are undifferentiated or anaplastic varieties. Extensive fibrosis can accompany the tumor, sometimes making it difficult to obtain diagnostic histology. The incidence peaks in the sixth or seventh decades, but in contrast to gallbladder carcinoma this tumor is more common in males. Bile duct carcinoma occurs with an increased incidence in patients with chronic ulcerative colitis. The mechanism of this association is not clear. When associated with ulcerative colitis, bile duct carcinoma tends to occur at a younger age (fourth or fifth decade), but usually only after the patients have had colitis for 15 to 20 years. The development of carcinoma is unrelated to the severity of colon symptoms and it may occur during remission of colitis or years after total colectomy. Other conditions associated with an increased incidence of bile duct carcinoma include choledochal cyst, papillomatosis of the biliary ducts, infestation with *Clonorchis sinesis,* and primary sclerosing cholangitis.

Most bile duct carcinomas arise in the extrahepatic ducts; 12 to 15 percent diffusely involve both the intra- and extrahepatic ducts. Carcinoma arising at the bifurcation of the intrahepatic ducts was described as a special clinical entity by Klatskin in 1965 and is often referred to as Klatskin tumor. In his description, Klatskin noted that this lesion tends to occur in a slightly younger age group, is easily overlooked at laparotomy, grows slowly by local extension, and is amenable to palliation by biliary diversion.

Three types of growth patterns may occur in bile duct carcinoma. The most common is an annular constricting lesion or localized stricture of the bile duct, whereas 12 to 15 percent are of the diffusely infiltrating variety and 2 to 3 percent are intraluminal polypoid or papillary lesions. Spread is by submucosal and lymphatic extension and local invasion. The most common mode of local extension is direct infiltration of the liver. In contrast to hepatoma, portal vein invasion usually does not occur until late in the course of the disease. Peritoneal seeding has been reported in 9

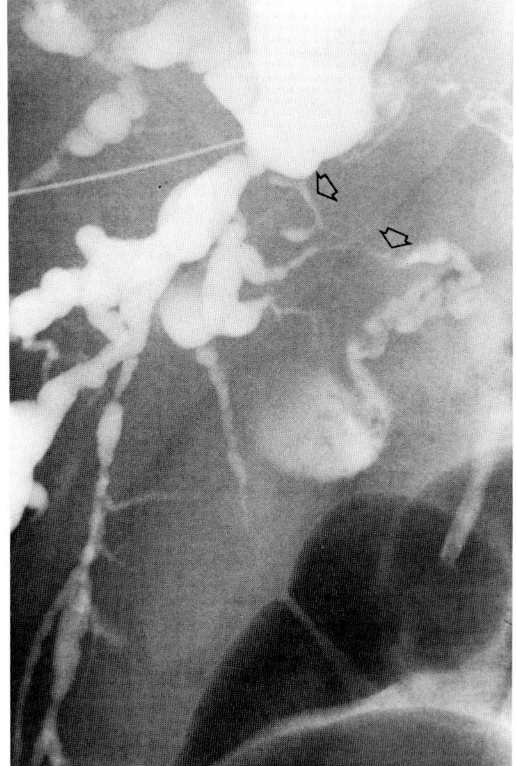

A

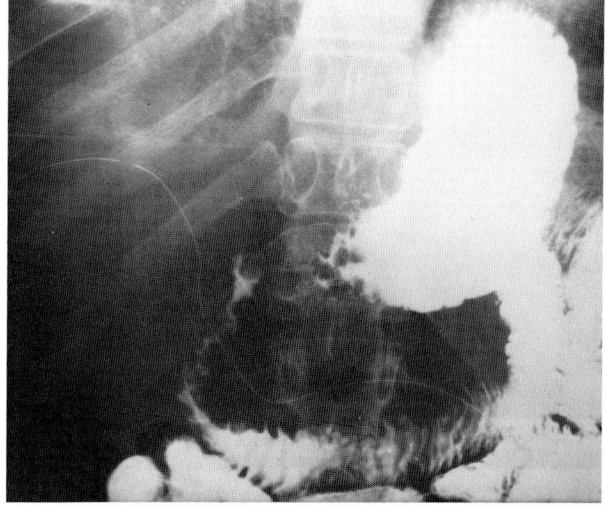

B

Fig. 6-25 (A) Bile duct carcinoma causing strictures at the bifurcation of the intrahepatic ducts *(arrows)*. (Williams SM, Harned RK: Bile duct carcinoma associated with chronic ulcerative colitis. Dis Colon Rectum 24:42, 1981.) **(B)** Cholangiocarcinomas can spread by direct extension. In this case the duodenum has been encased by the tumor.

percent of cases. Hematogenous metastasis are uncommon.

Periampullary bile duct carcinomas have the best chance of prolonged survival after radical resection. Unfortunately, most cholangiocarcinomas located more proximally are unresectable at the time of diagnosis. Because these tumors grow slowly, significant palliative benefit may be gained with endoscopic and percutaneous catheter biliary decompression, especially if internal biliary drainage is possible. Radiation therapy may slow tumor growth. One option currently under investigation involves placing ^{192}Ir through a decompression catheter to deliver a high radiation dose directly to the surface of the tumor.

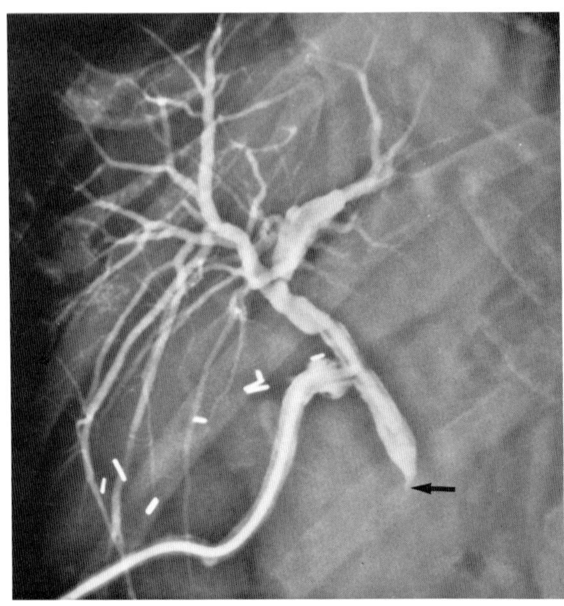

Fig. 6-27 Complete abrupt obstruction of the common bile duct *(arrow)* is characteristic of carcinoma of the pancreas.

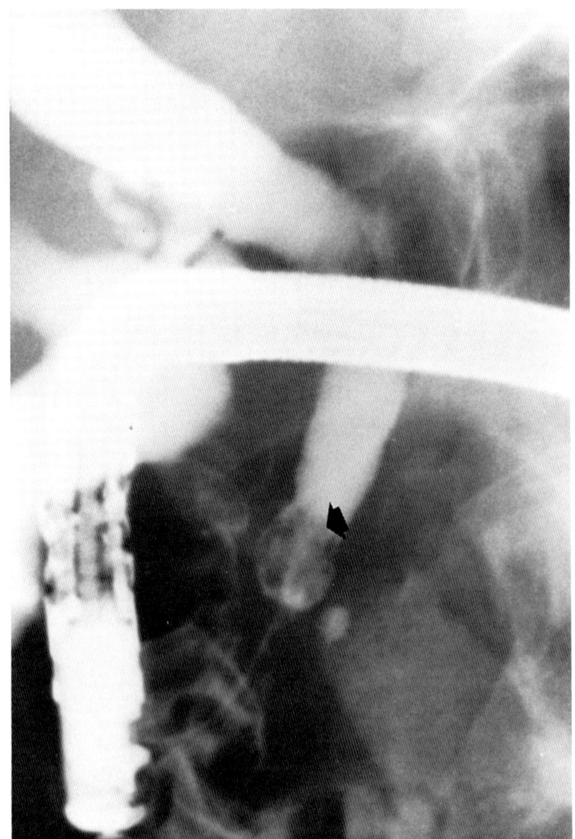

Fig. 6-26 A polypoid bile duct carcinoma *(arrowhead)* simulates a calculus at ERC. (Case courtesy of Dr. Joel Elson Clarkson Hospital, Omaha, Nebraska.)

Radiographically, the diagnostic features are best demonstrated by direct cholangiography, either PTC or ERC. The most common appearance is a localized stricture with variable dilatation of the proximal ducts. Occasionally, differentiation from pancreatic carcinoma, metastatic carcinoma, or benign stricture may not be possible. The appearance of the Klatskin type is quite characteristic (Fig. 6-25). Diffusely infiltrating scirrhous carcinoma may be especially difficult to differentiate from sclerosing cholangitis. Because of the extensive fibrosis accompanying both conditions, histologic differentiation is often a problem. The rare polypoid variety may be mistaken for an impacted calculus at the time of cholangiography (Fig. 6-26). Intrahepatic cholangiocarcinoma presents as a mass that can simulate primary hepatocellular carcinoma. Differentiation may be possible clinically, as heptocellular carcinoma tends to develop in patients with cirrhosis and is usually associated with elevated serum alpha-fetoprotein. Hepatocellular carcinomas have abundant neovascularity demonstrable by angiography, whereas cholangiocarcinoma tends to have only small neoplastic vessels often accompanied by arterial encasement.

Uncommon Bile Duct Malignancy

Primary biliary malignancy other than adenocarcinoma is uncommon. Rare cystadenocarcinoma has been reported. This tumor may be suspected at computed tomography or sonography when a cystic intrahepatic mass with internal papillary projections is identified. The differential diagnosis includes papillary cholangiocarcinoma, necrotic metastasis, liver abscess, or parasitic cyst. Rarely, leiomyosarcoma or melanosarcoma arise in the biliary ducts.

Secondary Malignancy Involving the Bile Ducts

Carcinoma of the head of the pancreas commonly obstructs the common bile duct. Complete, abrupt

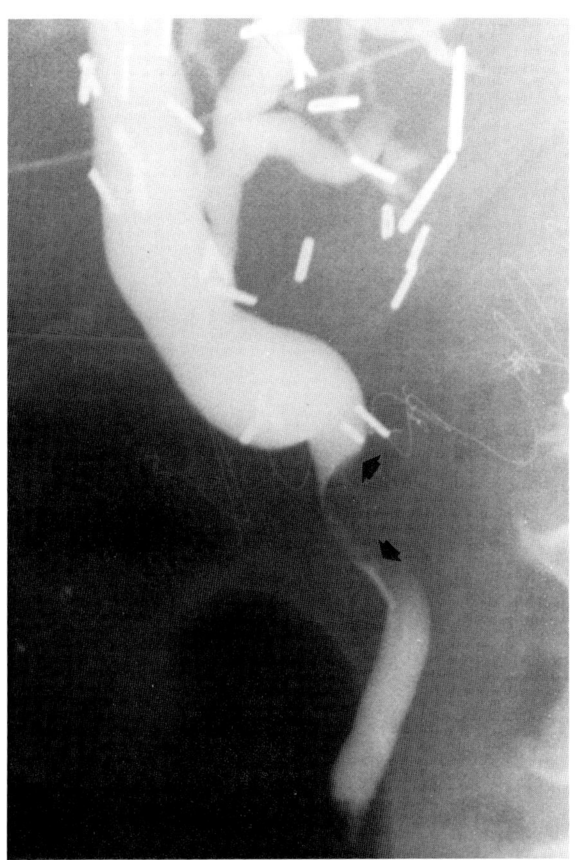

Fig. 6-28 A metastatic node in the porta hepatis is causing a smooth, extrinsic impression on the common hepatic duct (*arrowheads*).

obstruction of the intrapancreatic portion of the common duct is the usual finding at cholangiography (Fig. 6-27). The proximal ducts often become massively dilated. Carcinoma of the gallbladder also eventually extends to obstruct the extrahepatic ducts in most cases. Other malignancies that may metastasize to the portal area include carcinoma of the breast, stomach, and colon (Fig. 6-28). Lymphoma involving periportal nodes may cause jaundice by extrinsic compression of extrahepatic ducts.

BENIGN NEOPLASMS OF THE BILE DUCTS

Benign bile duct neoplasms are rare. Most are epithelial polyps, either adenomas or papillomas. A variety of mesenchymal tumors are even less common, but have been reported as isolated cases. Bile duct papillomas may have a multifocal origin and tend to recur after local excision. Progression of bile duct papillomatosis to invasive carcinoma has been reported.

Biliary cystadenoma is an uncommon, slowing growing, multilocular cystic neoplasm that may become quite large. The majority arise in the intrahepatic ducts and are most common in middle-aged females. The cystic mass is demonstrable by computed tomography or sonography, but sonography may be more useful to delineate the internal architecture. The lesions characteristically have thick walls with multiple mural nodules or papillary projections. The differential diagnosis includes necrotic metastasis, abscess, hematoma, and cystadenocarcinoma. Because malignant transformation of benign cystadenoma may occur, surgical excision is usually recommended.

Several uncommon lesions are of interest because of their propensity to arise in the cystic duct. The rare biliary granular cell myoblastoma has been reported to arise in the cystic duct, causing hydrops of the gallbladder. After cholecystectomy, regenerating nerves and scar in the cystic duct remnant occasionally cause a mass effect, which might be confused with neoplasm. This has been termed cystic duct neuroma, but is not a true neoplasm.

BENIGN STRICTURES OF THE BILE DUCT

Postoperative Stricture

The majority of benign biliary strictures occur postoperatively as a result of injury to the bile duct at the time of cholecystectomy. Extensive inflammation, fibrosis, or hemorrhage at the time of operation may cause difficulty in delineating the anatomy, making injury to the common duct more likely. Common duct exploration increases the probability of postoperative morbidity, especially if the T-tube is improperly positioned or becomes dislodged too soon postoperatively.

Clinically, postoperative strictures present with jaundice, chills, and fever, or biliary-cutaneous fistulas. The time of presentation varies from several days to many years after the initial operation. Radiographically, the site and extent of the stricture is best delineated by T-tube cholangiography, ERC, or PTC. The strictures are typically short and well defined. Retained or secondary calculi are not uncommon. Although the history of previous biliary operation aids the diagnosis, it may not be possible, in some cases, to radiographically differentiate benign stricture from malignancy.

Because repeated operations on the biliary tract are often technically difficult, owing to previous scarring and anatomic distortion, percutaneous or endoscopic stricture dilatation offers an attractive option for the management of benign strictures. The Gruentzig balloon catheter has been successfully used for this purpose. Specialized endoscopic balloon catheters are also available. Following dilatation, stints are usually left in place to insure patency with healing. There is no definite agreement as to how long such stints should remain in place. Long-term follow-up as to the continued patency of dilated strictures is not available. In many cases, repeated dilatations have been necessary. The best results seem to occur with localized strictures at sites of biliary-enteric anastomosis.

Chronic Pancreatitis

Approximately 2 to 10 percent of patients with chronic pancreatitis have been reported to develop some degree of biliary obstruction. Radiographically, the stricture is generally long and involves the intrapancreatic portion of the common bile duct. The associated manifestations of pancreatitis aid the radiographic diagnosis, although it may be difficult to exclude malignancy. Longstanding obstruction leads eventually to liver damage and biliary cirrhosis, so consideration should be given to surgical decompression of the biliary tract.

CYSTIC DISEASES OF THE BILIARY DUCTS

Choledochal Cyst

Cystic dilatation of the common bile duct is an infrequent condition most common in Orientals. More than one-third of the reported cases are from Japan. Among Western populations, it is more common in females. The diagnosis is usually made in childhood, or before the age of 30 years. Several types of cysts occur. A widely utilized classification scheme developed by Alonso-Lej identifies three types of choledochal cyst (Fig. 6-29). The most common, type A, is a localized, fusiform dilatation of the common bile duct. The second, type B, is an eccentric dilatation or diverticulum of the extrahepatic ducts. This type is quite rare and multiple diverticula may occur. The third type, a choledochocele, is a dilatation of the distal intramural portion of the common duct. The dilated segment prolapses into the duodenum in a manner similar to an ureterocele prolapsing into the urinary bladder. Choledochoceles are often lined with duodenal mucosa and probably have a different etiology than the other types. There is no definite agreement as to whether choledochocele represents a congenital or an acquired lesion. Variable degrees of intrahepatic duct dilatation are being recognized with increasing frequency in association with choledochal cysts. This has led several authors to expand the traditional classification to include subtypes with and without intrahepatic duct dilatation. Some also consider Caroli disease to be a part of the same spectrum of biliary cystic disease.

Because most cases appear in children or younger adults, choledochal cyst is felt to be either a congenital lesion or is acquired early in life. Wide speculation as to its etiology has led to multiple theories. One popular concept proposed by Babbitt suggests that the con-

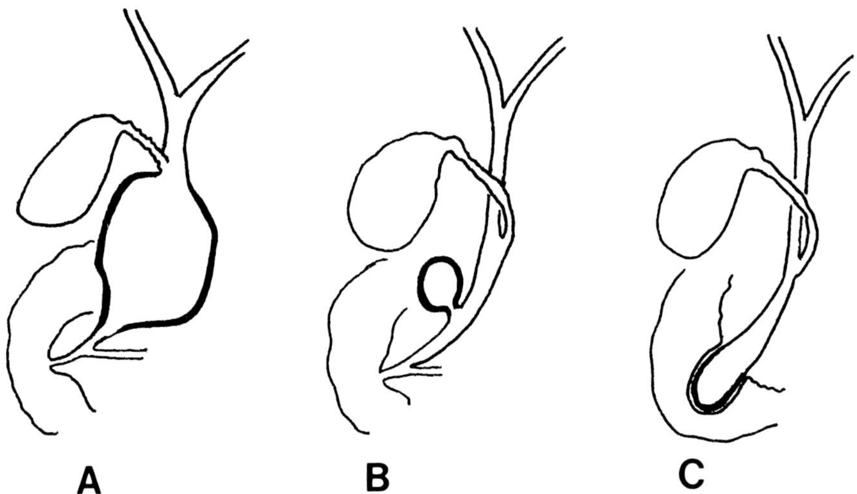

Fig. 6-29 The diagram illustrates three types of choledochal cyst. **(A)** Choledochal cyst. **(B)** Diverticulum. **(C)** Choleodochocele.

dition is related to an anomalous relationship of the common bile duct and main pancreatic duct with an unusually long common channel. This arrangement permits reflux of pancreatic enzymes into the biliary tree, causing cholangitis with secondary common duct dilatation. Another theory proposes that the entire spectrum of biliary cystic disease occurs as a result of infantile viral cholangitis.

The classic triad of clinical symptoms includes jaundice, abdominal pain, and palpable mass. Actually, the entire triad occurs in less than two-thirds of the cases. Newer imaging modalities have made preoperative diagnosis possible in almost all instances. The cystic segments can be identified by sonography or computed tomography. Because most cases are in children, sonography is probably the most valuable initial study. If a question exists as to the relationship of the cyst to the biliary tract, biliary communication is easily proven by ^{99m}Tc-IDA cholescintigraphy. Direct cholangiography via ERC, PTC, or operative cholangiography clearly delineates the anatomy. In the most common type of choledochal cyst, the proximal and distal margins of the dilated segment are abrupt (Fig. 6-30). The distal segment of the CBD is narrowed and a relatively long common channel is frequently demonstrated. As previously mentioned, associated intrahepatic duct dilatation is variable. The cystic duct is only rarely involved. Diagnosis of a choledochocele may be first suspected at a barium upper gastrointesti-

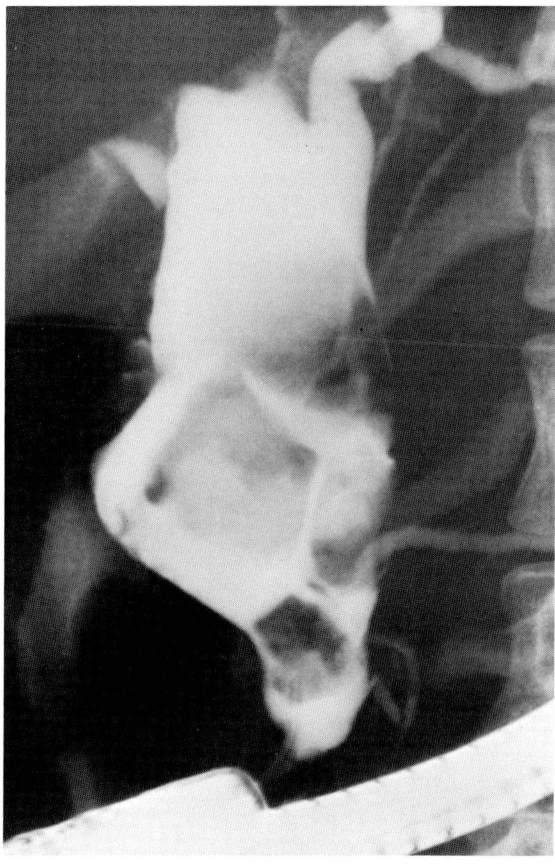

Fig. 6-30 A large choledochal cyst containing several calculi. (Case courtesy of Dr. Dennis Strauss, Nebraska Methodist Hospital.)

nal examination when a smooth intramural mass is identified at the level of the papilla of Vater (Fig. 6-31).

Rare complications of choledochal cyst include calculus formation within the cyst, biliary cirrhosis, rupture, hemorrhage, and portal vein obstruction. Carcinoma is reported to develop with an increased incidence in biliary cysts. Because of this risk, excision of the cyst is the preferred treatment. Biliary drainage is established by Roux-en-Y loop hepaticojejunostomy.

Caroli Disease

A rare syndrome of communicating cavernous ectasia of the intrahepatic ducts was described by Caroli in 1958. In this condition, bile stasis predisposes to intrahepatic calculi. Secondary pyogenic cholangitis develops and leads to intrahepatic abscesses and fistulas. Because periportal fibrosis is not a part of the typical syndrome, liver function is not impaired and portal hypertension does not develop. Death is usually due to sepsis. Renal tubular ectasia or medullary sponge kidney is frequently associated.

Caroli disease usually presents in young adults or children. Most authors consider it to be a unique clinical syndrome of familial congenital origin. However, occasional overlap with the features of choledochal cyst and hepatic fibrosis has led some authors to classify Caroli disease as a part of a wide spectrum of biliary cystic disease, possibly related to infantile cholangitis.

The typical clinical presentation is one of recurrent attacks of abdominal pain and fever. The cholangio-

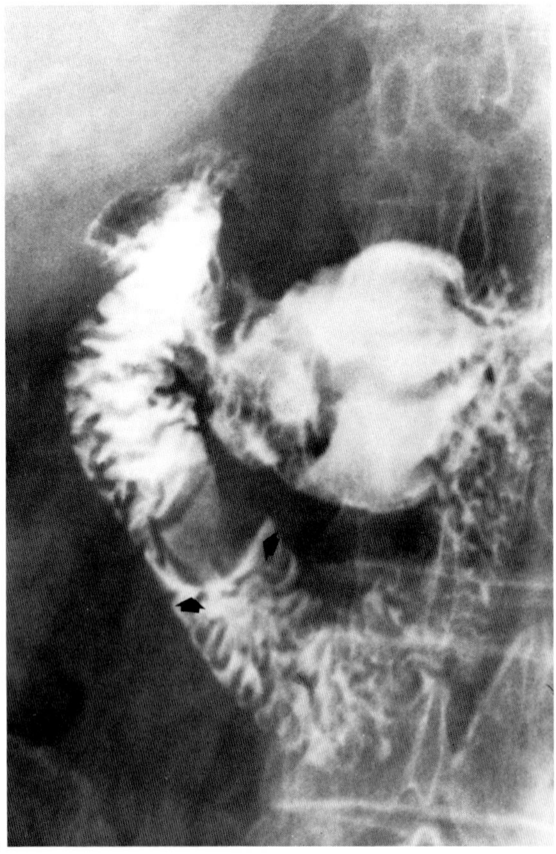
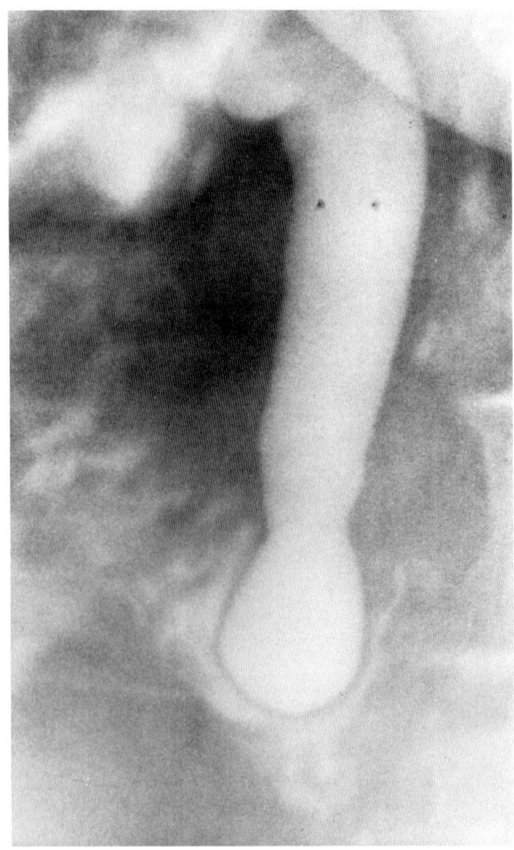

Fig. 6-31 (A) A smooth intramural mass in the duodenum is identified at upper gastrointestinal examination. **(B)** Cholangiogram confirms the diagnosis of choledochocele. (Case courtesy of Dr. James McGill, Creighton University.)

graphic findings are characteristic—i.e., saccular, beaded, intrahepatic ducts (Fig. 6-32). Ducts in both lobes of the liver are usually involved. Computed tomography and sonography visualize the branching tubular intrahepatic ducts with focal areas of ectasia and calculi, affording a noninvasive means of diagnosis in most cases.

Congenital Hepatic Fibrosis with Renal Tubular Ectasia

Cystic dilatation of tiny peripheral bile ducts associated with extensive periportal fibrosis is considered by some authors to be a variant of Caroli disease. Others consider this an individual entity or variant of renal cystic disease, since renal tubular ectasia is usually associated. This type is more common than pure Caroli disease without hepatic fibrosis. Cirrhosis and portal hypertension develop early in life and lead to death from bleeding varices or liver failure in

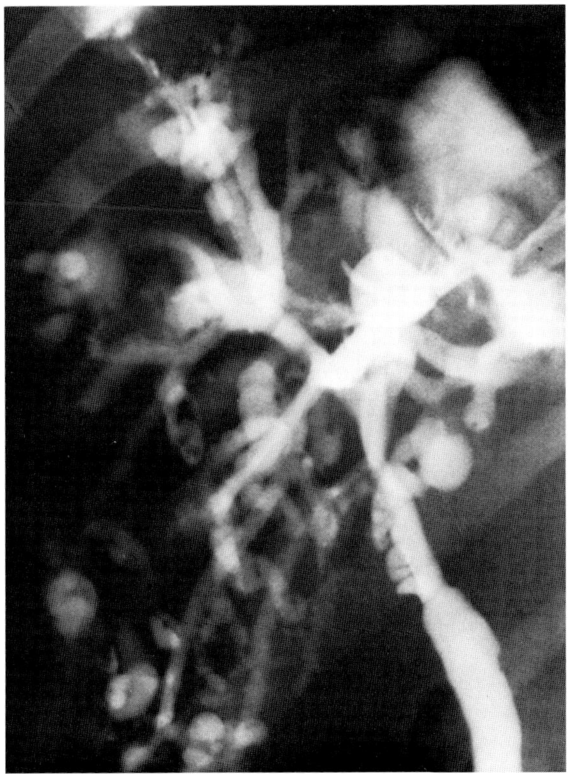

Fig. 6-32 Saccular intrahepatic ducts are characteristic of Caroli disease.

childhood. The dilated small bile ducts are usually too small to be recognized radiographically, but the fibrotic liver may be echodense at sonography. Note that this entity should not be confused with adult polycystic kidney disease. Liver cysts may occur in patients with polycystic kidneys, but they do not communicate with the bile ducts.

PAPILLARY STENOSIS AND BILIARY DYSKINESIA

Papillary stenosis is a poorly defined and incompletely understood clinical condition that continues to perplex and frustrate radiologists, clinicians, and patients. Precise diagnosis is frequently elusive. The patients typically present with a history of recurrent attacks of right upper quadrant or epigastric pain, usually postcholecystectomy. Laboratory evidence of pancreatitis or cholestasis may occur transiently. Radiographically, no morphologic basis for obstruction is evident; however, the common duct may be dilated and contrast emptying delayed. Delayed emptying has been defined as longer than 45 minutes in the absence of the gallbladder. Fibrosis or spasm of the sphincter of Oddi is the postulated etiology, but a consistant histologic basis for the stenosis is not always apparent in operated cases.

Recently, the availability of endoscopic manometry in some centers promises a better understanding of these conditions. Studies have shown that basal sphincter of Oddi pressures and gradients between the biliary and pancreatic ducts and the duodenum are elevated in symptomatic patients. Because endoscopic sphincterotomy has been shown to decrease sphincter of Oddi pressures for up to 2 years, this may become an option for treatment. Further controlled studies and long-term follow-up are necessary to more accurately define these disorders and to predict which patients might benefit from endoscopic sphincterotomy or operative sphincteroplasty.

SUGGESTED READING

Berk RN, Ferrucci JT, Leopold GR: Radiology of the Gallbladder and Bile Ducts. WB Saunders, Philadelphia, 1983

Berk RN, van der Vegt JH, Lichtenstein JE: The hyperplastic cholecystoses: Cholesterolosis and adenomyomatosis. Radiology 146:593, 1983

Berk RN, Cooperberg PL, Gold RP, et al: Radiography of the bile ducts. Radiology 145:1, 1982

Berk RN, Gerrucci JT, Fordtran JS, et al: The radiological diagnosis of gallbladder disease. Radiology 141:49, 1981

Ferrucci JT, Adson MA, Mueller PR, et al: Advances in the radiology of jaundice: A Symposium and review. AJR 141:1, 1983

Hatfield PM, Wise RE: Radiology of the Gallbladder and Bile Ducts. Williams & Wilkins, Baltimore, 1976

LaRusso NF, Wiesner RH, Ludwig J, MacCarty RL: Current concepts primary sclerosing cholangitis. N Engl J Med 310:899, 1984

7
Radiology of the Pancreas

Thomas S. Forrest
Mathis P. Frick

ANATOMY

The pancreas is a retroperitoneal organ situated in the anterior pararenal space. The gland crosses the upper abdomen at the level of the upper lumbar spine and is somewhat arbitrarily divided into head, body, and tail. The head of the pancreas is surrounded by the duodenum, where the posterior surface of the gland is in direct apposition with the inferior vena cava. The uncinate process is part of the pancreatic head and extends posteriorly between the superior mesenteric vessels and the aorta. The pancreatic body is located posterior to the stomach and is the most ventral portion, residing in a surprisingly anterior position as evidenced on cross-sectional display (Fig. 7-1). The body of the pancreas is ventral to the aorta, splenic vessels, and the origin of the superior mesenteric artery. The pancreatic tail curves posteriorly across the left kidney, ensheathed in the splenorenal and phrenicocolic ligaments, and extends to the splenic hilum.

The duodenojejunal junction (ligament of Treitz) is commonly used as a demarcation between the body and tail of the pancreas. The anterior surface of the pancreas is covered by the posterior parietal peritoneum. The parietal peritoneum forms the two leaves of the transverse mesocolon, which extends along the ventral surface of the entire pancreas. The root of the small bowel mesentery joins the transverse mesocolon at the junction of the pancreatic head and body and descends obliquely into the ileocecal junction.

The two excretory pathways of the pancreas are (1) the duct of Wirsung, which empties at the major papilla along with the common bile duct, and (2) the duct of Santorini, which empties at the minor papilla ventral from the origin of the major papilla. Generally, these ducts communicate with one another in the head of the pancreas, forming a single major duct that runs through the center of the body and tail of the pancreas. The duct of Wirsung serves as the main excretory duct in over 90 percent of patients. If the duct of Wirsung is the major drainage, it runs up, at first parallel with the common bile duct, ventrally toward the superior part of the head of the pancreas where it angles leftward so as to run horizontally, crossing the midline at the level of the upper lumbar vertebrae; thereafter, it is directed craniodorsally toward the hilum of the spleen. If the duct of Santorini is the main drainage, it takes a straightened course from the minor papilla to the tail of the pancreas. The maximum diameter of a main pancreatic duct varies

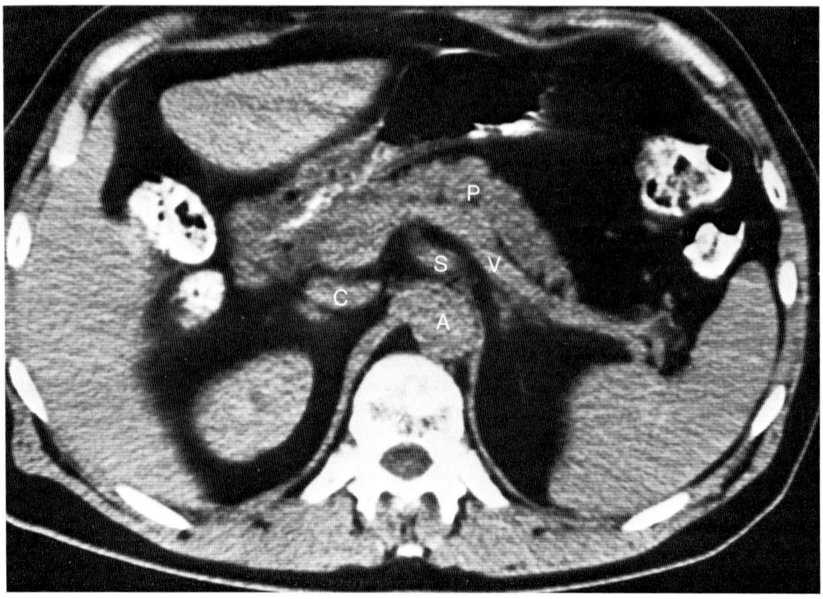

Fig. 7-1 Normal slightly atrophic pancreas in 72-year-old man. (*P*, pancreas; *A*, aorta; *S*, superior mesenteric artery; *C*, inferior vena cava; *V*, splenic vein.)

according to age. In young adults the maximal diameter ranges from 2.4 to 3.5 mm. In the elderly an allowable range varies from 3.0 to 5.5 mm.

SELECTION OF AN IMAGING MODALITY

Pancreatic disorders may be separated into several categories but are mainly inflammatory or neoplastic. Proper selection of the initial imaging procedure to evaluate pancreatic disease is crucial. A number of radiographic procedures are at the radiologist's disposal.

The abdominal plain film is often the initial examination in patients suspected of harboring acute pancreatic disease. Plain film radiography reliably displays normal and abnormal gas collections, large soft tissue masses, and calcifications. Occasionally, a sufficient number of findings are present to warrant a specific diagnosis in a particular clinical setting. However, a normal plain film of the abdomen does not exclude significant pancreatic pathology.

In patients with acute pancreatitis dilated and fluid-filled segments of bowel may be identified. Adynamic

ileus often accompanies acute pancreatic disease and may mimic mechanical small bowel obstruction. Focal adynamic ileus, also called the sentinel loop, commonly affects the duodenal loop and proximal jejunum. Differential diagnostic considerations of focal ileus include other causes of abdominal inflammatory disease such as appendicitis, cholecystitis, peritonitis, drugs, metabolic disorders, and trauma.

It is important to identify the exact location of upper abdominal gas, which may be extraluminal in certain clinical settings. Air may enter the biliary system through an incompetent sphincter after sphincterotomy, anomalous common bile duct insertion, or through a fistula caused by pancreatic disease. Focal gas collections within the pancreatic parenchyma may be secondary to the presence of a pancreatic abscess, fistulization of an inflammatory pancreatic mass with the intestinal tract, or dissociation of oxygen from hemoglobin in patients with hemorrhagic pancreatitis.

Pancreatic calcifications are often observed in patients with chronic pancreatitis (Fig. 7-2). In addition, hyperparathyroidism, hereditary pancreatitis, and various hypercalcemic states may result in pancreatic calcifications. Islet cell tumors and cystadenomas or cystadenocarcinomas may rarely contain calcifications.

Large masses in the pancreatic bed are rarely seen on plain radiographs. Such lesions are manifested by focal soft tissue density with displacement of adjacent bowel loops or distortion of the retroperitoneal fat planes.

Endoscopic retrograde cholangiopancreatography (ERCP) is a modality commonly in use and serves as a complimentary examination to computed tomography or ultrasound examination of the pancreas. Diagnostic uncertainties on computed tomographic and ultrasonographic examinations often relate to questions of subtle focal pancreatic enlargement (Fig. 7-3). In addition, diagnostic uncertainties arise from the need to exclude carcinoma in the presence of chronic pancreatitis or to distinguish pancreatic masses from peripancreatic lymphadenopathy in patients with known malignancy elsewhere. While both neoplastic and inflammatory disorders increase pancreatic size, measurement of the normal pancreas may occasionally exceed proposed normal limits because of variations in the pancreatic duct system or body build. In

these instances, ERCP often contributes significant diagnostic information by displaying a normal pancreatic ductal system.

In experienced hands, successful opacification of the pancreatic ductal system by ERCP can be achieved in an average of 70 to 75 percent of cases. The complication rate is low (1 percent) and is related to the occurrence of contrast-induced pancreatitis caused by the inadvertent opacification of the pancreatic parenchyma. Abnormal radiographic findings in the pancreatic ductal system include the presence of stenoses, obstruction, focal or diffuse dilatation, displacement, focal irregularities (encasement), and pseudocyst formation. A variety of ductal variations can normally occur.

Ultrasonography is an excellent and noninvasive modality for the identification of pancreatic pathology. The pancreas is equal to or slightly more echogenic than the liver. Echogenicity increases with advancing age, owing to fat deposition. There is considerable variation in the shape of the normal pancreas, as seen on ultrasound. At least three morphologic types have been described. The tadpolelike configuration of the pancreas is most common (44 percent), with the

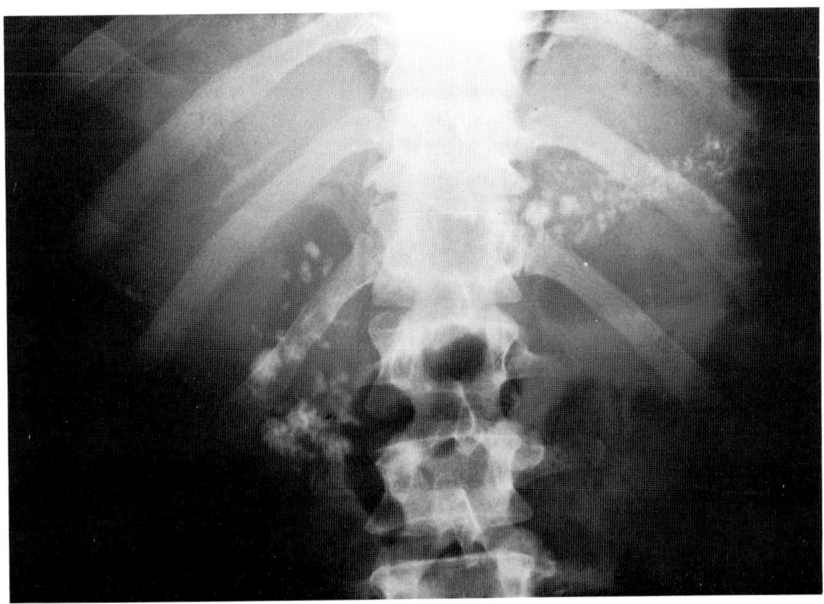

Fig. 7-2 Chronic pancreatitis resulting from ethanol abuse. Extensive amorphous calcifications involve the entire pancreas.

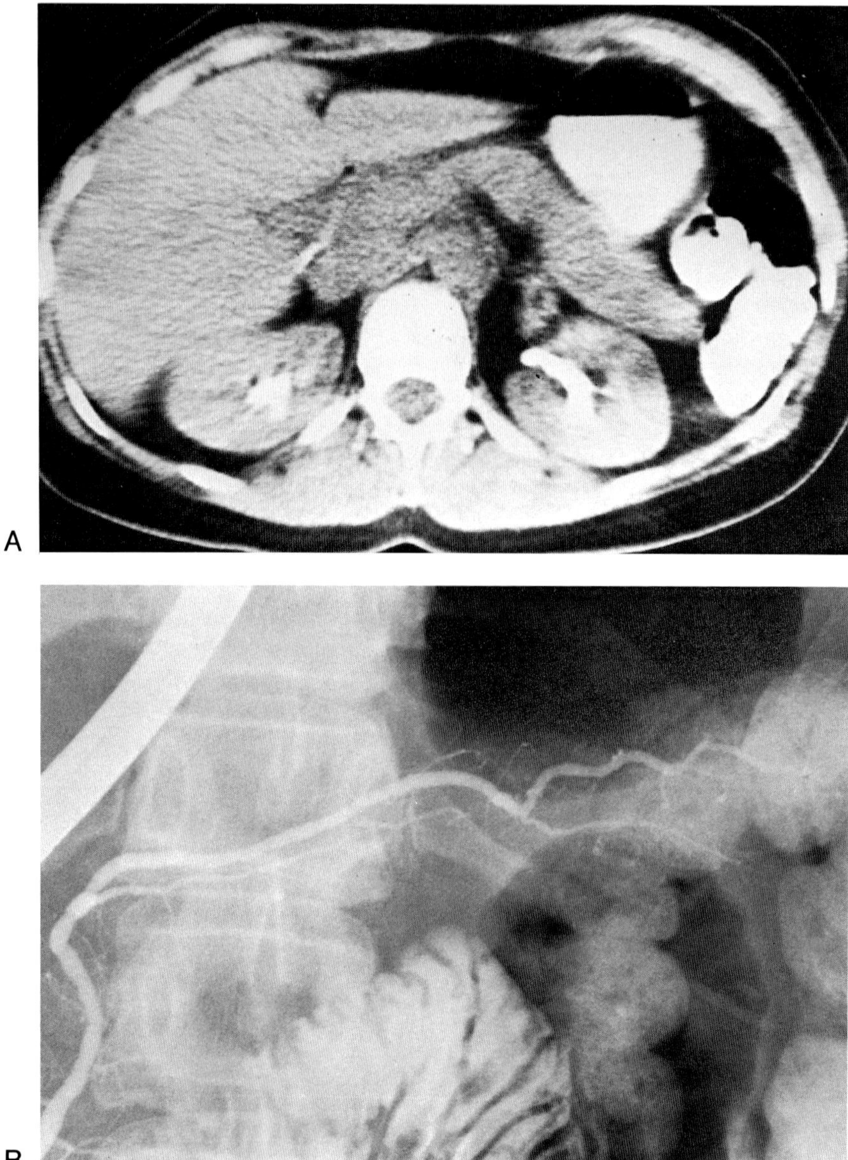

Fig. 7-3 Normal pancreatic ductal variant mimicking pancreatic mass. **(A)** CT scan. Prominent pancreatic tail. **(B)** On ERCP, prominence of the pancreatic tail was shown to be secondary to an accessory duct, which is a normal variant. (Frick MP, Feinberg JB, Goodale RL: The value of retrograde cholangiopancreatography in patients with suspected carcinoma of the pancreas and indeterminate computed tomographic results. Surg Gynecol Obstet 155:177, 1982. Reprinted by permission from Surgery, Gynecology Obstetrics.)

thickness of the gland decreasing gradually from head to tail. The next most common type is the dumbbell shape (33 percent), with the head and tail of the pancreas appearing thicker than the body. The third type is the sausage shape (23 percent)—the head, body, and tail are of equal width. Blunting or rounding of the apex of the triangular-shaped uncinate process generally indicates the presence of pathology.

Imaging the pancreas with ultrasound is a technical challenge. The sonologist must aggressively apply various techniques to improve visualization of the pancreas. The tail of the pancreas is frequently difficult to image, owing to gas in the stomach and small bowel. A combination of prone or decubitus scanning and water distension of the upper gastrointestinal tract may decrease the number of indeterminate examinations (Fig. 7-4). Marked obesity, large amounts of bowel gas, or both may occasionally lead to complete nonvisualization of the pancreas. When the pancreas is adequately imaged, the echo texture of the pancreas can be evaluated. Any abnormalities in the pancreas may be characterized as diffuse or focal, with increased or decreased echogenicity. Any disproportionate enlargement of a portion of the gland, or a width more than 3 cm in diameter should raise the suspicion of a pancreatic mass. Using the 3.5 or 5.0 MHz transducer, the normal pancreatic duct can be evaluated in most patients. Any focal or diffuse ectasia of the pancreatic duct is considered abnormal.

Abdominal computed tomography readily displays the size, shape, and texture of the pancreas as well as the adjacent anatomy. There are few limitations with regard to optimal computed tomographic imaging. These include paucity of intraabdominal and retroperitoneal fat, incomplete opacification of the upper gastrointestinal tract, metallic artifacts in the upper abdomen, and poor patient cooperation (patient motion).

Computed tomographic evaluation of the pancreas requires the introduction of both oral and intravenous contrast agents. Aggressive technique using intravenously injected contrast agents provides optimal visualization of the peripancreatic vascular anatomy. Computed tomographic angiography (CTA) is reserved for the detection of small hypervascular pancreatic neoplasms such as islet cell tumors. Normal pancreatic tissue is slightly enhanced after the intravenous injection of contrast material. Since pancreatic adenocarcinomas are typically hypovascular, an isodense pancreatic carcinoma may be uncovered by the lack of normal contrast enhancement during routine dynamic scanning. The normal vascularity of the pancreas causes transient opacification, whereas the hypovascular neoplasm remains relatively unenhanced. After detection, further characterization of a mass is often possible by defining its contour and density (attenuation coefficient). CT detection of intrapancreatic air or calcifications may suggest a more specific diagnosis of inflammatory disease.

There is considerable overlap between lesions of different origins. Solid neoplasms may undergo necrosis

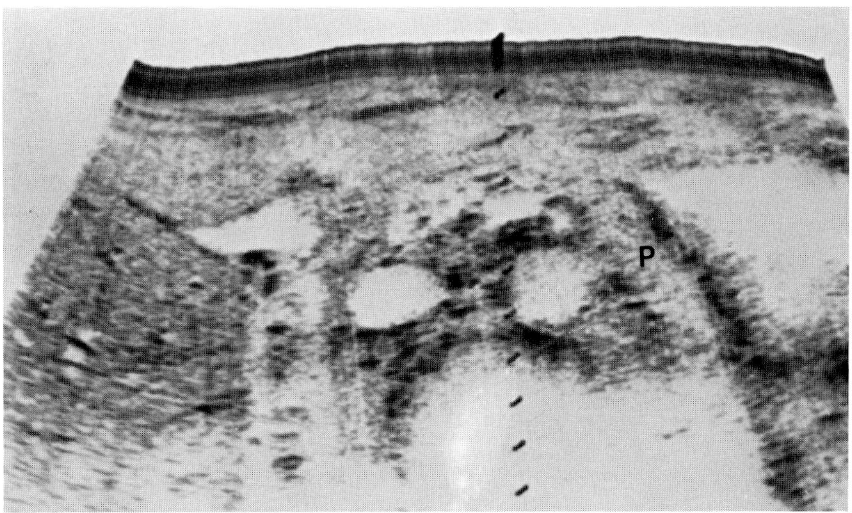

Fig. 7-4 Normal pancreatic tail. Ultrasound scan, transverse projection. Fluid-filled stomach acts as a sonic window (*P*, pancreas).

or hemorrhage and appear cystlike. Pseudocysts may exhibit increased density caused by internal hemorrhage or high protein content. Pancreatitis may coexist with a more distally located obstructing carcinoma. In any questionable instance, a CT-guided fine-needle aspiration biopsy (FNAB) may be extremely useful; with FNAB, mass lesions and fluid collections can be evaluated more specifically — i.e., tissue specimens can be removed from masses for histologic study and aspirated fluids can be examined biochemically and microbiologically. The ability to obtain a tissue specimen by simple nonoperative percutaneous technique is a low-risk procedure that frequently prevents unnecessary exploratory laparotomy.

PANCREATITIS

Acute pancreatitis is a term used to describe pancreatic inflammation associated with a variety of etiologic factors, pathologic findings, and clinical features. The physiology of pancreatitis is poorly understood, and its exact etiology is unknown; however, a twofold process is felt to occur. Initially, normal pancreatic defense mechanisms are broken down and subsequently an inflammatory response is initiated.

Eventually necrosis and hemorrhage develop in severe cases. A number of conditions predispose to the development of pancreatitis. Most patients (66 percent) have biliary tract disease or a history of alcohol abuse. Other predisposing conditions include hyperparathyroidism, trauma, infection, surgery, hereditary defects, hyperlipidemia, drugs, and pregnancy. An idiopathic category, in which no etiology can be identified, occurs in approximately 20 percent of patients.

Pancreatitis may be acute, subacute, or chronic and may or may not be associated with a variety of complications that include intra- or peripancreatic fluid accumulations. Pathologic examination of the pancreas specifically reveals pancreatic edema, interstitial inflammation, and often frank hemorrhage and necrosis. The broad clinical spectrum ranges from self-limiting disease to a lethal course. Approximately three-fourths of all patients with acute pancreatitis recover uneventfully with conservative medical man-

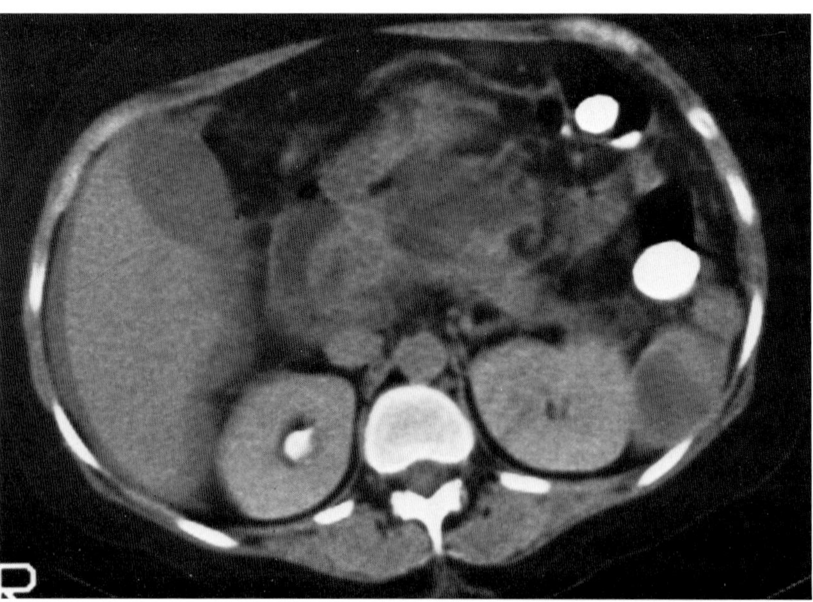

Fig. 7-5 Acute pancreatitis with phlegmon. The pancreas is enlarged, ill-marginated, and contains areas of lower and higher density. Note ascites along the lateral liver margin.

agement. The remainder of the patients develop more serious, often life-threatening complications.

The complications of pancreatitis include phlegmon, pseudocyst, and abscess formation. These entities may coexist. They cannot always be radiographically differentiated from one another. A phlegmon, a solid inflammatory mass, may involve the entire pancreas or it may be localized in any portion of the gland. These inflammatory masses occur in approximately one-fifth of patients with acute pancreatitis and generally resolve within several weeks. However, they may progress to pseudocyst or abscess formation. When localized, phlegmons may resemble carcinoma. Computed tomography demonstrates a poorly defined solid pancreatic mass (Fig. 7-5). The surrounding peripancreatic fat becomes streaky and indistinct owing to the surrounding inflammation. Ultrasound demonstrates a poorly defined, focal hypoechoic mass (Fig. 7-6).

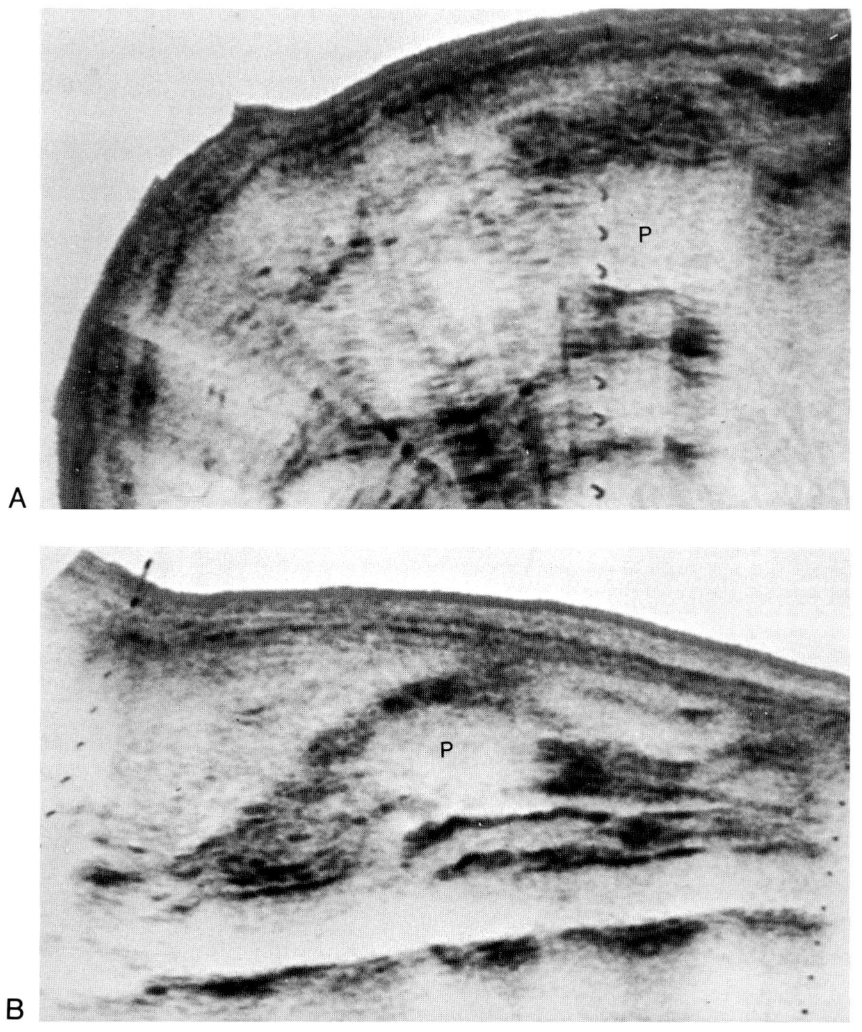

Fig. 7-6 Acute edematous pancreatitis. **(A)** Ultrasound scan in transverse and **(B)** parasagittal projections. The pancreatic head and body are enlarged and poorly defined, with decreased echogenicity (*P*, pancreas).

Pseudocysts represent collections of necrotic tissue and/or pancreatic secretions that result from autodigestion of the gland by pancreatic enzymes. The fluid accumulates in necrotic portions of the pancreas. The walls of pseudocysts are nonepithelialized, hence the term pseudocyst. Growth of a pseudocyst is caused by the osmotic influx of fluid in response to tissue necrosis. So-called ectopic pseudocysts are extensions of pancreatic fluid collections from the pancreas into the abdomen, pelvis, or mediastinum. Pseudocysts may evolve over a period of days or weeks after the clinical onset of acute pancreatitis. The majority of pseudocysts resolve spontaneously. The rest decompress into the abdomen (pancreatic ascites) or adjacent bowel.

Ultrasound and CT have had a significant impact on the diagnosis and potential percutaneous drainage of pseudocysts and on the differentiation of these lesions from neoplasms (Fig. 7-7). Ultrasonographically, pseudocysts are anechoic or hypoechoic fluid collections. On CT they appear as homogeneous, almost water-density lesions. Densities greater than water may represent hemorrhage or debris in the pseudocyst (Fig. 7-8). Septations or increased density in cystic lesions of the pancreas should lead one to suspect cystic neoplasms.

ERCP procedures have the potential of flaring pancreatitis and are not indicated in patients with a clinical diagnosis of acute pancreatitis or its complications. (In patients with gallstone disease, however, ERCP may be obtained primarily to study the biliary ductal system.) There is a distinct possibility that sepsis will develop if a pseudocyst is filled during ERCP.

Pancreatic fluid collections are not always confined to the gland itself. They may rupture beyond the thin fibrous sheath surrounding the pancreas and the parietal peritoneum anteriorly to enter the lesser sac, creating an inflammatory mass effect along the posterior wall of the stomach, or they may extend posteriorly into other retroperitoneal spaces. Inflammatory pancreatic fluid collections may present in any of the three retroperitoneal spaces—i.e., the anterior pararenal space, the perirenal space, or the posterior pararenal space.

Extrapancreatic fluid collections frequently elicit an inflammatory mass effect on structures adjacent to

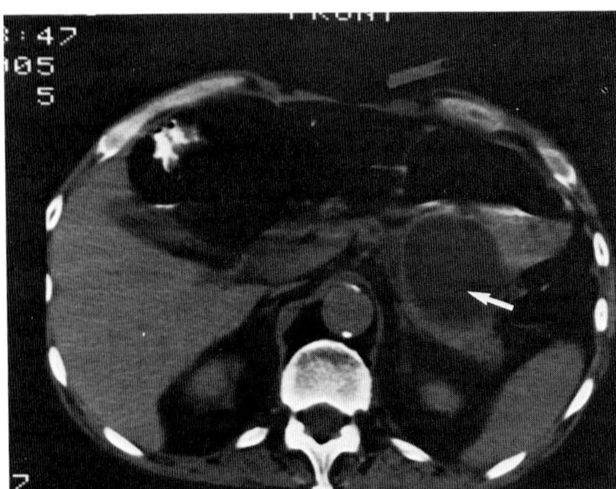

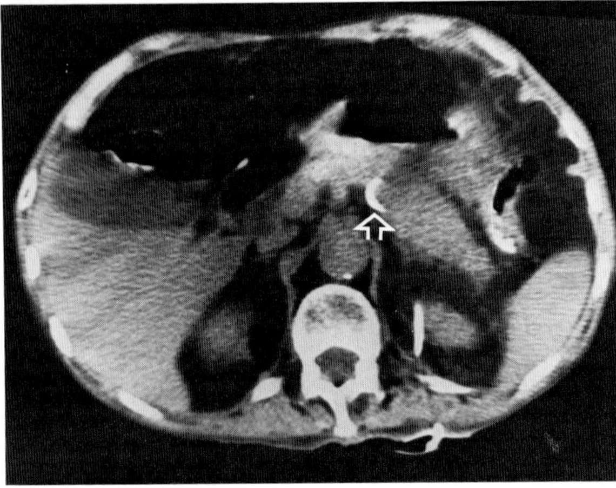

Fig. 7-7 Chronic pancreatitis with pseudocyst. Well-marginated, low density mass lesion in the pancreatic tail is consistent with a pseudocyst *(arrow)*. After successful drainage, using CT guidance and placement of a drainage catheter *(open arrow)*, the patient improved symptomatically without complications.

them. In the anterior pararenal space, the duodenum and the ascending and descending portions of the colon may be involved. As the inflammatory enzymatic exudate spreads across Gerota's fascia, inflammation in the perirenal space may cause obstruction of either of the two kidneys. The exudate can also spread along the transverse mesocolon to involve the entire length or a localized segment of the transverse colon, or it may spread along the small bowel mesentery to the ileocecal region.

Pancreatic abscesses can result secondary to infection of devitalized pancreatic tissues or to infection of pre-

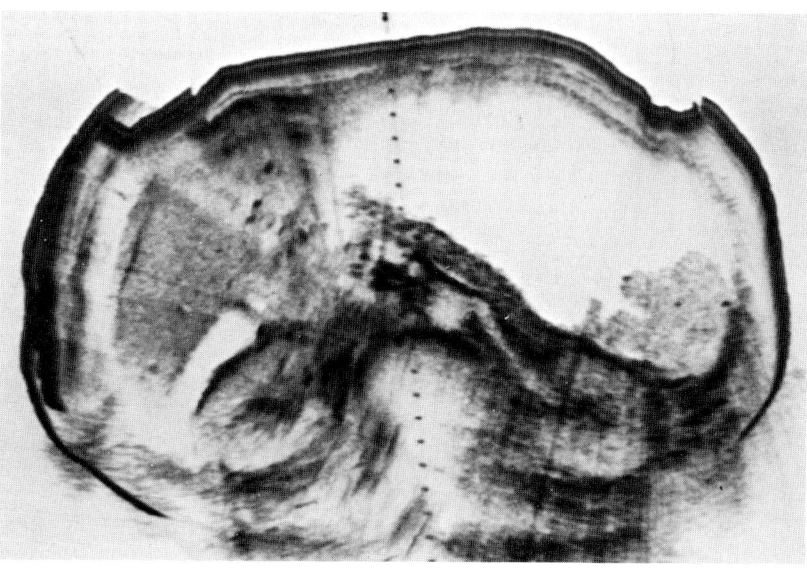

Fig. 7-8 Pancreatitis with pseudocyst. Ultrasound scan, transverse projection. The large pseudocyst contains gravity-dependent debris. Note fluid collection in subphrenic and posterior subhepatic space (Morison's pouch), representing pancreatic ascites.

viously existing pseudocysts. Approximately 10 percent of patients with acute pancreatitis will develop a pancreatic abscess. The most common infectious agents are *Escherichia coli, Staphylococcus, Enterococcus, Klebsiella,* and *Pseudomonas.* Recognition of a pancreatic abscess is important because abscesses generally require surgical or percutaneous drainage. When gas-forming organisms are present, occasionally extraluminal upper abdominal gas collections can be identified on plain radiographs of the abdomen. Optimally, however, computed tomography is the technique of choice in demonstrating the presence and extent of abscess formation (Fig. 7-9). Ultrasound is also useful in patients with pancreatic abscesses; however, the examination may frequently be limited by the presence of adynamic ileus or by gas in the abscess itself.

There may be compromise of the biliary system with compression of the distal common bile duct as it courses through the head of the pancreas. Spontaneous hemorrhage, caused by erosion of the inflammatory exudate into the wall of adjacent arteries, is not an uncommon complication. The splenic artery is the most common source of UGI bleeding, with lesser involvement occurring in the pancreaticoduodenal, gastroduodenal, and gastric arteries. Pseudoaneurysm

formation can occur in approximately 9 percent of the patients. The major venous complication is thrombosis involving the splenic vein, portal vein or, less frequently, the superior mesenteric and gastric veins. Splenic vein occlusion is frequently associated with splenomegaly and gastric or esophageal varices, or both. (Esophageal varices may not be present if collateral pathways circumvent the obstruction between the spleen and portal vein.) Portal venous thrombosis can be identified as an isolated finding or result from the propagation of thrombus, spreading from the splenic vein, superior mesenteric vein, or gastric vein. In the latter cases, gastrointestinal bleeding and bowel infarction are more likely to occur.

Pleuroparenchymal complications of acute pancreatitis are not uncommon. Most patients with acute pancreatitis have some form of respiratory insufficiency; some abnormality is identified on chest radiographs in as many as 49 percent of patients. The most common abnormalities include pneumonia, atelectasis, and pleural effusions. Other less common complications include pulmonary infarction, pulmonary edema, empyema, mediastinal abscess formation, bronchopancreatic fistula, bronchopleural fistula, pericarditis, and adult respiratory distress syndrome.

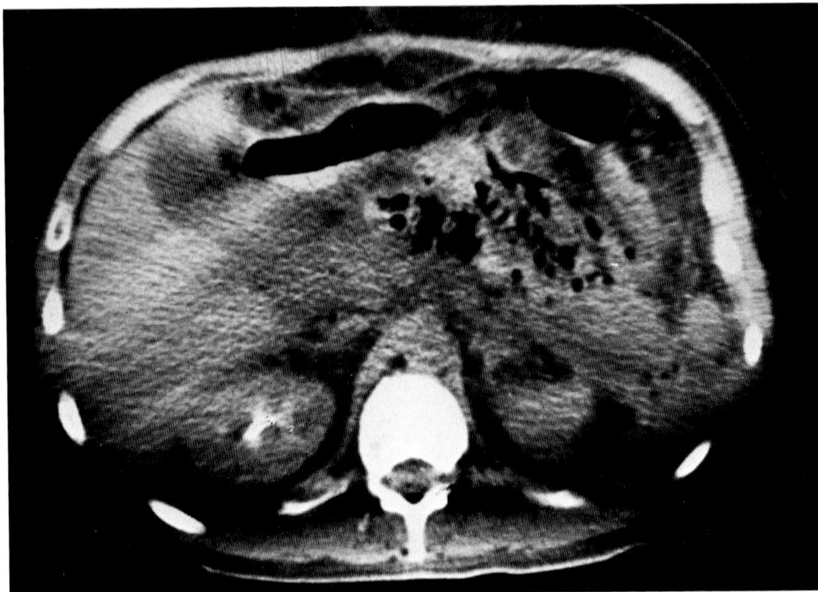

Fig. 7-9 Pancreatic abscess. CT scan. The pancreas is massively enlarged, ill-marginated, and contains air bubbles. Needle aspiration was positive for *Escherichia coli*. Note adynamic ileus adjacent to the pancreas.

The complications are caused by postulated pulmonary changes from the indirect or direct action of disseminated intravascular pancreatic enzymes. A second mechanism is a postulated pulmonary vasoconstrictive agent released from the damaged pancreas. Effusions are felt to be secondary to sympathetic transportation of amylase-rich fluid from below the diaphragm, through the lymphatics, and into the pleural cavity.

Disseminated fat necrosis is also considered a complication of acute pancreatitis. Patients may have widespread fat necrosis in the mediastinum, liver, subcutaneous tissues, and periarticular tissues. The pathophysiology is secondary to compromised microcirculation and eventual ischemic necrosis associated with the dissemination of intravascular pancreatic enzymes. Another theory suggests dissemination of fat from fat necrosis in the pancreas, embolizing to small end arteries.

CHRONIC PANCREATITIS

Chronic pancreatitis is a common disease. Pain is its principal symptom, and alcohol abuse its most common etiologic factor. In addition to alcohol-induced pancreatitis, chronic familial pancreatitis, calcifying pancreatitis secondary to insufficient protein intake, chronic pancreatitis associated with biliary tract disease, and idiopathic chronic pancreatitis have been differentiated.

Pathologically, chronic pancreatitis is initially characterized by parenchymal fibrosis with a mild degree of tissue destruction. Associated with the parenchymal disease is the precipitation of protein-linked calcium in the excretory system. Calculus formation in secondary radicles and in the main pancreatic duct disseminate throughout the organ, or may be present focally. The role of radiology in patients with chronic pancreatitis is limited to the exclusion or diagnosis of underlying carcinoma and to the definition of the pancreas prior to surgical intervention.

The CT findings associated with chronic pancreatitis include focal or diffuse enlargement of the gland (33 percent), pseudocyst or abscess formation (30 percent), calcifications (40 percent), atrophy (15 percent), ductal dilatation (5 to 8 percent), and normal gland contour (20 percent) (Fig. 7-10).

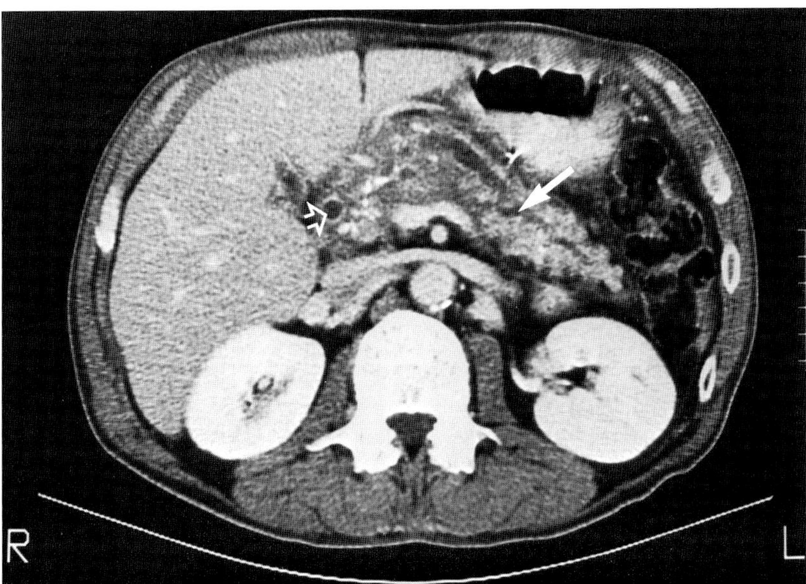

Fig. 7-10 Chronic pancreatitis CT scan. Note the dilated pancreatic *(arrow)* and common bile *(open arrow)* ducts, scattered calcifications in the pancreatic head and irregular outline of the gland. (Excellent demonstration of the peripancreatic vascular anatomy after intravenous contrast administration.)

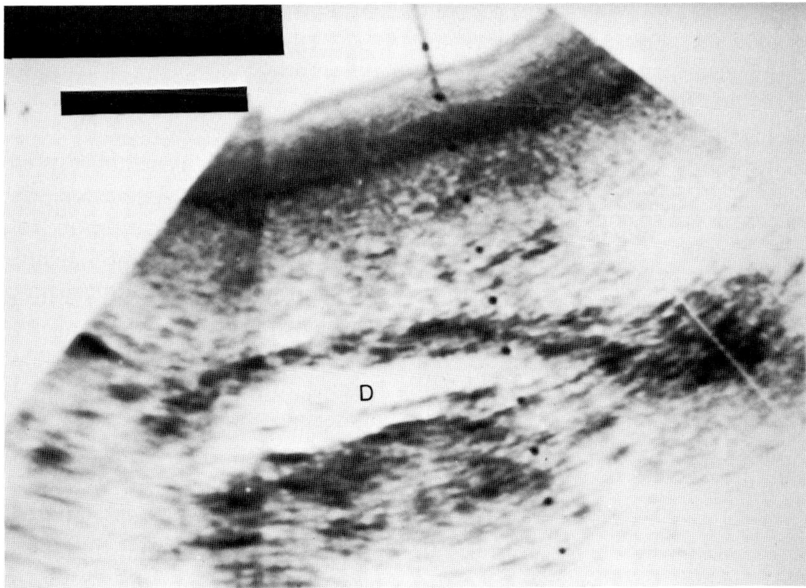

Fig. 7-11 Chronic pancreatitis. Ultrasound scan, transverse projection. Note pancreatic atrophy and massively dilated main pancreatic duct *(D)* anterior to the splenic vein (findings confirmed by ERCP).

The ultrasonographic appearance of chronic pancreatitis also varies. The echogenicity of the gland is usually increased; however, as stated previously this is quite variable and is usually associated with fatty infiltration. Increased echogenicity cannot be used as a reliable sign of chronic pancreatitis. More reliable signs include irregular gland contour, scattered calcifications with shadowing, atrophy, and pancreatic ductal ectasia (Fig. 7-11).

A main contribution of ERCP in patients with chronic pancreatitis is in the preoperative planning of ductal drainage procedures and pancreatectomy rather than in excluding suspected superimposed carcinoma. In select instances, ERCP may be useful in identifying biliary strictures of the distal common bile duct and in the diagnosis of previously unsuspected choledocholithiasis. Associated with pancreatitis ERCP findings are well known. They consist of multiple strictures and areas of intermittent dilatation of the pancreatic duct (chain-of-lakes appearance) as well as dilatation of secondary branches.

NEOPLASMS

Adenocarcinoma

Despite a variety of modern imaging techniques to visualize the pancreas, the diagnosis of a pancreatic neoplasm is usually a difficult one. Although computed tomography and ultrasound are accurate methods of diagnosing pancreatic neoplasms, currently there is no evidence indicating that these modalities have had a favorable influence on the high mortality rate of pancreatic cancer.

There are many types of pancreatic tumors. By far, the most common is pancreatic adenocarcinoma (95 percent). Tumors other than adenocarcinomas include the functioning and nonfunctioning islet cell tumors and cystic pancreatic neoplasms, which will be discussed later.

Pancreatic adenocarcinoma probably arises from the ductal system and presents as a mass distorting the normal pancreatic contour (Fig. 7-12). Nonfocal enlargement of the pancreas caused by infiltrative pancreatic carcinoma also occurs, but is less common.

Any focal increase in size or any change in the shape of the pancreas should cause one to suspect a pancreatic neoplasm. Since the attenuation coefficient of a pancreatic adenocarcinoma is similar to that of the normal pancreas, focal contour defects may present the only sign of pathology. Adenocarcinomas do not calcify. Disproportionate prominence of a part of an atrophied pancreas in an older person is suspicious for neoplastic degeneration, even though absolute measurements may be deceptive and are, therefore, sometimes inaccurate (Fig. 7-13). Areas of poorly marginated, decreased attenuation in the carcinoma may indicate necrosis or cystic degeneration. If a carcinoma of the pancreas is suspected, a search for additional features of carcinoma is initiated. Since the majority (60 percent) of carcinomas occur in the head of the pancreas, the main pancreatic duct, the common bile duct, or both ducts may be dilated. Combined ductal dilatation (the double-duct sign) strongly suggests ampullary or pancreatic head pathology, even when the tumor itself cannot be identified (note: double-duct sign is not specific and can also be seen in patients with pancreatitis) (Fig. 7-14). Other indirect signs of pancreatic carcinoma are related to the obstructive, and often subsequent, inflammatory responses in the pancreas, such as pseudocyst formation and edema. Other findings include obliteration of the peripancreatic fat planes that surround the superior mesenteric vessels (Fig. 7-15), the celiac trunk, and aorta; retroperitoneal and porta hepatis adenopathy; and hepatic metastases. These criteria indicate surgical unresectability.

If a focal mass is noted on computed tomography or ultrasound and it does not resolve, or actually enlarges on follow-up examinations, fine-needle biopsy can assist in the diagnosis. Positive results can be obtained in more than three-quarters of patients with adenocarcinoma. The absence of a positive cytology, however, does not exclude the presence of neoplasia; the utility of percutaneous biopsy is solely in the detection of neoplasia, not in its exclusion.

On ultrasound, pancreatic adenocarcinoma typically presents as a focal, solid, hypoechoic mass with decreased through-transmission of sound (Fig. 7-16). Rarely, a carcinomatous lesion may appear partially cystic with increased through-transmission. This reflects liquefaction of the tumor secondary to necrosis.

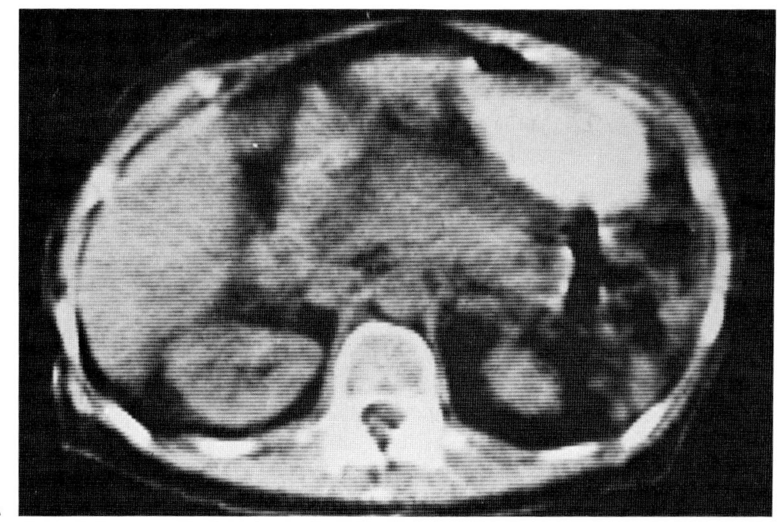

Fig. 7-12 Carcinoma of the pancreas with direct extension into the transverse colon. **(A)** Pancreatic mass involving the body of the pancreas with anterior extension into transverse colon. **(B)** Single contrast barium enema. Solitary intramural nonobstructing filling defect typically involving the lower margin of the transverse colon.

If a lesion suspicious for carcinoma is detected, biliary and pancreatic ducts are carefully evaluated. Conversely, any dilated pancreatic duct requires that a pancreatic carcinoma be excluded. If a pancreatic mass is documented, the presence or absence of related abnormalities, such as liver metastases, lymphadenopathy, or ascites, are documented.

Gastrointestinal contrast studies play a secondary role in the evaluation of pancreatic adenocarcinoma. Radiologic obstruction of the duodenum may result from an inflammatory or a neoplastic pancreatic process. The findings include effacement of the duodenal folds and widening of the duodenal sweep. Pancreatic tumor extension into the duodenum may result in the typical "inverted three" (Frostberg sign) appearance. Invasion ultimately leads to ulcer formation as well as mass effect, commonly along the medial aspect of the second portion of the duodenum (Fig. 7-17).

ERCP displays the ductal system from which most pancreatic adenocarcinomas arise. Carcinomas may be diagnosed if the double-duct sign or a complete main pancreatic duct obstruction are found in the absence of additional signs of chronic pancreatitis. In the absence of radiographic findings of chronic pancreatitis,

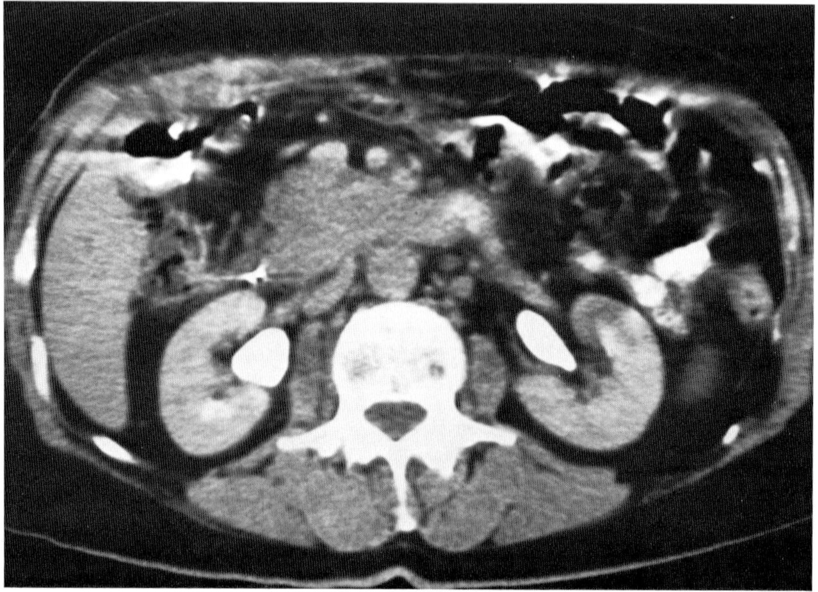

Fig. 7-13 Adenocarcinoma of the head of the pancreas. The pancreatic head is mildly enlarged and well-marginated. There is atrophy of the body and tail of the pancreas (surgical proof).

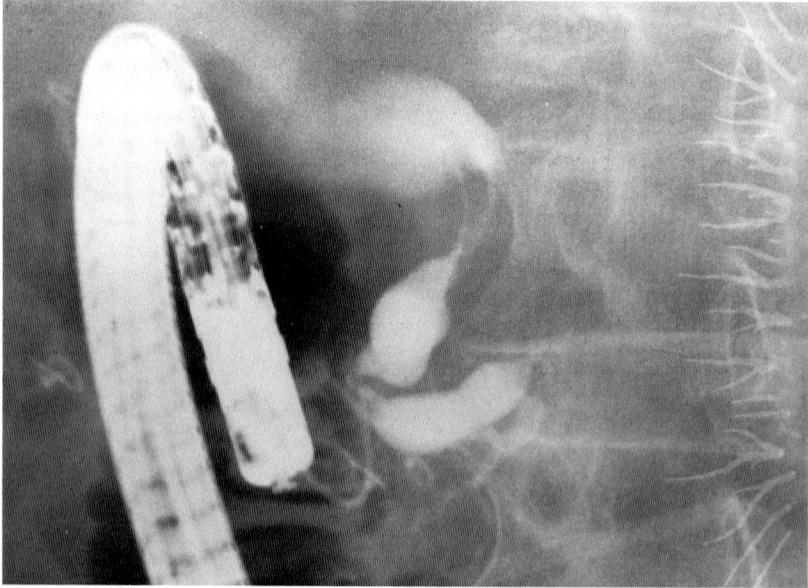

Fig. 7-14 Pancreatic adenocarcinoma ERCP. High-grade obstruction and encasement of both main pancreatic duct and distal common bile duct (double-duct sign) as a result of adenocarcinoma involving the head of the pancreas.

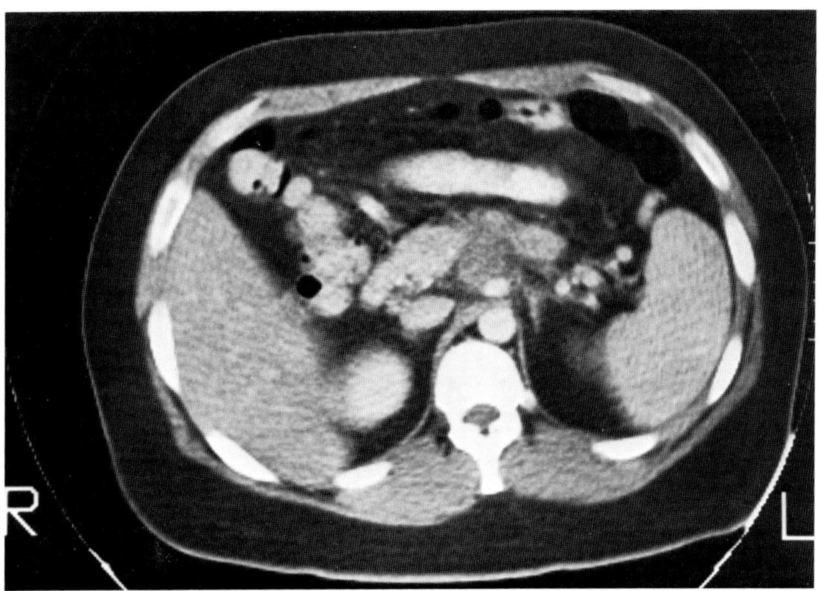

Fig. 7-15 Adenocarcinoma of the pancreas. Posterior tumor extension with encasement of the superior mesenteric vessels indicates nonresectability.

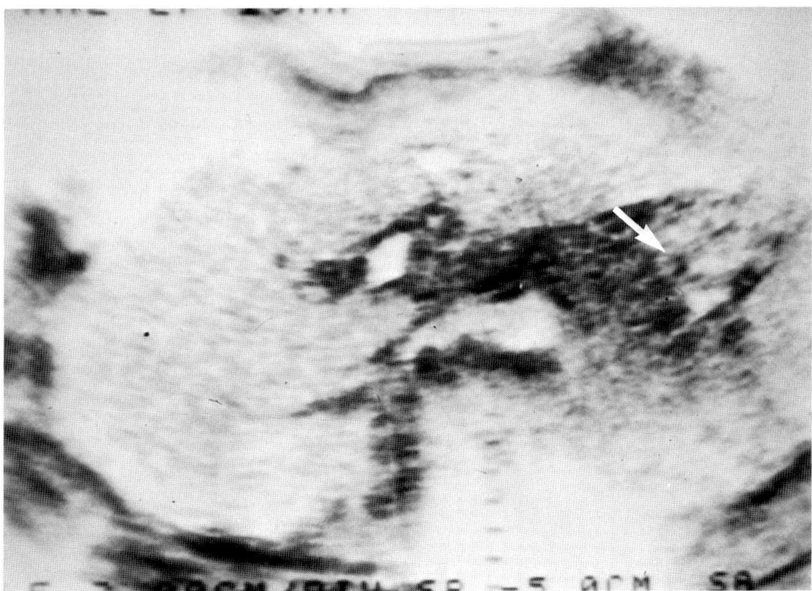

Fig. 7-16 Adenocarcinoma of the pancreatic tail. Ultrasound scan, transverse projection. Hypoechoic mass *(arrow)* contrasts with normal more echogenic pancreatic tissue (surgical proof).

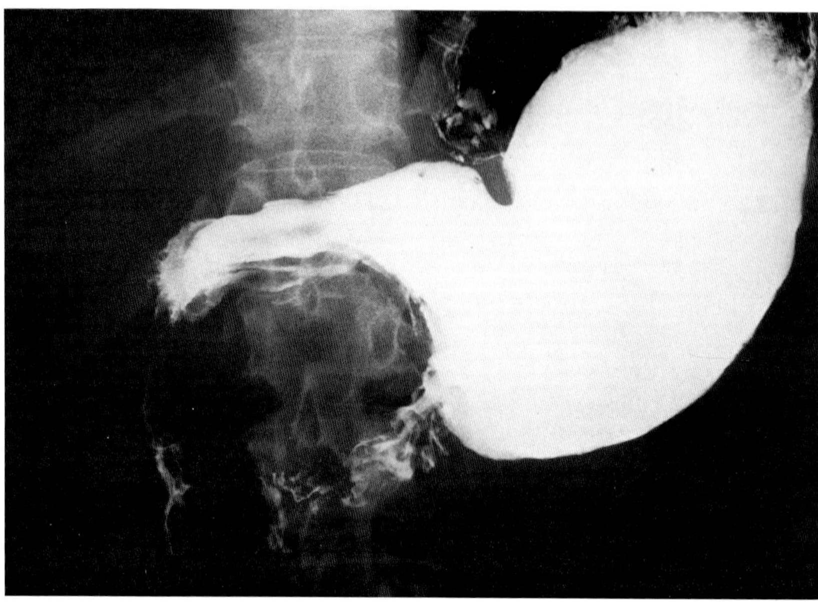

Fig. 7-17 Adenocarcinoma of the pancreas. There is extrinsic mass effect on the greater curvature of the antrum and encasement of the duodenal sweep with mucosal irregularity. Findings are consistent with pancreatic carcinoma (surgical proof).

ERCP is accurate in diagnosing pancreatic carcinoma. It is less helpful in evaluating patients with clinically suspected pancreatic carcinoma and concurrent pancreatitis. In these patients, additional studies should be obtained, including cytologic sampling during ERCP (Fig. 7-18). The use of angiography to evaluate patients suspected of harboring a pancreatic adenocarcinoma has been steadily declining. Adenocarcinomas are usually avascular. Thus, their demonstration depends on indirect evidence of mass effect, vessel encasement, vascular compression or displacement, and intrapancreatic capillary staining. Many of these angiographic findings are also seen in chronic pancreatitis and certain congenital variations. Angiography has been advocated as a useful tool in mapping the parenchymal and collateral blood flow of the pancreas prior to surgery.

Islet Cell Tumors

Islet cells represent approximately 1.0 g of tissue and produce at least 12 different hormones. The number of functioning (secretory) islet cell tumors is small compared with that of nonfunctioning tumors of the same histologic appearance found incidentally at autopsy. Because of the discovery and isolation of new hormonal polypeptides and the development of new morophologic techniques, an increased number of cell types has been identified in the pancreatic islets. There are A cells producing glucagon, B cells producing insulin, and D cells producing somatostatin. In addition, at least 12 additional hormones are being produced by at least five or more types of islet cells, as documented by immunocytochemistry.

The APUD-cell concept helps in the understanding of various pancreatic endocrine systems and neoplasms. According to this concept, there is a common embryologic origin (neural crest) for pancreatic islet cells that produce peptide hormones. Islet cell tumors may generally be termed APUD-omas (tumors composed of Amine Precursor Uptake and Decarboxylation cells). Typically, individual neoplasms have been named after the hormone produced, such as insulinoma (B cells), gastrinoma producing the Zollinger-Ellison syndrome (G cells), glucagonoma (A cells) and somatostatinoma (A cells). Since the discovery of many hormones, the term nonfunctioning islet cell tumor has become somewhat tenuous and should be replaced by "functioning but not clinically apparent."

Insulinomas are the most common islet cell tumors and occur as solitary (85 percent) or multiple (15 percent) adenomatous tumors. Ninety percent of these lesions are benign and are usually treated by simple enucleation. Ten percent of insulinomas are malignant. Insulinomas are often small and difficult to detect by computed tomography or ultrasound. During angiography, insulinomas appear typically as discrete areas of blush with a delayed capillary phase.

When insulinomas are detected, multiple endocrine adenopathy (MEA) type I should be excluded, especially if there is a family history of endocrine disorders. In differentiating benign from malignant insulinomas, detection of metastases (usually in the liver) is probably the only certain evidence for proving malignancy.

The gastrinoma is the second most common islet cell tumor. Typically, it leads to gastric hypersection and multiple, often atypically located, gastroduodenal ulcers as a part of the Zollinger-Ellison syndrome. Gastroduodenal ulcerations may penetrate into the pancreas, secondarily causing pancreatitis. The diagnosis of gastrinoma is often suspected radiographically on UGI studies that demonstrate hypertrophic gastric mucosa, multiple gastric or duodenojejunal ulcerations, and a prominent hypersecretory small bowel pattern. After subtotal gastric resection, anastomotic ulcers are common. In patients with gastrinomas, the location of the neoplasm rather than its specific diagnosis is the most valuable contribution of diagnostic imaging.

On computed tomography, the only feature that distinguishes the islet cell tumor from pancreatic adenocarcinoma is focal, prominent contrast enhancement on dynamic scanning or computed tomographic angiography (CTA). The islet cell tumor, in distinction to adenocarcinoma, is usually located in the body and tail of the pancreas and may become calcified or cystlike (Fig. 7-18). The diagnosis of islet cell tumors is aided by the patient's clinical presentation and laboratory

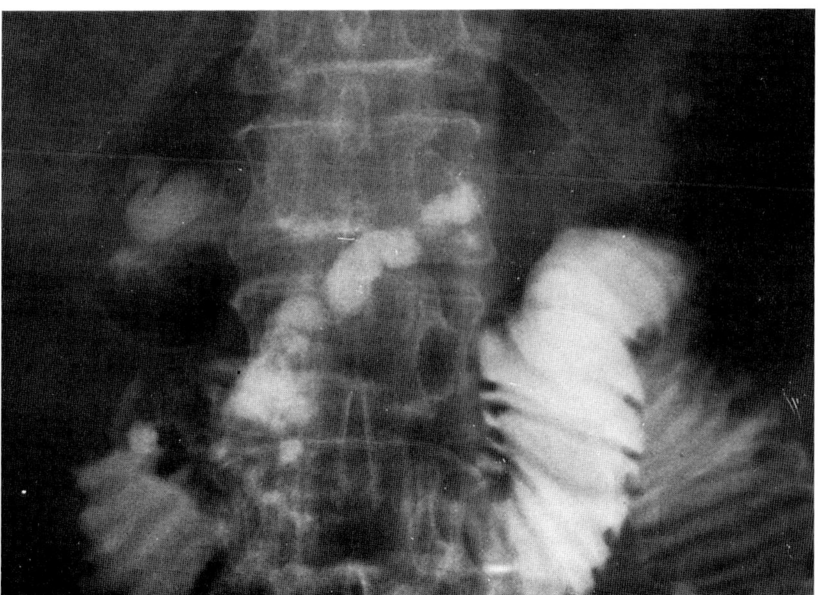

Fig. 7-18 Longstanding chronic pancreatitis and pancreatic adenocarcinoma of the pancreatic tail. On ERCP, note a grossly abnormal main pancreatic duct with areas of strictures and dilatation and the absence of secondary radicals consistent with chronic pancreatitis. Percutaneous biopsy of the proximal pancreatic lesion verified the presence of an adenocarcinoma.

findings. The 5-year survival of patients with malignant islet cell tumors is usually increased, compared with adenocarcinoma.

CYSTIC NEOPLASMS

Rare cystic neoplasms of the pancreas are composed of two groups. The first group is the macrocystic adenoma/adenocarcinoma (formerly cystadenoma/cystadenocarcinoma) and the microcystic adenoma (glycogen-rich cystadenoma).

Macrocystic neoplasms occur in the body and tail of the pancreas. They are generally large and are composed of multiloculated cystic spaces. The septa may calcify. Occasionally, these lesions are unilocular and have a strong malignant potential (Fig. 7-19).

Microcystic adenomas are benign and occur predominantly in the head of the pancreas. They are generally small — less than 2 cm in diameter — and contain multiple small cysts. Radiating strands of connective tissue may calcify, creating a "sunburst" appearance (Fig. 7-20).

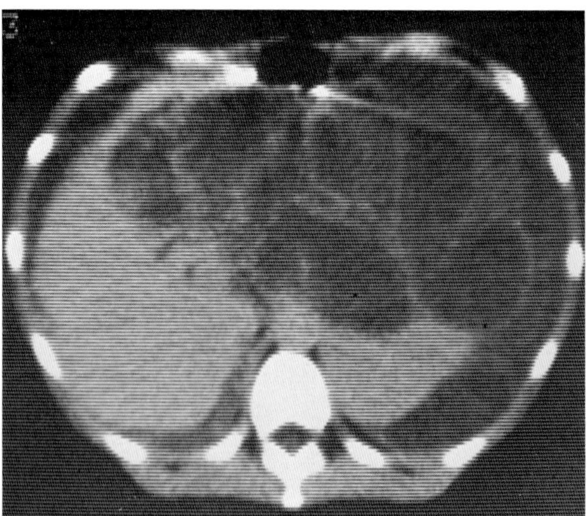

Fig. 7-19 Cystadenocarcinoma of the pancreas, CT scan. A large septated cystic mass has replaced virtually the entire pancreas.

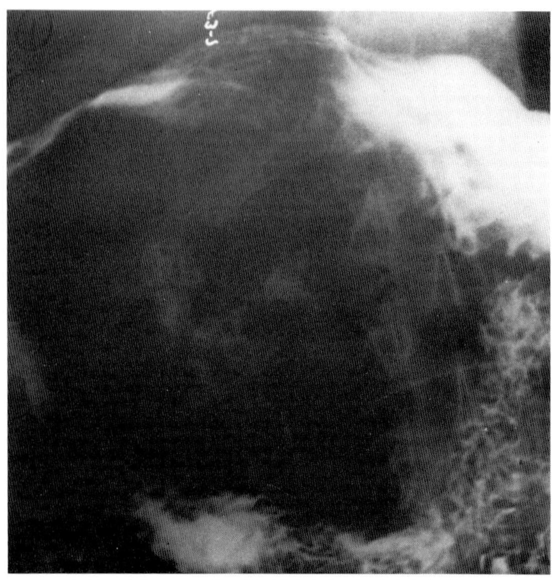

Fig. 7-20 Microcytic adenoma of the pancreas. Upper gastrointestinal contrast study. Large mass in the head of the pancreas with typical sunburst calcifications (surgical proof).

The differential diagnostic considerations include pancreatitis, with pseudocyst formation and cystic degeneration of pancreatic adenocarcinoma.

METASTASES

Apparent enlargement of the pancreatic gland may be caused by local invasion of an adjacent carcinoma of the stomach, duodenum, or hepatobiliary system, including the gallbladder. Computed tomography reliably demonstrates peripancreatic anatomy, including its adjacent organ systems, lymph nodes, and vascular structures. Retroperitoneal or mesenteric lymphadenopathy is often the result of a carcinoma or lymphoma. Located near the pancreatic bed, lymphadenopathy may mimic pancreatic enlargement (Fig. 7-21). Peripancreatic lymphadenopathy associated with carcinomatosis or inflammatory disorders may encase the superior mesenteric vessels, infiltrate the mesentery, or both. The root of the mesentery is usually not obliterated by lymphomatous lymphadenopathy. Lymphomatous deposits typically exhibit a hypoechoic pattern on ultrasonography compared

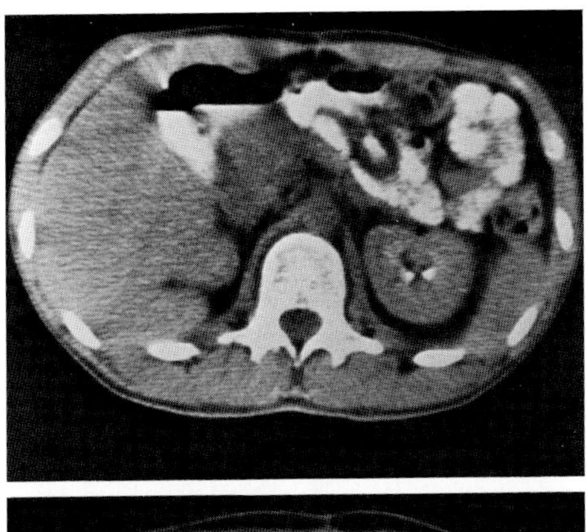
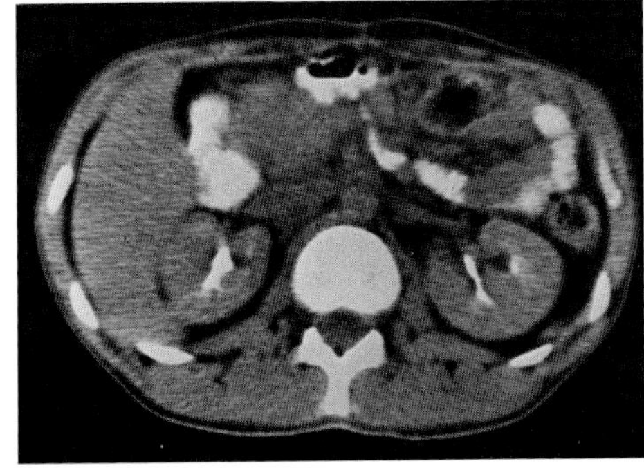
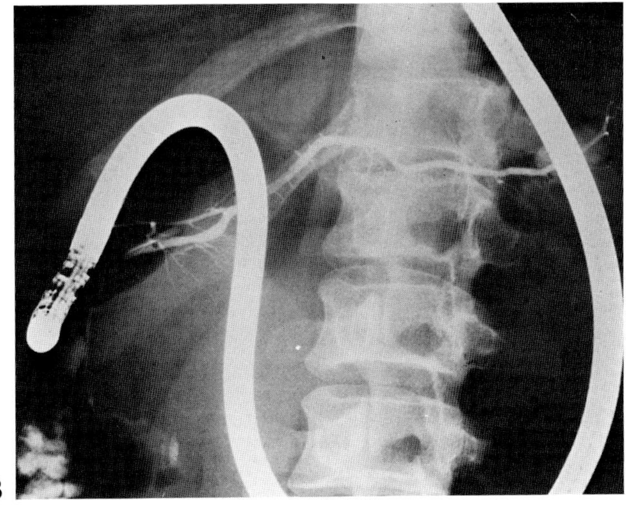

Fig. 7-21 (A) On CT, enlargement of peripancreatic lymph nodes mimics enlargement of the pancreatic head. **(B)** Endoscopic retrograde pancreatography shows normal pancreatic ductal system, excluding chronic pancreatitis and pancreatic carcinoma (surgical proof).

with other causes of lymphadenopathy because of the more homogeneous cell structure.

RARE PANCREATIC NEOPLASMS

Most pancreatic neoplasms arise from ductal epithelium or islet cells. Any of various other tissues (fibrous capsule, adipose tissue, blood vessels, nerves) may undergo neoplastic transformation to result in exceedingly rare lesions such as fibromas, sarcomas, lipomas, hemangiomas, and neurofibromas.

CONGENITAL ABNORMALITIES AND NORMAL VARIANTS

Pancreas Divisum

Pancreas divisum is an embryologic variation of pancreatic development in which the dorsal and ventral portions remain separate. The dorsal pancreas normally develops from the duodenum toward the spleen in an area that later becomes the posterior wall of the lesser sac. The ventral pancreas is part of the liver bud from which the gallbladder, liver, and common bile duct arise. In most instances, the ventral pancreas rotates clockwise and fuses with the dorsal pancreas to form the uncinate process. This occurs between the sixth and seventh weeks of intrauterine life. The pancreatic ductal system from the dorsal and ventral portions join to create a common excretory system into the duodenum.

In pancreas divisum, there is absent or incomplete fusion of two embryologic pancreatic segments (Fig. 7-22). The duct of Santorini remains completely independent of the duct of Wirsung. The former may resemble the main excretory route of the pancreas, and the latter may be totally absent.

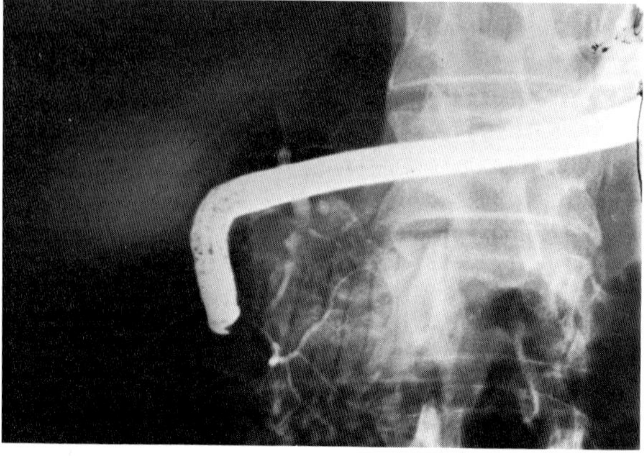

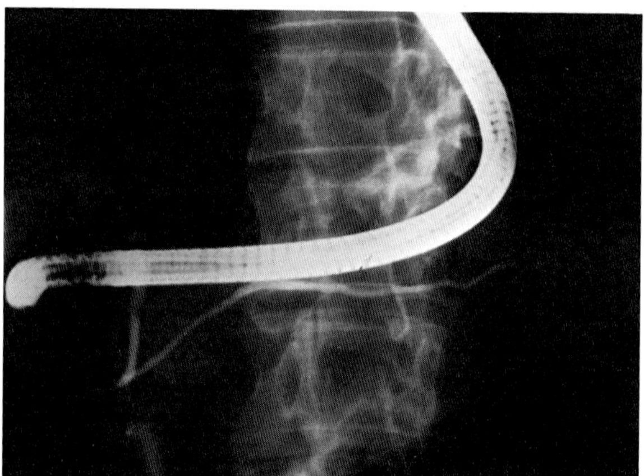

Fig. 7-22 Normal pancreatic variant, nonfusion. Endoscopic retrograde pancreatography demonstrates filling of a small main pancreatic duct *(above)*. Filling of a more prominent duct of Santorini *(below)* showed no communication with the main pancreatic duct. Incidence of this normal variant is 2 percent.

It is unclear whether a pancreas divisum, with its complete separation of the ducts of Wirsung and Santorini is in itself a cause of pancreatitis. In the general population the incidence of pancreas divisum is 4 percent. Of these, approximately one-fourth will develop pancreatitis. Pancreas divisum may mimic a pancreatic mass on computed tomography and ultrasound, but is readily diagnosed on ERCP.

Ectopic Pancreas

Pancreatic tissue may be found remote from the pancreas. Ectopic pancreas occurs in 1 to 13 percent of patients typically within the stomach (antral area) or

the duodenum (Fig. 7-23). It presents as a smooth, submucosal mass, often with a central umbilication. The umbilication represents a remnant of the pancreatic duct. Differential diagnosis of this incidental finding includes other intramural lesions such as leiomyoma, Brunner's gland adenoma, and metastases (see Chapter 2).

Annular Pancreas

Annular pancreas is a result of abnormal migration of the ventral pancreas. This congenital anomaly results in a partial or complete band of pancreatic parenchyma, surrounding and partially obstructing the descending duodenum. On gastrointestinal contrast examinations, annular pancreas is characterized in the adult patient by a smooth, concentric narrowing and intact duodenal mucosa. Definite proof is provided by ERCP showing the main pancreatic duct encircling the descending limb of the duodenum. This abnormality is best treated with a gastro- or duodenojejunostomy.

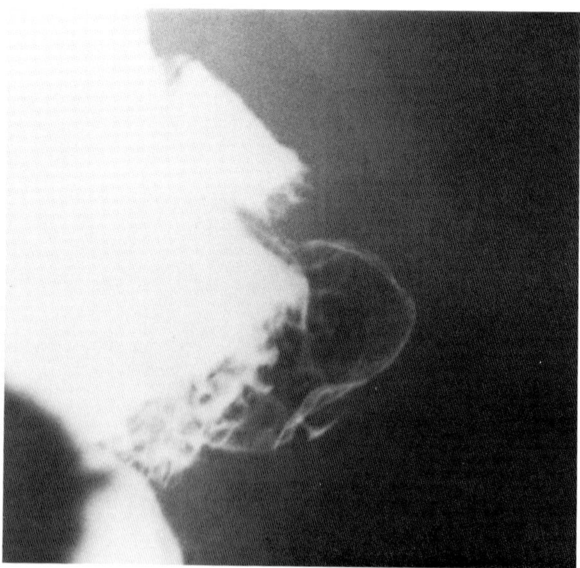

Fig. 7-23 Aberrant pancreas. Barium study of the stomach. Note a well-marginated 1.5 cm intramural filling defect along the greater curvature of the antrum. A central umbilication is typical and represents a small pancreatic duct, best seen in tangential projection.

PANCREATIC TRAUMA

Traumatic pancreatitis is a surgical term that describes pancreatic lesions resulting from external trauma. The injury may consist of laceration, perforation, simple contusion with hematoma formation, or severe contusion with devitalization of portions of the pancreas.

Pancreatic injuries exhibit little bleeding. Because of the location, injuries of adjacent organs are commonly associated with the pancreatic damage. These typically involve the stomach, duodenum, ascending and descending limbs of the colon, liver, and spleen. In pancreatic trauma, major vessels, such as the aorta; inferior vena cava; as well as the hepatic, splenic, and superior mesenteric vessels are of particular importance. In patients suspected of significant upper abdominal injury, computed tomography is probably the modality of choice.

The most common complications of pancreatic injury are the formation of a pancreatic pseudocyst, fistula, or abscess similar to the complications associated with inflammatory pancreatic disorders.

SUGGESTED READINGS

Frick MP, Feinberg JB, Goodale RL: The value of endoscopic retrograde cholangiopancreatography in patients with suspected carcinoma of the pancreas and indeterminate computed tomographic results. Surg Gynecol Obstet 155:177, 1982

Gedgaudas RK, Rice RP: Radiological evaluation of complicated pancreatitis. Critical Reviews in Diagnostic Imaging 15:319, 1981

Kurtz AB, Goldberg BB: Pancreas, p. 163. In Goldberg BB (ed): Abdominal Ultrasound. 2nd Ed. John Wiley, New York, 1984

Neumann CH, Hessel SJ: CT of the pancreatic tail. AJR 135:741, 1980

Sarti DA, King W: The ultrasonic findings in inflammatory pancreatic disease. Semin Ultrasound 1:178, 1980

Siegelmann SS, Copeland BE, Saba GP, et al: CT of fluid collections associated with pancreatitis. AJR 134:1121, 1980

Taylor KJW, Buchin PJ, Viscomi GN, et al: Ultrasonic scanning of the pancreas. Radiology 138:211, 1981

Ward EM, Stephens DH, Sheedy PF: Computed tomographic characteristic of pancreatic carcinoma analysis of 100 cases. Radiographics 3:547, 1983

Weinstein BJ, Weinstein DP: Sonographic anatomy of the pancreas. Semin Ultrasound 1:156, 1980

Wittenberg J, Simeone JE, Ferrucci JT, et al: Nonfocal enlargement in pancreatic carcinoma. Radiology 144:131, 1982

Index

Page numbers followed by *f* represent figures; those followed by *t* represent tables.